DISPOSITION OF THE AIR FORCE HEALTH STUDY

Committee on the Disposition of the Air Force Health Study
Board on Population Health and Public Health Practice

INSTITUTE OF MEDICINE
OF THE NATIONAL ACADEMIES

THE NATIONAL ACADEMIES PRESS
Washington, D.C.
www.nap.edu

THE NATIONAL ACADEMIES PRESS 500 Fifth Street, N.W. Washington, DC 20001

NOTICE: The project that is the subject of this report was approved by the Governing Board of the National Research Council, whose members are drawn from the councils of the National Academy of Sciences, the National Academy of Engineering, and the Institute of Medicine. The members of the committee responsible for the report were chosen for their special competences and with regard for appropriate balance.

This study was supported by Contract No. V101(93)P-2154 between the National Academy of Sciences and US Department of Veterans Affairs. Any opinions, findings, conclusions, or recommendations expressed in this publication are those of the author(s) and do not necessarily reflect the view of the organizations or agencies that provided support for this project.

International Standard Book Number 0-309-10099-2 (BOOK)
International Standard Book Number 0-309-65685-0 (PDF)
Library of Congress Control Number: 2006923463

Additional copies of this report are available from the National Academies Press, 500 Fifth Street, N.W., Lockbox 285, Washington, DC 20055; (800) 624-6242 or (202) 334-3313 (in the Washington metropolitan area); Internet, http://www.nap.edu.

For more information about the Institute of Medicine, visit the IOM home page at: **www.iom.edu**.

Cover image: © Corbis Corporation.

Printed in the United States of America.

The serpent has been a symbol of long life, healing, and knowledge among almost all cultures and religions since the beginning of recorded history. The serpent adopted as a logotype by the Institute of Medicine is a relief carving from ancient Greece, now held by the Staatliche Museen in Berlin.

"Knowing is not enough; we must apply.
Willing is not enough; we must do."
—Goethe

THE NATIONAL ACADEMIES

Advisers to the Nation on Science, Engineering, and Medicine

The **National Academy of Sciences** is a private, nonprofit, self-perpetuating society of distinguished scholars engaged in scientific and engineering research, dedicated to the furtherance of science and technology and to their use for the general welfare. Upon the authority of the charter granted to it by the Congress in 1863, the Academy has a mandate that requires it to advise the federal government on scientific and technical matters. Dr. Ralph J. Cicerone is president of the National Academy of Sciences.

The **National Academy of Engineering** was established in 1964, under the charter of the National Academy of Sciences, as a parallel organization of outstanding engineers. It is autonomous in its administration and in the selection of its members, sharing with the National Academy of Sciences the responsibility for advising the federal government. The National Academy of Engineering also sponsors engineering programs aimed at meeting national needs, encourages education and research, and recognizes the superior achievements of engineers. Dr. Wm. A. Wulf is president of the National Academy of Engineering.

The **Institute of Medicine** was established in 1970 by the National Academy of Sciences to secure the services of eminent members of appropriate professions in the examination of policy matters pertaining to the health of the public. The Institute acts under the responsibility given to the National Academy of Sciences by its congressional charter to be an adviser to the federal government and, upon its own initiative, to identify issues of medical care, research, and education. Dr. Harvey V. Fineberg is president of the Institute of Medicine.

The **National Research Council** was organized by the National Academy of Sciences in 1916 to associate the broad community of science and technology with the Academy's purposes of furthering knowledge and advising the federal government. Functioning in accordance with general policies determined by the Academy, the Council has become the principal operating agency of both the National Academy of Sciences and the National Academy of Engineering in providing services to the government, the public, and the scientific and engineering communities. The Council is administered jointly by both Academies and the Institute of Medicine. Dr. Ralph J. Cicerone and Dr. Wm. A. Wulf are chair and vice chair, respectively, of the National Research Council.

www.national-academies.org

COMMITTEE ON THE DISPOSITION OF THE AIR FORCE HEALTH STUDY

DAVID J. TOLLERUD, M.D., M.P.H., (*Chair*), Professor and Chair, Department of Environmental & Occupational Health Sciences, University of Louisville, Louisville, Kentucky

DAN G. BLAZER, M.D., Ph.D., M.P.H., Professor of Psychiatry, Duke University Medical Center, Duke University, Durham, North Carolina

ELLEN WRIGHT CLAYTON, M.D., J.D., Professor, Center for Genetics and Health Policy, Vanderbilt University, Nashville, Tennessee

MANNING FEINLEIB, M.D., M.P.H., Dr.P.H., Professor, Bloomberg School of Public Health, The Johns Hopkins University, Baltimore, Maryland

MARK S. GOLDBERG, Ph.D., Associate Professor, Department of Medicine, McGill University, Quebec, Canada

SUSAN E. HANKINSON, Sc.D., M.P.H., Associate Professor, Department of Epidemiology, Harvard School of Public Health, Boston, Massachusetts

DAVID A. KALMAN, Ph.D., Professor and Chair, Department of Environmental and Occupational Health Sciences, University of Washington, Seattle, Washington

DEJURAN RICHARDSON, Ph.D., Professor of Mathematics, Lake Forest College, Chicago, Illinois

REGINA SANTELLA, Ph.D., Professor, Mailman School of Public Health, Columbia University, New York City, New York

CONSULTANTS TO THE COMMITTEE

JAMES G. HODGE, JR., J.D., L.L.M., Associate Professor, Bloomberg School of Public Health, The Johns Hopkins University, Baltimore, Maryland

VICTOR PONTES, M.S., Senior Data Manager, The Channing Laboratory, Brigham and Women's Hospital and Harvard Medical School, Boston, Massachusetts

STAFF

David A. Butler, Ph.D., Study Director

Amy O'Connor, M.P.H. candidate, Research Associate

Sonia J. Cheruvillil, M.P.H., Senior Program Assistant

Michael Saulle, B.S., Staff Intern

Rose Marie Martinez, Sc.D., Director, Board on Population Health and Public Health Practices

Reviewers

This report has been reviewed in draft form by individuals chosen for their diverse perspectives and technical expertise, in accordance with procedures approved by the NRC's Report Review Committee. The purpose of this independent review is to provide candid and critical comments that will assist the institution in making its published report as sound as possible and to ensure that the report meets institutional standards for objectivity, evidence, and responsiveness to the study charge. The review comments and draft manuscript remain confidential to protect the integrity of the deliberative process. We wish to thank the following individuals for their review of this report:

Christine B. Ambrosone, Ph.D., Director, Epidemiology; Department of Cancer Prevention and Population Sciences; Roswell Park Cancer Institute

Garnet L. Anderson, Ph.D., Co-Principal Investigator; Fred Hutchinson Cancer Research Center

Erik W. Austin, Acting Director, Assistant Director of ICPSR and Director of Collection Development, and Archivist; Inter-university Consortium for Political and Social Research (ICPSR), Institute for Social Research; University of Michigan

Tee L. Guidotti, M.D., M.P.H., Professor and Chair, Department of Environmental and Occupational Health; School of Public Health and Health Services; The George Washington University Medical Center

Stephen W. Lagakos, Ph.D., Henry Pickering Walcott Professor of Biostatistics and Chair, Department of Biostatistics; Harvard School of Public Health

Mark A. Rothstein, J.D., Herbert F. Boehl Chair of Law and Medicine and Director, Institute for Bioethics, Health Policy and Law; University of Louisville

Louise Ryan, Ph.D., Professor of Biostatistics, Department of Biostatistics; Harvard School of Public Health

Robert D. Sparks, M.D., Senior Associate; California Medical Association Foundation

David S. Strogatz, Ph.D., M.S.P.H., Associate Professor and Chair, Department of Epidemiology and Biostatistics; School of Public Health; University at Albany, State University of New York

Although the reviewers listed above have provided many constructive comments and suggestions, they were not asked to endorse the conclusions or recommendations nor did they see the final draft of the report before its release. The review of this report was overseen by **M. Donald Whorton, M.D.**, WorkCare, Inc. and **Stephen E. Fienberg, Ph.D.**, Carnegie Mellon University. Appointed by the National Research Council and Institute of Medicine, they were responsible for making certain that an independent examination of this report was carried out in accordance with institutional procedures and that all review comments were carefully considered. Responsibility for the final content of this report rests entirely with the authoring committee and the institution.

Contents

DISPOSITION OF THE AIR FORCE HEALTH STUDY

Executive Summary

The last three decades have seen an often acrimonious debate about the effects of the military use of herbicides in Vietnam and, in particular, the potential adverse long-term health effects on those who may have been exposed to these herbicides. The Vietnam War was fought in a jungle environment that provided cover to the enemy and made battlefield observations difficult. Military strategists decided to use herbicides to remove foliage along key roads and waterways, defoliate areas surrounding enemy bases and supply and communications routes, improve visibility in heavily canopied hardwood forests and coastal mangrove forests, and destroy enemy subsistence crops such as rice.

Herbicide missions were executed primarily by U.S. Air Force (USAF) personnel involved in *Operation Ranch Hand* using specially modified C-123 aircraft. From 1962 to 1971, Operation Ranch Hand disseminated over 19 million gallons of herbicides in Vietnam, of which at least 12 million gallons were *Agent Orange*, the name given to a 50:50 mixture of the herbicides 2,4-D and 2,4,5-T. Health concerns over Agent Orange exposure have centered on a contaminant of 2,4,5-T: 2,3,7,8-tetrachlorodibenzo-*p*-dioxin; often abbreviated as *TCDD* and colloquially referred to as *dioxin*. Operation Ranch Hand was the first (and only) large-scale experience with chemical defoliants in U.S. military operations.

Based on the assumption that Ranch Hand personnel were likely to have been among the most highly herbicide-exposed U.S. service members in Vietnam, this group was deemed desirable as a study cohort for the evaluation of the frequency and nature of adverse health effects related to Agent Orange and other military herbicide exposures. The USAF made a commitment to Congress and the White House in 1979 to conduct an epidemiologic study of this group. Dubbed the *Air Force Health Study* (AFHS), it comprises the Ranch Hand veterans as well as a comparison group of USAF personnel who were also in the Vietnam theater, but who were presumed not to have been exposed to herbicides. The study includes a morbidity component with periodic physical examinations and other data collection, a companion examination of reproductive outcomes in subjects' offspring, and a records-based mortality-only component.

AFHS funding has been provided by direct congressional appropriation as a line item in the Department of Defense budget. Approximately $143 million has been spent or allocated for the study.

Major data gathering activities for the AFHS have been completed, and investigators are finishing research projects. The study is currently scheduled to end on September 30, 2006.

INTENT AND GOALS OF THE NATIONAL ACADEMIES STUDY

Public Law 108-183, the Veterans Benefits Act of 2003, directed the Secretary of Veterans Affairs to contract with the National Academy of Sciences (NAS) to address several questions regarding the appropriate disposition of the AFHS.

Section 602(c) of the law charged the NAS to evaluate the following:

> (1) The scientific merit of retaining and maintaining the medical records, other study data, and laboratory specimens collected in the course of the Air Force Health Study after the currently scheduled termination date of the study in 2006.
>
> (2) Whether or not any obstacles exist to retaining and maintaining the medical records, other study data, and laboratory specimens referred to in paragraph (1), including privacy concerns.
>
> (3) The advisability of providing independent oversight of the medical records, other study data, and laboratory specimens referred to in paragraph (1), and of any further study of such records, data, and specimens, and, if so, the mechanism for providing such oversight.
>
> (4) The advisability of extending the Air Force Health Study, including the potential value and relevance of extending the study, the potential cost of extending the study, and the federal or nonfederal entity best suited to continue the study if extended.
>
> (5) The advisability of making the laboratory specimens of the Air Force Health Study available for independent research, including the potential value and relevance of such research, and the potential cost of such research.

This report, prepared by the Committee on the Disposition of the Air Force Health Study, provides responses to these charges.

CHARACTERISTICS OF THE AFHS DATA ASSETS

Most of the AFHS research is focused on the morbidity component of the study, where exceptionally detailed data gathering took place. The initial physical examination and surveying of AFHS subjects (Cycle 1) was conducted in 1982 and subsequent cycles were conducted in 1985, 1987, 1992, 1997, and 2002. Data from the physical examinations include blood draws, urine and semen collections, skin and fat biopsies, stool smears, spirometry, chest X rays, electrocardiograms (ECGs), dermatology and peripheral vascular examinations, neurological assessments, psychological testing, and many other clinical endpoints. Subjects were asked to provide their medical records, as well as those of their children (up to age 17), their present partner, and any previous partner. Questionnaires eliciting information on education; employment; income; marital and fertility history; child and family health; health habits; recreation, leisure, and physical activities; toxic substances exposure; military experience; and wartime herbicide exposure were also administered. In 1982, 1,046 of the so-called *Ranch Hands* and 1,223 comparison subjects participated in the first of the physical exam cycles. Twenty years later, 777 Ranch Hands and 1,174 comparison subjects completed the sixth cycle. In all, 2,758 subjects participated in at least one cycle exam. Reproductive data were gathered and coded on 9,921 conceptions and 8,100 live births. The mortality component of the study has followed over 20,000 Vietnam War-era veterans with service in Southeast Asia for nearly 25 years.

More than 86,000 biologic specimens have been collected over the course of the study; approximately half of these are serum. Blood was collected in all six cycles and serum stored; semen was obtained in the first cycle and urine in Cycles 1–3 (1982, 1985, and 1987). Adipose tissues collected during Cycle 5 are currently held at UC Davis. In the last (sixth) cycle, whole blood was also stored.

Participation rates in the morbidity study have been relatively high, particularly among Ranch Hand subjects, ranging from 87 percent at the baseline examination to 74 percent at the fifth follow-up. All told, the AFHS has more data points and a higher rate of follow-up than the Framingham Heart Study.

Chapter 2 of the report provides background information on Operation Ranch Hand and on the origins, development, implementation, findings, and impact of the AFHS. It also briefly summarizes the results of AFHS reports and papers.

FINDINGS, CONCLUSIONS, AND RECOMMENDATIONS

Box ES-1 summarizes the committee's response to the charge contained in the Veterans Benefits Act of 2003. Specifics are discussed below.

BOX ES-1
Summary of the Committee's Response to the Charge

There is scientific merit in retaining and maintaining the medical records, other study data, and laboratory specimens collected in the course of the Air Force Health Study after the study's currently scheduled termination date: no other epidemiologic dataset on Vietnam veterans contains as detailed information over as long a time period, the data appear to be of high quality and the specimens well preserved, and analysis of the assets has contributed to the literature addressing the health of Vietnam veterans.

Obstacles exist to retaining and maintaining the AFHS data assets. These relate to factors intrinsic to the study's design, resulting from implementation decisions made by the investigators, relating to documentation and organization of the data assets, and addressing the preservation of the privacy of the study subjects and the confidentiality of their personal information. The committee believes that the identified obstacles are surmountable.

Further study of the AFHS medical records, other study data, and laboratory specimens is advisable. This should be accomplished by making these materials available for research via a custodian that takes an active role in fostering use of the assets. Five years after the chosen custodian assumes responsibility, a committee should be convened to evaluate whether any further support should be extended to the maintenance of access to the data or the biospecimens.

The potential value and relevance of further study of the AFHS data assets rest in the application of the results of future health research on the data assets. This research could encompass using novel analysis approaches, employing new technology and techniques, and examining data and outcomes not evaluated to date. The cost of such work will vary greatly, depending on the research question that is addressed.

The committee cannot offer a specific recommendation on the federal or nonfederal entity best suited to continue the study of the AFHS data assets but has identified a number of options that could be pursued successfully.

Independent oversight of future research using the AFHS data assets is advisable, and should be provided through the review of proposals for scientific merit and adherence to ethical, legal, and related considerations by an Institutional Review Board and, separately, an advisory and oversight board. Additionally, research should be carried out in a manner transparent to study subjects, through systematic communication of research plans and results.

The Database and Specimens Repository

Chapter 3 describes the elements comprising AFHS data holdings and their accessibility to outside researchers; Chapter 4 details the AFHS specimen collection, including information related to specimen gathering, processing, and storage, and obstacles and limitations to the collection's future use. Together, these two chapters recapitulate and expand on the text of the committee's interim letter report, which was issued in November 2005.

The committee found that while the medical records, other study data, and laboratory specimens collected in the course of the AFHS have been properly maintained, they are not currently organized and documented in a manner that allows them to be easily understood, evaluated, managed, or analyzed by persons outside of the AFHS. It therefore concluded that the present state of the documentation and organization of these assets was an obstacle to retaining and maintaining them. The committee recommended that action be taken prior to the currently scheduled termination date to reorganize and document the study's medical records, other study data, and laboratory specimens in a form and format that allows them to be easily understood, evaluated, managed, or analyzed by persons outside of the AFHS. Several specific actions to address the shortcomings are detailed in these chapters. Reorganization and documentation of the data assets is a crucial prerequisite to their future use.

The committee believes that it is incumbent on the USAF as the current custodian of the research materials to ensure their proper documentation and organization. It therefore recommended that, if available AFHS program funds are not sufficient to accomplish the actions it proposes, then supplemental funding be provided to carry out such work in a complete and timely manner.

Value of the Research Assets

Chapter 5 builds on the material presented in the earlier chapters to address the scientific merit of retaining and maintaining the AFHS data and specimen holdings. The following three general conclusions are drawn:

1. The AFHS data assets are unique: no other epidemiologic dataset on Vietnam veterans contains as detailed information over as long a time period.
2. The data collected by the AFHS appear to be of high quality and the specimens appear to be well preserved.
3. Analysis of the AFHS data assets has contributed to the literature addressing the health of Vietnam veterans.

It follows that there is scientific merit in retaining and maintaining these resources after the study's currently scheduled termination date.

Some limitations to the further use of AFHS materials were identified, including those related to the design and execution of the study, and to privacy, security, and other ethical, legal, and social issues. The committee concluded that these concerns and issues are not an intrinsic obstacle to retaining and maintaining the assets after the currently scheduled termination date. However, attention to such concerns and issues must play a central role in decisions regarding their future disposition.

Because there is scientific merit in retaining and maintaining these assets and the identified obstacles to these are believed to be surmountable, the committee concluded that further study of the AFHS medical records, other study data, and laboratory specimens is advisable.

To date, research results published by study investigators have been largely limited to outcomes related to the examination of the possible long-term health effects of wartime exposure to the herbicides used in Vietnam. However, the data assets can be used to examine a far broader range of health questions. The potential value and relevance of extending the study of the AFHS data assets rest in taking full advantage of the available information and in the application of the results of future research on the assets. This research could encompass

- reanalysis of outcomes examined by the AFHS using different assumptions and approaches than have been applied to date,
- new analyses of the medical records and other study data that examine questions that were not addressed in the AFHS,
- new studies of the collected biospecimens that take advantage of advances in technology and science to conduct analyses that were not contemplated in the AFHS protocol,
- expansion of the study's period of analysis through follow-up of the cohorts using publicly available information, and
- additional follow-up of health outcomes in AFHS participants.

The AFHS dataset has several weaknesses that limit its utility as a means of evaluating the health impacts of Agent Orange exposure. These include the inherently small size of the cohort,[1] the fact that the cohort is unrepresentative of in-theater veterans, lack of any biomarkers of herbicide exposure other than TCDD, little information on subjects' locations in the theater of operations, unavailability of detailed exposure histories, and possible herbicide exposures in the comparison population. It would thus be a mistake to view the committee's conclusions as an indication that the AFHS data assets are a definitive source of information on this topic. Instead, the data and specimens are pieces of evidence that can be

[1]The reproductive outcomes and mortality-only components of the study have larger sample populations but far less detailed data on the subjects.

put to use in the effort to understand the determinants of good and ill health in Vietnam veterans and to address other scientific questions. Some of these may not be directly related to herbicide exposure but may still be important for furthering knowledge about veterans' health and the natural history and risks of disease.

While some analyses of AFHS data assets have been carried out by outside researchers, the capacity of the assets to inform the study of other health issues is largely untapped and unknown. Until they are made available to the research community, their worth as a source of information on veterans' and men's health will remain open to question.

Options and Recommendations for Further Study

The committee took a broad view of what constituted extension of the AFHS. In Chapter 6, it offers a number of options and recommendations regarding the further study of the data assets. These include observations on the maintenance and use of the assets, the protection of the interests of the study subjects, the characteristics of a good future custodian of the assets, mechanisms for providing oversight of prospective research, alternatives for the management of the assets, and the costs associated with the assets' maintenance and use. Throughout, it addresses the obstacles to conducting further research and possible means of overcoming them.

The two primary considerations in evaluating the disposition of the AFHS hard copy records are compliance with the Federal Records Act and retention for further research purposes. Many of the hard copy records have been scanned and the images stored in electronic files in Portable Document Format (PDF) that were subjected to quality control checks for readability. The committee recommends that the hard copy originals of these saved documents be destroyed unless the National Archivist concludes that they must be maintained or they are subject to other records retention requirements. No matter what decision is made by the National Archives regarding the retention of the records, the committee recommends that a separate electronic copy of these records should be kept for possible placement with another custodian.

Recommendations intended to facilitate the future use of other nonelectronic assets are also presented. In brief, the committee believes that such data assets should be written to electronic form where a mature technology exists to do so and where the assets have future research value. The X-ray films can be readily converted to digital format—this should be done with acceptable quality control, the resource properly documented, and thereafter the original films disposed of according to standard practices. As no widespread technology exists for ECG strip digitization, the originals should be retained. The AFHS should consult with the National Institute of Dental and Craniofacial Research on whether the video tapes of subjects' teeth collected in the course of the study have future research value—if the decision is made to retain them, they should be digitized for ease of long-term management and storage.

Five alternatives for the future of the AFHS data assets were identified:

1. Render the data assets to the National Archives for evaluation and possible retention.
2. Identify or establish a research entity for the management and dissemination of existing data assets.
3. Have that entity also continue passive data collection on AFHS subjects.
4. Have the entity maintain contact with the AFHS subjects and conduct or facilitate further active data collection.
5. Extend the AFHS as it is presently constituted.

The medical records and other study data collected in the course of the AFHS will be rendered to the National Archives for evaluation because this is required by statute. Should the National Archives choose to retain them, the records and other study data may be made available to the public *as is* at some point in the future. The Archives does not, however, have exclusive rights to the data. No matter what it decides, copies of the data may be made available through other channels. If these assets, along with the study's biospecimen collection, are transferred to a new custodian, other alternatives that would enhance access to the assets would be possible. A custodian could offer research support of various forms that would facilitate their use; or the custodian or outside researchers could supplement the assets with data from publicly available sources or the study participants themselves.

The committee concludes that it is advisable to extend the AFHS by making the database and associated biospecimen collection available for study via a custodian that should take an active role in fostering research on the assets. The committee is thus not recommending that the AFHS be extended in its current form as a research study characterized by periodic, cohort-wide data and biospecimen collection, and analysis by a dedicated team of researchers. Instead, the committee believes that the present data assets should be made available to the whole of the research community. This will allow them to continue to be used to help understand the health consequences of service in Vietnam and also to address other scientific questions related to the health of veterans as well as aging persons.

The committee also concludes that it is advisable to allow for the *possibility* of collecting additional data and specimens, work that could be conducted by the custodian or by independent researchers. The committee does not explicitly endorse the collection of further morbidity or mortality data but believes that it is appropriate to leave the option open should both the need and support for such work be identified. Developing a future research agenda or setting research priorities is beyond the charge of the committee.

The committee identified several characteristics of a good custodian of the assets. Among these is the ability to satisfy operational requirements related to the supervision of and access to the data and biological materials. Also important is a commitment to address the complex ethical, legal, social, and related issues that arise when managing epidemiologic records and associated biospecimens. The committee specifically recommends that the successor custodian be able to demonstrate in advance its capacity to protect the privacy and security of the research participants and their data to the greatest extent possible. The custodian also should comply with the information and publication restrictions in Section 308(d) of the Public Health Act and should seek a certificate of confidentiality under Section 301(d) of the Act.

The concept of individual informed consent is particularly salient in the setting of the AFHS where thousands of research participants devoted a great deal of time and underwent significant inconvenience and discomfort to contribute to the study. Their wishes must be considered in deciding whether and how to use these data in future research. In recognition of this, the committee recommends that prior to the end of the study, the AFHS should notify the study participants of the following:

- The study, as currently constituted, is ending.
- The assets will be transferred to a successor custodian, the characteristics of which will be described to the extent feasible.
- The successor custodian will seek additional consent for future research involving identifiable data from the research participants, which will cover the topics enumerated below, prior to conducting any research.

This notification should offer the participants the opportunity to decide that information and specimens relating to them should not be transferred.

The committee also recommends that the successor custodian obtain new informed consent that includes

- their identity;
- notice of the types of participant data and samples that will be maintained by the custodian;
- the procedural protections that will be provided for the data and specimens, including access policies, and oversight;
- the specific privacy and security protections that will protect the data and specimens;
- the types of studies that the participant is willing to have his data and specimens used for;
- whether the participant is willing to be approached in the future by investigators to seek participation in additional studies, including information regarding notice and recontact criteria; and
- which individual study results the participant will and will not receive.

If health information regarding the partners and children of the AFHS research participants is made available for future research, consent, and where appropriate, parental permission and assent, must be sought from these individuals. Conducting future research on the data assets is predicated on gaining permission for such work from the subjects. If a significant number of subjects choose not to make their information available, it will greatly limit the future usefulness of the assets.

The committee believes that independent oversight of the AFHS data assets is advisable. Specifically, it recommends that the successor custodian of the AFHS data and biospecimens should commit to reviews of future research involving the assets by an Institutional Review Board constituted in accordance with the Common Rule, create and maintain an independent advisory and oversight board to provide guidance on the conduct of future research and to review and evaluate proposals for use of the data and biologic samples, and develop and implement strategies for apprising the research subjects about the ways in which their information is used and the scientific discoveries that result. These commitments should be a prerequisite to the transfer of the assets. The committee suggests that the advisory and oversight board's membership consist of 8–12 established scientists representing a range of appropriate disciplines such as herbicide exposure health effects, military health, epidemiology, and aging. Two lay members—study subjects if possible—should be included to provide insights from the participant and veteran perspectives.

The committee identified the following seven options for future management of the data assets:

1. Use the National Archives data management and distribution mechanisms.
2. Use the existing AFHS infrastructure within the USAF.
3. Use Department of Defense (DOD) epidemiologic data management and distribution mechanisms.
4. Use Department of Veterans Affairs or VA-affiliated epidemiologic data management and distribution mechanisms.
5. Use National Institutes of Health or Centers for Disease Control and Prevention epidemiologic data management and distribution mechanisms.
6. Use the Institute of Medicine (IOM) Medical Follow-up Agency.
7. Identify a new custodian through a competitive process.

The committee does not offer a recommendation on the specific federal or nonfederal entity best suited to assume responsibility for the AFHS data assets. All of the listed options have advantages and disadvantages, and all could be made to work with the appropriate provision of funds, commitment on the part of the custodian, and implementation of the recommendations offered in the report. The committee believes that the AFHS data would be unlikely to realize their research potential if they were only available from the National Archives, which would neither promote their use nor supported analysis of them and which could not be a home for the specimens. The USAF and DOD manage and analyze other epidemiologic data assets comprising military populations but have not expressed an interest in the AFHS materials, which address a population that is no longer on active duty and exposures that are unlikely to be an issue for future operations. The CDC and NIH have extensive infrastructures in place to manage the dissemination of epidemiologic data and biospecimens in a manner that protects the interests of research subjects. It is unclear, however, whether these bodies would like to assume custody of the data assets or whether the AFHS subjects would be comfortable with any shift in focus in the use of their materials that might be occasioned by a CDC or NIH custodianship. Using a competitive process to identify a new custodian would ensure that a motivated party with an explicit data management plan would assume responsibility for the assets. It would, though, present logistical challenges to carry out this process in a timely manner.

The Department of Veterans Affairs maintains Epidemiological Research and Information Centers (ERICs) under their Cooperative Studies Program. The committee considers two of the centers—the Massachusetts Veterans Epidemiology Research and Information Center (MAVERIC) and the Seattle Epidemiologic Research and Information Center (Seattle ERIC)—to be good candidates for custodianship, in part because they manage data assets that are in some respects similar to AFHS's and make these assets available to independent, outside researchers under controlled circumstances. The IOM's Medical Follow-up Agency (MFUA) is also identified as a good candidate. MFUA conducts epidemiologic studies of military and veterans' health, focusing on records-based research—primarily retrospective cohort studies of morbidity outcomes and mortality. It also maintains a collection of data on study populations of former military personnel that it makes available to independent researchers.

These three candidates share several positive attributes. MAVERIC, Seattle ERIC, and MFUA all have prior experience in veterans' health studies, collecting and storing epidemiologic data, disseminating it to independent researchers, fostering collaborations with those researchers, maintaining quality control over the studies that use their datasets, and publishing results in the peer-reviewed literature. All have military or veteran health issues as the central focus of their operations, but also conduct other types of studies with their data assets. To the committee's knowledge, none has experienced a breach in their system of protecting subjects' privacy and the security of their data. These entities are not, however, without weaknesses. Among the concerns noted by the committee is whether the ERICs have the interest or ability to take on the additional responsibility of the AFHS data assets and how MFUA would manage the biospecimens in the absence of its own repository.

A common issue for these potential custodians is a secure source of funding. Assigning responsibility for the assets to a government entity without also providing a budget allocation would sap funds in a time of constrained resources, and MFUA or other nongovernment entities could not take on the assets without financial support.

The committee was asked to consider the costs of extending the study of the AFHS data assets. These comprise the costs of maintaining and providing access to the assets and the costs of doing research on them. The primary physical costs of maintaining AFHS's medical records and other study data and making them available to researchers are associated with storage and handling of the electronic materials. Personnel expenses related to database management are best expressed in terms of workforce needs, as the allocations required to cover direct and indirect costs vary by location and type of institution (government, nonprofit, or commercial) as well as over time. Typical needs would be for time from a principal investigator or project director, data manager, programmers, clerical personnel, and perhaps a webmaster or participant liaison. With the possible exception of a data manager, none of these persons would need to devote their full time to these tasks. The cost for physical maintenance of the AFHS biospecimens will vary considerably, again depending upon the type of institution in which the collection is housed and whether an existing facility is used or a new one created.

It is difficult for the committee to present a bottom-line estimate for the total cost of implementing its recommendations because of the number of uncertainties and variables involved. *Roughly speaking*, the committee estimates that $150,000–300,000 per year would be required to support the custodian's database management responsibilities and an additional $200,000 or more per year for proper maintenance of the biospecimens. The actual amount would depend critically on the custodian chosen and the number and type of studies proposed for and conducted with the data assets. First year costs would be higher because a number of one-time-only tasks would have to be performed to set up the operation. The committee assumes that the custodian will impose fees for the provision of database and biospecimen access to recover at least some their costs. It is important, especially in the early years of this new phase in the life of the AFHS resources, that such fees be set at a level that will facilitate use of the resource.

The cost of conducting new studies using the AFHS data assets will greatly depend on their scope and whether they require the use of other databases, analyze biospecimens, or contact subjects. Pilot studies and empirical analyses of the existing AFHS dataset could have relatively modest needs for support—tens of thousands of dollars—while investigations that include collecting additional data and specimens could potentially cost millions of dollars. However, with the exception of the program proposed below, these costs will be the responsibility of prospective researchers, who will need to obtain their own support from funding sources.

The committee believes that funds are needed to establish the AFHS data assets as a resource for external researchers. Its judgment is that a limited-life, small grant program is the best way to accomplish this goal. The committee anticipates that this program will stimulate prospective researchers to also seek external funding from other existing sources for further or more in-depth projects. The committee therefore recommends that Congress should allocate a minimum of $250,000 per year for three years to cover the direct costs of small grants for secondary data analysis or pilot projects using the data assets of the AFHS. This allocation would provide seed money for one to three investigations each year. These funds should be *in addition to* previously planned or contemplated support of Vietnam veterans' health research—funding should not be diverted from other research efforts for this initiative.

Although the committee is enthusiastic about the potential for future studies of the AFHS data assets, it understands that the viability of such work is not assured. It therefore believes that it is appropriate to revisit the question of support for further work after the committee's recommendations have been implemented and have had time to play out in the research realm. A 5-year commitment—that is, two years after the last small grants proposed above are made—should be sufficient to establish whether the AFHS resources have value and relevance as a resource. The committee therefore recommends that five years after the chosen custodian assumes responsibility a committee should be convened to evaluate the potential value and relevance of extending further support to the maintenance of access to the data or the biospecimens collected in the course of the AFHS.

The costs of properly documenting the data assets, making them available to the research community, and implementing the proposed 5-year program to encourage their use are small in comparison with the government's investment of ~$143 million to date. The potential benefits of these actions, while subject to considerable uncertainty, appear to greatly outweigh the costs.

1

Introduction

INTENT AND GOALS OF THE STUDY

Public Law 108-183, the Veterans Benefits Act of 2003, directed the Secretary of Veterans Affairs to contract with the National Academy of Sciences (NAS) to address several questions regarding the appropriate disposition of the Air Force Health Study (AFHS). The AFHS is an epidemiologic study of U.S. Air Force (USAF) personnel who were responsible for conducting aerial spray missions of herbicides during the Vietnam era—called *Ranch Hands* because the spray program was designated *Operation Ranch Hand*—and a matched cohort of comparison subjects who performed similar duties in Southeast Asia during the same time period but who were not involved with herbicide spraying. The study's first of six cycles of physical examinations were conducted in 1982 on 1,046 Ranch Hands and 1,223 comparison subjects (Michalek, 2005).

Section 602(c) of Pub. L. 108-183 charged the NAS to evaluate the following:

> (1) The scientific merit of retaining and maintaining the medical records, other study data, and laboratory specimens collected in the course of the Air Force Health Study after the currently scheduled termination date of the study in 2006.
>
> (2) Whether or not any obstacles exist to retaining and maintaining the medical records, other study data, and laboratory specimens referred to in paragraph (1), including privacy concerns.
>
> (3) The advisability of providing independent oversight of the medical records, other study data, and laboratory specimens referred to in paragraph (1), and of any further study of such records, data, and specimens, and, if so, the mechanism for providing such oversight.

(4) The advisability of extending the Air Force Health Study, including the potential value and relevance of extending the study, the potential cost of extending the study, and the federal or nonfederal entity best suited to continue the study if extended.

(5) The advisability of making the laboratory specimens of the Air Force Health Study available for independent research, including the potential value and relevance of such research, and the potential cost of such research.

In response to a request by the Secretary of Veterans Affairs, the Institute of Medicine (IOM) of the National Academies constituted the Committee on the Disposition of the Air Force Health Study to tackle these issues.

INFORMATION GATHERING BY THE COMMITTEE

The committee conducted four meetings. During the first meeting, the committee received its charge from Dr. Mark Brown, the director of the Environmental Agents Service of the Department of Veterans Affairs (VA). The committee was also briefed on the study design, protocol, and results of the AFHS by the study's then principal investigator, Dr. Joel E. Michalek. The second and third meetings included workshop sessions with presentations from experts in the conduct of longitudinal epidemiologic studies and the management and dissemination of epidemiologic data and biospecimens. Representatives of veterans service organizations also presented information for the consideration of the committee. Appendix A lists the workshop speakers and presentation topics. The final meeting was a closed session where committee members concluded their deliberations and finalized their findings, conclusions, and recommendations.

In addition to the meetings and workshops, the committee engaged in an extensive effort to collect other information on topics relevant to its charge. As part of this effort, four members of the committee—Drs. Blazer, Hankinson, Kalman, and Richardson—conducted a site visit to the AFHS research facility at Brooks City-Base, San Antonio, Texas, on May 27, 2005. Accompanying them were IOM study staff and Mr. Victor Pontes, a consultant to the committee on issues related to SAS datasets.[1] The intent of the visit was to evaluate the state of the documentation of the study's data assets, examine how they were stored, and assess the ease of access to them. Working groups were established to focus on the electronically stored data and the specimens. Their findings are summarized in the committee's interim letter report (IOM, 2005a).

The committee's information gathering was greatly aided by AFHS staff members, who were helpful in answering the committee's many questions. The committee thanks them for their cooperation.

[1]SAS is a software database management and analysis system. AFHS uses SAS to electronically store and analyze data collected over the course of the study.

THE COMMITTEE'S INTERIM LETTER REPORT

The committee produced an interim letter report in October 2005 (IOM, 2005a). The purpose of this report was to address a component of the charge that had a bearing on the conduct of the AFHS in the time leading up to its scheduled termination date of September 30, 2006. Specifically, the committee applied the information it learned in a May 2005 site visit to the AFHS research facility to the question of "whether or not any obstacles exist to retaining and maintaining the medical records, other study data, and laboratory specimens" collected in the course of the study. The committee believed that it was important to offer findings, conclusions, and recommendations on this topic in advance of its final report to allow for their timely consideration, as the availability of the investigators most familiar with the AFHS data assets and the funding to support them cannot be assured after the end of fiscal year 2006.

The findings, conclusions, and recommendations contained in the interim letter report are recapitulated in Chapters 3 and 4 of this report.

RELATED INSTITUTE OF MEDICINE REPORTS

Three IOM reports in the Veterans and Agent Orange (VAO) series have addressed issues directly related to this study. *Veterans and Agent Orange: Update 2000* (IOM, 2001) is the first of these. Based on their evaluation of available information, the committee responsible for that report stated:

> There is scientific merit in retaining and maintaining [AFHS] medical records and samples, so that—with proper respect for the privacy of the study participants—they could be available for future research. It therefore recommends that the federal government examine whether and how the various forms of data and specimens collected in the course of the AFHS could be retained and maintained, and what form of oversight should be established for their future use. The committee further recommends that consideration be given to whether it is appropriate to continue the study past its planned completion date. (p. 161)

Veterans and Agent Orange: Update 2002 (IOM, 2003) reiterated the findings and recommendations related to retaining and maintaining the data assets and making them available for future research. It went on to state:

> The committee recommends continuing the study past its planned completion date. . . . Given the increased incidence of such diseases as amyotrophic lateral sclerosis, Parkinson's disease, prostatic cancer, and brain cancer in aging populations and the increasing age of the Vietnam-veteran cohort, research should specifically examine those diseases in the Vietnam veterans. (p. 542)

The most recent (as of 2005) report in the series, *Veterans and Agent Orange: Update 2004* (IOM, 2005b), was being conducted during the time this study was initiated. It noted, "Previous VAO committees have recommended extending the AFHS, and this committee encourages the newly appointed AFHS review committee to consider those recommendations in the course of its deliberation" (p. 492). The legislative history of the Veterans Benefits Act of 2003 does not indicate whether the *Update 2000* recommendations to consider whether the AFHS should be extended and examine the disposition of its data assets were influential in the decision to mandate the formation of this committee. To the best of the committee's knowledge, no other actions were taken in response to the previous committees' recommendations. This committee is aware of the previous committees' findings and recommendations but operated completely independent of them and reached its own conclusions based on its own evaluation of the available information.[2]

ORGANIZATION OF THE REPORT

The balance of this report is organized in five chapters and supporting appendixes. Chapter 2 provides background material for several aspects related to the committee's charge. It chronicles the development of the military herbicide program and *Operation Ranch Hand*—specifically, the ensuing controversy and the creation, implementation, findings, and impact of the AFHS. Chapter 3 describes not only the elements comprised by the AFHS data holdings collected and assembled during the course of the study but their accessibility to outside researchers as well. Chapter 4 details the AFHS specimen collection including elements related to specimen gathering, processing, storage, and their potential application to future research. Chapter 5 builds on the material presented in Chapters 2 through 4 related to the scientific merit of retaining and maintaining AFHS data and specimen holdings and discusses some of the associated ethical, legal, and social issues. Chapter 6 contains the committee's conclusions and recommendations regarding the disposition of the specimen and data assets collected in the course of the AFHS subsequent to its currently scheduled termination date.

Agendas from all public meetings held by the Committee on the Disposition of the Air Force Health Study through June 2005 are provided in Appendix A. Appendix B contains 16 tables pertaining to the endpoints analyzed, covariates included in analyses, and laboratory tests performed as part of AFHS physical examinations. Appendix C comprises a list of the epidemiologic studies related to Vietnam veterans' health reviewed in the IOM's VAO series. Appendix D presents an analysis of the statistical power to detect excess relative risks among the AFHS population in a follow-up mortality study. Appendix E—which is excerpted from the IOM report *Vaccine Safety Research, Data Access, and Public*

[2]None of the committee members responsible for this report served on the committees responsible for the 2000, 2002, or 2004 updates. Dr. David Tollerud—the chair of this committee—did serve on previous Veterans and Agent Orange committees.

Trust (IOM, 2005c)—contains summary information from existing repositories on procedures for asset access application, processing, and associated fees. A final Appendix (F) provides biographic information on the committee members, consultants, and staff responsible for this project.

REFERENCES

IOM (Institute of Medicine). 2001. *Veterans and Agent Orange: Update 2000.* Washington, DC: National Academy Press.

IOM. 2003. *Veterans and Agent Orange: Update 2002.* Washington, DC: The National Academies Press.

IOM. 2005a. *Disposition of the Air Force Health Study—Interim Letter Report.* Washington, DC: The National Academies Press. [Online]. Available: http://www.nap.edu/catalog/11483.html [accessed December 1, 2005].

IOM. 2005b. *Veterans and Agent Orange: Update 2004.* Washington, DC: The National Academies Press.

IOM. 2005c. *Vaccine Safety Research, Data Access, and Public Trust.* Washington, DC: The National Academies Press.

Michalek JE. 2005 (January 5). *The Air Force Health Study: An Overview and Update.* PowerPoint presentation before the Committee on the Disposition of the Air Force Health Study, Washington, DC.

2

Background

This chapter provides background information on a number of topics related to the committee's charge. It begins with accounts of the development of a military aerial herbicide delivery system and the Operation Ranch Hand spray program during the Vietnam War. The early history of the Agent Orange controversy is then reviewed along with the first studies of Vietnam veterans' health. A detailed description of the Air Force Health Study (AFHS) follows—its origins, the development of the protocol, identification of the exposed and comparison cohorts, means by which exposure was characterized, collection and analysis of data, results of the research,[1] and cost of conducting the study. The Department of Veterans Affairs (VA) compensation policy for health problems deemed to be associated with wartime exposure to herbicides is also outlined. The chapter concludes with a discussion of the Institute of Medicine's (IOM) comprehensive reviews of the literature regarding adverse health outcomes and herbicide and dioxin exposure, as well as the role of AFHS reports and papers in that work.

This information forms the foundation for many of the committee's findings, conclusions, and recommendations in succeeding chapters.

DEVELOPMENT OF A MILITARY AERIAL HERBICIDE DELIVERY SYSTEM

It has been said that the seeds of the Agent Orange controversy were planted during World War II (WWII) when the conquest of islands in the Pacific theater

[1]This chapter is not intended to provide a critical review of the research results—a task outside of the committee's charge—but rather to recap the content of the reports and papers prepared by the investigators over the years.

of operations exacted enormous human tolls on the U.S. Army and Marine Corps units mounting first-wave beach assaults (Galston, 2001). At the time, high explosives designed expressly for tree destruction had been used by the military as one tactical option to eliminate the enemy advantage afforded by the dense indigenous vegetation. This tactic was eventually abandoned, as fallen trees could still provide effective cover and concealment for defensive enemy positions along targeted beachheads (Minarik, 1964).

Prior to WWII, the U.S. Army Air Corps had assembled the basic physical apparatus of aerial chemical delivery systems as part of its chemical warfare research and development effort (Buckingham, 1982). Methods for low-altitude application were well beyond preliminary developmental stages, and the atmospheric conditions necessary for the delivery of effective chemical concentrations to targets had also been characterized (Buckingham, 1982). Despite their availability during WWII, aerial chemical delivery systems for herbicide application were not widely implemented in the Pacific theater.[2] The technology was, however, employed at many locations including Morotai, Palau, Iwo Jima, and Okinawa in an effort to rid regions of strategic importance of disease-carrying vectors (Cecil, 1986).[3] In the 1950s, the British military effectively used aerially disseminated herbicides,[4] a fact that did not go unnoticed by U.S. military planners and the State Department as the situation grew more volatile in Southeast Asia (SEA) during the late 1950s and early 1960s (Buckingham, 1997).

By the time President Kennedy took office in 1961, the U.S. military possessed a fairly well-developed arsenal of herbicidal agents. Three years prior to Kennedy's inauguration, an efficient large-capacity system for the delivery of liquid agents had become standard U.S. Air Force (USAF) inventory (Buckingham, 1982). This system, referred to as the MC-1 Hourglass, comprised a 1,000-gallon tank, pump, and pipe assembly with six nozzles and emergency dumping capabilities (IOM, 1994). The MC-1 was the forerunner of the spray system that was ultimately fitted to the Fairchild C-123s flown in Vietnam.

Meanwhile, in 1959, an H-21 helicopter was successfully used for aerial delivery of herbicides to clear a grove of nuisance sugar maples from an artillery firing range at Camp Drum, New York.[5] The herbicide used at Camp Drum was a 50:50 mixture of two phenoxyacetic acids: 2,4-dichlorophenoxyacetic acid

---

[2]Limited aerial spray tests did occur on some Japanese-controlled islands to demarcate navigation points and to remove dense tropical foliage (Buckingham, 1997).

[3]Vector-borne disease (malaria, dengue, filariasis, and fly-borne dysentery) was the major cause of lost man-hours for the Army Air Corps in the Pacific during WWII. Copper acetate arsenite (*Paris Green* dust) and dichlorodiphenyltrichloroethane (DDT) were among the insecticides used in the Pacific to destroy adult and larval vector populations (Cecil, 1986).

[4]During the Malayan Emergency (1953–1954) the British used helicopters and some fixed-wing aircraft for successful aerial delivery of sodium arsenate, and later, a mixture of trioxene and diesolene to agricultural targets (Buckingham, 1982).

[5]Known today as *Fort Drum*.

(2,4-D) and 2,4,5-trichlorophenoxyacetic acid (2,4,5-T).[6] The herbicide application achieved the desired effect: within one month, treated trees were undergoing abscission (falling) of leaves and significant regrowth was not observed the following year (Warren, 1968).

The organic acid mixture used at Camp Drum was only one herbicidal candidate of more than 1,000 compounds tested during and after WWII at the Army Chemical Corps laboratories at Fort Detrick, Maryland (Midwest Research Institute, 1967). Early synthetic pesticides were mainly inorganic compounds. The emergence of organic compounds as effective herbicidal agents can be attributed to the isolation and ultimate synthesis of compounds during the 1930s that were found to act as chemical messengers (hormones) in plants (Butler, 2005).[7] Defoliants are a subclass of herbicides that induce abscission.[8] Their application can, but does not necessarily, destroy the entire plant (Buckingham, 1982). Both 2,4-D and 2,4,5-T act as plant hormones, and application of species-appropriate concentrations ultimately induces abscission.

By the end of WWII, 2,4-D had found widespread use in the agricultural and forestry industries. More than 5 million pounds of 2,4-D were produced in 1945 and *Weedone*, which was released that same year, was the first 2,4-D-containing weed killer marketed in the United States for general use (Cecil, 1986). Both civilian and military WWII-era research efforts led to the same conclusion with respect to chlorophenoxy herbicides: formulations containing a combination of 2,4-D and 2,4,5-T were found to exhibit the most effective level of selective herbicidal activity for both broad-leafed and woody plants.[9] Thus, the herbicides used in Vietnam were not novel compounds. Just one year prior to the launch of herbicidal missions in Vietnam, hundreds of thousands of miles of U.S. roads, railways, and utility easements as well as tens of millions of acres of agricultural land had been treated with chlorophenoxy herbicides, an appreciable percentage of which had been disseminated aerially (Buckingham, 1982).

---

[6]The mixture tested at Camp Drum in 1959 was actually Agent Purple, which was a 50:30:20 mixture of n-butyl 2,4-D, n-butyl 2,4,5-T, and isobutyl 2,4,5-T (Stellman et al., 2003).

[7]Butler (2005) summarizes the history of the development of 2,4-D and 2,4,5-T and the subsequent discovery of 2,3,7,8-tetrachlorodibenzo-*p*-dioxin as a 2,4,5-T contaminant.

[8]Abscission is typically governed by changes in diurnal cycle duration and occurs when auxin (3-indoleacetic acid) levels increase, ultimately leading to the production of enzymes that digest the structural plant material that secures the leaf to the plant stem. Both 2,4-D and 2,4,5-T trigger this same chain of chemical events (Galston, 2001).

[9]The selectivity of these compounds is based, in part, on leaf surface area in the horizontal plane, meaning horizontally planar leaves make better herbicide collection areas than leaves that grow predominately in the vertical plane (Buckingham, 1982). Selectivity holds true up to a certain threshold concentration (Cecil, 1986) and is also governed by variation in plant growth, absorption, and metabolism rates (Lavy, 1987).

OPERATION RANCH HAND

The defoliation initiative that eventually became known as *Operation Ranch Hand* officially began in January 1962 (Buckingham, 1982). Aerial defoliants were used in Vietnam to efficiently clear vegetation providing concealment for enemy movements, bunkers, and other structures (McConnell, 1970). Major supply and communication routes vital to the U.S. mission, and therefore to the safety of U.S. military personnel, were under constant threat of guerrilla ambush as the Viet Cong had in many areas established complex networks of tunnels, caves, and trenches that under the cover of the dense jungle canopy were difficult, if not impossible, to detect from the air. These conditions put U.S. ground forces at a great disadvantage (Cecil, 1986). Defoliant operations in a much-reduced capacity also targeted agricultural concerns considered to be potential food sources for enemy troops.[10] Although the Army Corps of Chemical Engineers and the Navy were also involved in defoliant missions,[11] the bulk of defoliation efforts in *Operation Trail Dust*[12] were undertaken by a largely volunteer group of Air Force personnel who eventually became known as the *Ranch Hands*.

In July of 1961, before the Ranch Hands arrived in South Vietnam, the Combat Development and Test Center at Saigon received its first shipments of defoliant chemicals from the United States (Buckingham, 1982) and, beginning in August of that same year, spray tests were conducted by the (South) Viet Nam Air Force using H-34 helicopter dissemination of *Dinoxol*, *Trinoxol*, and *Concentrate 48*[13] (Cecil, 1986). Two months earlier, the Office of the Secretary of Defense tasked researchers at Ft. Detrick with a feasibility study of Vietnamese jungle defoliation (Young and Reggiani, 1988). Eighteen spray tests formed the basis of their analyses and in weighing the costs and strategic benefits, researchers determined that the most effective defoliant regimen for the region would involve the application of two distinct classes of herbicides—chlorophenoxy acids and cacodylic acids (Young and Reggiani, 1988).

The original unit, officially named *Tactical Air Force Transport Squadron Provisional 1* (Buckingham, 1982) began trial operations in Vietnam in 1962 with three modified C-123 aircraft (McConnell, 1970). The unit initially com-

---

[10]*Farmgate* was the operational code name for the food deprivation project (Stellman et al., 2003).

[11]Ground delivery of herbicides also took place to a much lesser degree. Truck- and trailer-mounted sprayer units called "Buffalo" turbines as well as hand-held and backpack sprayers were used for treatment of roadsides and base perimeters (Stellman et al., 2003; Young and Reggiani, 1988). The "brown water Navy" treated the banks of inland rivers (Bullman et al., 1994).

[12]*Operation Trail Dust* was the code name of the U.S.–Vietnam allied herbicide program and *Operation Ranch Hand* referred specifically to the C-123 mission (Stellman et al., 2003).

[13]Dinoxol was a 50:50 formulation of butoxyethanol esters of 2,4-D and 2,4,5-T. The active ingredient in Trinoxol was 2,4,5-T. Concentrate 48 (Weedone) contained the ethyl ester of 2,4-D (Cecil, 1986).

prised six pilots and 12 enlisted personnel (Buckingham, 1982) and was later supplemented with volunteers from Pope Air Force Base (AFB), North Carolina. At Pope AFB, Capt. Carl W. Marshall recruited from a pool of Air Force personnel who had volunteered for an earlier USAF counterinsurgency mission codenamed *Jungle Jim* (Buckingham, 1982). USAF personnel from this pool readily volunteered for the new mission, which had been packaged as a 120-day temporary duty assignment to SEA during which unit members would don civilian attire and fly unmarked aircraft. Potential volunteers were also informed that if captured, the U.S. military would renounce any affiliation with them. Ultimately, six spray aircraft and 69 USAF personnel left for SEA in November 1961 as the first defoliation unit deployment (Buckingham, 1982) and arrived at Clark AFB in the Philippines on December 6. The first three spray-ready planes were ordered to Saigon on January 7, 1962 (Buckingham, 1982) and a shipment of Agents Blue and Purple arrived at Tan Son Nhut Air Base on January 9 (Young and Reggiani, 1988). The initial choice of Agents Blue—a water-soluble liquid containing the active ingredient hydroxydimethylarsine oxide (cacodylic acid)—and Purple—a 50:30:20 mixture of n-butyl 2,4-D, n-butyl 2,4,5-T, and isobutyl 2,4,5-T—was consistent with the recommendation that had been made by Ft. Detrick researchers a year earlier. On January 10, 1962, Ranch Hands flew their first spray mission using Agent Purple. While the application was ineffective—which was later thought to be attributable to the delivery of a suboptimal concentration of herbicide—Ranch Hand crews discovered that the herbicide destroyed the rubber seals of the Hourglass spray system (Buckingham, 1982). Thus, the Ranch Hands, operating under the call signs *Cowboy* and later *Hades*,[14] were required to develop their own operational tactics tailored to indigenous conditions during their first year in Vietnam. By June 1962, the Ranch Hands were ready to fly their first tactical missions.

In 1968 the Special Aerial Spray Flight received the new unit designation of 12th Special Operations Squadron (McConnell, 1970). Generally, excepting missions associated with Operation Mule Train, Operation Flyswatter, and the Tet Offensive,[15] the 12th Special Operations Squadron was engaged exclusively in the execution of defoliant operations. Over time, the unit developed a group persona that, like their mission, made them somewhat unique among their fellow service members. Contrary to initial plans of anonymity, the Ranch Hands wore

---

[14]In 1966 the 12th Air Commando Squadron moved from Tan Son Nhut to Ben Hoa. The change in call sign accompanied the move (Cecil, 1986).

[15]Operation Mule Train comprised logistical missions in 1962 and 1963, which the Special Aerial Spray Flight supported. Operation Flyswatter missions were carried out to kill malaria-carrying mosquitoes and other insects. The Ranch Hands flew airlift support missions during the 1968 Tet Offensive (Cecil, 1986).

special insignia as well as purple scarves[16] that were a source of controversy[17] among USAF commanders and which would eventually come to be recognized as a unit symbol (Cecil, 1986). Like the purple scarf, the Chinese character for *purple* at the center of the Ranch Hand unit insignia echoed the namesake of one of the earliest herbicide agents used in Vietnam (Cecil, 1986).

Prior to each Ranch Hand mission, a flight mechanic or a crew chief facilitated herbicide loading. Herbicides were not loaded directly from the 18-gauge, 205-liter steel drums that were used for transport by all of the 11 companies[18] that manufactured herbicides for the military (Young and Reggiani, 1988). Drums were offloaded from cargo vessels, transported to Ranch Hand unit locations, and then herbicide was transferred from drums to F-6 trailer tanks.[19] An assembly of pumps, pipes, and hoses allowed the F-6 to remain stationary during aircraft tank filling. Residuals (2–5 liters per drum) were collected from inverted drums in a drip pan and used to treat base perimeters. It was common for military personnel to utilize discarded drums to fortify defensive positions and to construct barriers (Young and Reggiani, 1988).

Three to six C-123s typically made up a tactical formation (Meek, 1981). When mission[20] requirements were at their highest levels between 1967 and 1969, more than 10 C-123s would fly in a single formation (Boyne, 2000; Cecil, 1986). C-123s normally at or above their weight limit were required to fly "low and slow," typically at 150 feet and 130 knots for targets to be effectively treated. This meant that Ranch Hand aircraft were extremely vulnerable to enemy fire. Early formations flew at an altitude of 3,000 feet on target approach and then went into a 2,500 feet per second dive to the optimum spray delivery altitude of 150 feet. It was soon discovered that the high altitude approach was costing the aviators the element of surprise. A reverse approach was later used and formations would fly as low as 20 feet and then abruptly climb to the optimum spray altitude (Boyne, 2000). Shortly after a ground fire incident that disabled the hy-

---

[16]The purple scarf became part of the Ranch Hand uniform after a violet scarf had been presented to one of the flight commanders by South Vietnam Prime Minister Nguyen Cao Ky, who had accompanied the Ranch Hands on some of their early missions (Cecil, 1986).

[17]Policy coming from (commander of U.S. forces) General William Westmoreland's office forbade the wearing of the purple scarves. However, threats made by Prime Minister Ky to close Tan Son Nhut over the wearing of the purple scarves resulted in an exception to the USAF uniform policy for Ranch Hands (Cecil, 1986).

[18]In a class action lawsuit initiated in 2004, more than 30 Agent Orange manufacturers are named (de Sola, 2004).

[19]Each F-6 tank could accommodate approximately 78 drums of herbicide (Young and Reggiani, 1988).

[20]Each single aircraft take-off/landing cycle was termed a *sortie*; a *mission* was the collective reference to sorties flown with a common target. A *project* was all missions related to a specific target (Lavy, 1987; Young and Reggiani, 1988).

draulic system of one C-123, which controlled the spray pump and herbicide shut-off valve, the decision was made to fly future missions with the rear cargo door open so that if an onboard flare was ignited by incoming fire it could be shuttled out the back door (Buckingham, 1982). Although the open rear door reduced the risk of injury to crew members and of damage to the spray system from internal fire and potential onboard herbicide combustion or leakage, in cases where the hydraulic lines suffered direct hits from enemy fire, the cargo area and flight mechanic could be sprayed with herbicide. Bottles of distilled water were installed in the cargo bay to flush eyes after such events (Buckingham, 1982). The open aft door of the fuselage also allowed the flight mechanic who operated the spray console to drop smoke grenades marking enemy positions for fire-support aircraft (Meek, 1981). Additionally, both cockpit side windows remained open for ventilation during missions (Meek, 1981) and to prevent crew injury resulting from flying Plexiglas shards should a window sustain a direct hit (RHAC, 2000). These operational conditions resulted in a situation where the crews of lead aircraft of the formation were exposed to spray mist carried forward by the internal aft-forward airflow created by the open door and windows. Aircraft in positions other than the lead were not only flying directly into the spray paths of aircraft before them in the formation (Cecil, 1986), but they were also drawing into the fuselage some of their own spray mist (Meek, 1981; Wilcox, 1989).

Other conditions under which Ranch Hands were subject to herbicide exposure included the use of herbicides as hand cleaners (efficient for grease and oil removal), during the removal of debris from nozzles (rubber bits from dissolved seals), and through the maintenance of the herbicide tank valve (the maintenance person was required to actually enter the tank to lubricate the dump valve) (RHAC, 2000).

Flight conditions for the Ranch Hands improved with the introduction of a new spray system and jet-powered aircraft. In July of 1966 the MC-1 Hourglass system was replaced by the A/A45Y-1 spray system (Cecil, 1986). The A/A45Y-1 provided a flow rate of 250 gallons per minute, improved spray pattern evenness, and allowed the entire herbicide payload to be dumped in just 30 seconds in emergency situations (Cecil, 1986). The introduction of the C-123K—the *K* in the nomenclature referred to the jet version of the C-123—in 1968 reduced hits from enemy fire by 28 percent (Cecil, 1986). This reduction was attributed in part to the greater number of targets that the enemy had to fire at—formation numbers increased to as high as 12 aircraft on some missions (Cecil, 1986). The new jet-equipped C-123Ks had also undergone some structural improvements to better protect the engines from enemy fire and to reduce windshield shattering. They were fitted with larger spray pumps that were able to maintain a constant spray flow rate (3 gallons per acre) during airspeed fluctuations (Cecil, 1986).

By the time that the jet-equipped C-123Ks arrived in 1968, the Ranch Hand mission, technically, had already peaked; mission requirements had steadily in-

TABLE 2-1 Herbicides Used in Vietnam Between 1961 and 1971

Herbicide Designation	Years Used	Millions of Gallons Potentially Used in Vietnam[a]	Active Ingredient(s)[b,c]
Agent Pink	1961; 1965	0.013	n-butyl, isobutyl esters of 2,4,5-T
Agent Green	1961–1965[d]	0.008	n-butyl ester of 2,4,5-T
Agent Purple	1962–1965	0.499	n-butyl ester of 2,4-D; n-butyl and isobutyl esters of 2,4,5-T
Agent Orange I[e]	1965–1970	12.054	n-butyl esters of 2,4-D and 2,4,5-T
Agent Orange II	1968–?	0.948	n-butyl ester of 2,4-D and isooctyl ester of 2,4,5-T
Agent White	1966–1971	5.425	Picloram
Agent Blue[f]	1962–1971	1.251	Cacodylic acid

[a]In some instances procurement records are represented versus spray volumes (Stellman et al., 2003).

[b]Young and Reggiani, 1988.

[c]Stellman et al., 2003.

[d]Estimated to be within the Agent Pink usage time frame.

[e]There were two Agent Orange formulas used in Vietnam. The original formula was a 50:50 mixture of 2,4-D and the n-butyl ester of 2,4,5-T. In the formula known as Agent Orange II the isooctyl ester of 2,4,5-T was used. Improved production methods allowed synthesis to occur at lower temperatures, ultimately reducing levels of TCDD contamination in the 2,4,5-T component of Agent Orange II (Stellman et al., 2003).

[f]Two herbicides were referred to as Agent Blue. One was a powder (cacodylic acid/sodium chloride mix) and the other was a water-based solution (cacodylic acid/sodium cacodylate) (Stellman et al., 2003).

SOURCE: Adapted from Stellman et al., 2003.

creased through 1967 and then gradually began to decline (Buckingham, 1997). By the end of 1970 President Nixon had issued an order to phase out the herbicide mission (Cecil, 1986). Between 1962 and 1971 Ranch Hands flew 19,977 sorties (IOM, 2003b), and herbicides had been sprayed on nearly 10 percent of the South Vietnamese landmass (Table 2-1) (Alcott, 1995). The last fixed-wing application of herbicides took place on January 7, 1971[21] (Buckingham, 1982). It has been claimed (Gough, 1986) that the Ranch Hand mission resembled civilian crop-dusting to some degree—both required excellent piloting skills for extremely

[21]The last helicopter application took place on October 31, 1971 (Buckingham, 1982).

low-altitude flight, but Ranch Hand C-123s were generally dangerously overweight during takeoff, were far less maneuverable than civilian crop dusting aircraft (110-foot wingspan), and when pilots were required to execute the most difficult of maneuvers (60° banks at treetop level), they normally did so under enemy fire (Boyne, 2000). Largely due to the receipt of the Purple Heart, the Ranch Hand unit ended up being the most highly decorated USAF unit in Vietnam (Gough, 1986).

THE AGENT ORANGE CONTROVERSY

Initial Concerns over the Use of Herbicides in Vietnam

As early as 1963 the American public was made aware through media reports of the use of herbicides in Vietnam (Buckingham, 1997). As media coverage continued to draw attention to the potential legal, political, and ethical consequences of the defoliant operations, concerns about ecological and human health impacts were also mounting. The year before the first missions disseminating Agent Orange were flown in Vietnam (March 1965) (Cecil, 1986), the Federation of American Scientists publicly condemned the use of herbicide in Vietnam, marking the beginning of a concerted campaign against U.S. military use of defoliants (Young and Reggiani, 1988). Several scientific organizations petitioned for the cessation of spraying and for the investigation of the short- and long-term consequences of the military's herbicide use. Under increasing pressure from the scientific community and in response to increasing media coverage of what was rapidly becoming a major domestic controversy, the Department of Defense (DOD) commissioned a series of studies related to herbicide exposure. Two studies were instrumental in the eventual modification of U.S. military policy governing the use of herbicides. The first was a literature survey carried out by the Midwest Research Institute (MRI) that resulted in a recommendation of further Agent Blue (an arsenical) research, but did not specifically address the major herbicidal mixtures (Agents Purple and Orange) used in Vietnam (Butler, 2005). Additionally, the MRI study was not able to draw definitive conclusions regarding the long-term effects of herbicide exposure (Young and Reggiani, 1988).The second study, conducted by Bionetics Research Laboratories under contract from the National Cancer Institute, evaluated the potential teratogenic effects of 2,4,5-T exposure (Galston, 2001). Results from the Bionetics study, reported in 1968, indicated that 2,4,5-T exposure could elicit teratogenic outcomes in some species. In response to these results, as well as increasing media reports implicating Agent Orange as a causative agent for myriad health problems, the use of 2,4,5-T was domestically restricted on April 15, 1970, and the DOD concomitantly suspended 2,4,5-T's military use (Butler, 2005).

Later that year, Congress requested (Pub. L. 91-441) the National Academy of Sciences (NAS) to form a committee whose task would be to conduct a comprehensive evaluation of the physiological and ecological impacts of herbicidal operations in Vietnam (NAS, 1974). In their report published in 1974, the committee stated that they could not determine whether exposure to herbicides in Vietnam was responsible for any deleterious health outcomes among war veterans or civilian populations. The committee also noted that when defoliant operations were initiated in Vietnam, it was not widely known[22] that the 2,4,5-T stores were contaminated with 2,3,7,8-tetrachlorodibenzo-*p*-dioxin (TCDD). Records were reviewed from three Saigon hospitals, but no convincing association between birth defects and herbicidal exposure was found.[23] The committee, in conclusion, suggested that Congress fund further evaluation of potential adverse ecological and physiological outcomes associated with defoliant operations in Vietnam.

Early Studies of Vietnam Veterans' Health

In 1979, Pub. L. 96-151 was endorsed by President Carter and required the Veterans Administration—known today as the Department of Veterans Affairs—to conduct studies of adverse health outcomes among Vietnam veterans exposed to TCDD-containing herbicides (Young and Reggiani, 1988). In the same year, the Agent Orange Working Group (AOWG) was established. The AOWG comprised several governmental entities under the executive branch with a vested interest in the health effects associated with exposure to Agent Orange. In 1980, the congressional Office of Technology Assessment (OTA) became an active member of the AOWG, and in 1981 President Reagan incorporated the AOWG into the Cabinet Council on Human Resources, greatly increasing the influence of the AOWG (Young and Reggiani, 1988). By congressional mandate, the VA was required to produce a study protocol within 180 days of the passage of Pub. L. 96-151. The VA failed to meet this deadline, and the protocol that finally made its way to the OTA was declared inadequate. It was not until 1982 that the VA submitted a protocol for review that was approved by the OTA. However, by that time, the AOWG's priorities had shifted to the study of the Vietnam experience; i.e., in the health status of Vietnam veterans vs. non-Vietnam veterans. This resulted in pressure on the VA to shift from a study of the health effects of Agent Orange to a study of the Vietnam experience. Ultimately, Congress decided to transfer the responsibility for the execution of such studies from the VA to the

---

[22]German researchers Georg Sorge and Karl Schulz had, in the 1950s, isolated TCDD from 2,4,5-T samples and in 1957 published three papers in scientific journals (in German) relating the occurrence of chloracne with TCDD exposure in occupational settings (Butler, 2005).

[23]The committee did cite in their report the existence of a series of unconfirmed reports of respiratory illness among Montagnard (inhabitants of the highland regions of southern Vietnam) children that warranted further investigation (NAS, 1974).

Centers for Disease Control (CDC)—known today as the Centers for Disease Control and Prevention.

The CDC, instead of choosing between a study of Agent Orange or the Vietnam experience, decided to conduct both studies (Young and Reggiani, 1988). The Vietnam Experience Study was eventually conducted, but researchers ran into difficulties trying to carry out the Agent Orange Study. In short, the CDC had formulated an exposure index based on the assumptions that all members of a battalion were located at the centroid of the reported locations of their component units and that the entire battalion was considered to be exposed if that "average" location was within 2 kilometers of an active spray tract (OTA, 1983). The OTA rejected the CDC's proposed exposure model, noting that as the model was designed, it was an inadequate representation of actual troop locations, and as such, could not establish the magnitude of exposure at even the battalion level.[24] A year later the CDC developed an assay (Patterson et al., 1987) for measuring serum 2,3,7,8-TCDD levels—hereafter referred to as simply serum TCDD—which presumably could serve as a biomarker of Agent Orange exposure. With the advent of the serum TCDD assay, the CDC conducted the Agent Orange Validation Study to determine the feasibility of an Agent Orange study using both military records and serum TCDD levels as surrogates of in-theater herbicide exposure (VA, 2003). Serum TCDD levels were measured for 696 ground troops who had served in Vietnam and 97 Vietnam veterans who had not served in the theater of conflict. Mean serum TCDD levels were "nearly identical"[25] for both groups. Additionally, serum TCDD measures could not be correlated with exposure indices based on existing military records or self-reports of Agent Orange exposure. The CDC, with the assent of the AOWG and the OTA as well as the Science Panel of the Domestic Policy Council, cancelled the planned Agent Orange Study (VA, 2003).[26] By the time the CDC Agent Orange study was cancelled, CDC and AFHS investigators had already begun collaboration on a serum TCDD assay pilot study of Ranch Hand sera (RHAC, 2000). A detailed overview of Vietnam veterans' studies is provided in Appendix E.

---

[24]The CDC presented as an example a calculated centroid battalion location with an associated range of ~40 kilometers. OTA concluded that it was impossible to know how battalion members were distributed within the circumscribed area and that individuals could have been as far as ~20 kilometers from the centroid (OTA, 1983).

[25]Mean serum TCDD levels were approximately 4 ppt for both groups (CDC, 1988).

[26]A proposed UCLA Agent Orange study was also cancelled as its protocol was deemed inadequate by President Reagan's AOWG (Cecil, 1986).

THE AIR FORCE HEALTH STUDY

Origins and Protocol Development

On June 5, 1979, the *Washington Post* reported[27] that a commitment had been made by the USAF in consultation with the White House to study the potential adverse health outcomes of service members involved in Operation Ranch Hand. Five months before the announcement, a class action suit had been filed by the organization Agent Orange Victims International seeking compensation from Dow and other chemical companies for a series of illnesses ranging from cancer to skin disorders that plaintiffs believed to be attributable to Agent Orange exposure (Schuck, 1987). In the midst of a groundswell of controversy surrounding Agent Orange and in partial response to an increasing number of congressional inquiries, in 1979, independent of the mandates of Pub. L. 96-151, the USAF initiated an epidemiologic study of USAF personnel involved in defoliant operations in Vietnam.

On June 6, 1979, the USAF officially began development of its Agent Orange study protocol. The University of Texas School of Public Health in Houston first reviewed the USAF protocol. Following the university's review, the protocol underwent two additional reviews—first by an USAF scientific advisory board and then by a subcommittee of the Armed Forces Epidemiologic Board. Subsequent to a series of review-prescribed revisions, the NAS was asked by USAF investigators to review the study protocol—version 6 of November 28, 1979 (AFHS, 1982). Although this request does not mark the origins of Academy involvement with Agent Orange (NAS, 1974), it does mark the beginning of the Academy's association with the USAF's Agent Orange study.

In December of 1979, the NAS Panel on the Proposed Air Force Study of Herbicide Orange convened to review the proposed protocol, and their final report was issued on May 6, 1980 (NRC, 1980). Within the context of the health, political, and legal goals of the study, as stated by the USAF, the panel's objective was to assess the scientific merit of the protocol as it related to toxicological, epidemiologic, and statistical relevance and validity. The protocol, as then proposed, was divided into three major study components: a retrospective mortality study, a retrospective morbidity study, and a 5-year prospective follow-up study

[27]The decision by the USAF at the time was contrary to existing Pentagon policy, which can be characterized by Major General Garth Dettinger's (Deputy Surgeon General of the Air Force) 1978 testimony before the House Veterans Affairs subcommittee where he testified that there was "no evidence of any lasting health damage to anyone" involved in defoliant operations (*500 vets*, 1978). Prior to the USAF announcement, follow-up study of Vietnam veterans exposed to chemical defoliants had been recommended by the General Accounting Office in their 1979 report conducted at the request of Rep. Bennett M. Stewart (D-IL) on the subject (*Herbicide victim study*, 1979).

of original study participants (Ranch Hand and C-130 cargo crews). In their report, the NAS panel commended USAF investigators on their thorough consideration and acknowledgement of inherent protocol limitations, specifically those imparted by the relatively small size of the exposed cohort (n ≈ 1,200). From its protocol analysis and the methodological weaknesses therein identified, the panel arrived at the following four primary recommendations:

1. Lengthen the follow-up period beyond the proposed 3- and 5-year points.
2. Limit outcome measures and focus in greater detail on reproductive outcomes as well as hepatic, nervous system, and immune system dysfunction.
3. Identify additional subjects (U.S. Army and Marine Corps) for possible inclusion in the cohort.
4. Revise the protocol, and again, seek outside peer review of the revised protocol.

The panel also discussed potential credibility issues likely to emerge resulting from primary study administration by the USAF. It noted that, while not lacking proficiency as the investigating body, the USAF might generally be considered to be lacking in impartiality.

One minority opinion was included in the final report in which dissent was expressed with panel recommendations regarding the need for major methodological revision of the proposed protocol, but concurrence was stated regarding the recommendations of the panel to investigate reproductive outcomes and to extend the follow-up period.

The NAS protocol review recommendations for the evaluation of reproductive outcomes and extended follow-up period were assimilated into the seventh version of the protocol dated October 8, 1980. The USAF rejected the suggestion of cohort expansion through the inclusion of military members from other branches of service and attributed the issues of suboptimal study power not "to the epidemiologic design, but to the vagaries of history" and postulated that "the Marine group probably received an herbicide exposure three orders of magnitude less than the Ranch Hand cohort" (Lathrop, 1980).[28] Four additional protocol revisions over the next 15 months refined information on the study cohorts and expanded discussions of key issues (AFHS, 1982).

The implemented protocol (version 11), which called for a 20-year follow-up of the cohort and up to six physical examination cycles, was completed in January 1982 (AFHS, 1982). By that time, the effort—which was originally called the

---

[28]In the 1980 NAS protocol review, the panel suggested both Army and Marine Corps members for potential cohort inclusion. A Marine Corps group numbering 5,900 was specifically mentioned as they were known to have been less than one kilometer away from spray tracts on the days that the tracts were sprayed (NRC, 1980).

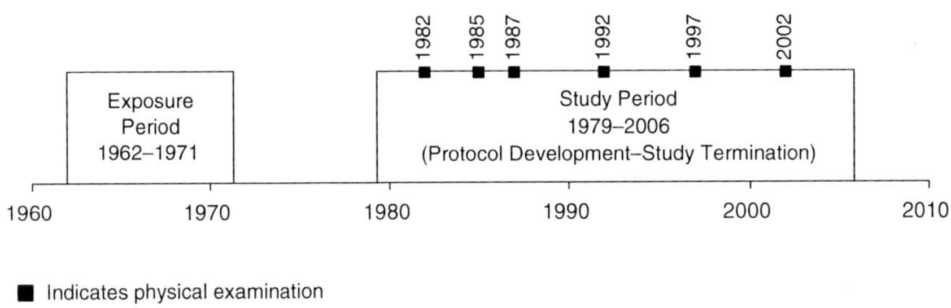

FIGURE 2-1 Air Force Health Study time line.

Ranch Hand II Study—had been given its present name: the *Air Force Health Study* (AFHS). Colloquially, it is referred to as the *Ranch Hand Study*.

The physical examination cycles correspond to years 1, 3, 5, 10, 15, and 20 of the study. AFHS investigators refer to the 1982 baseline morbidity evaluation as Cycle 1, the first follow-up (1985) as Cycle 2, the second (1987) as Cycle 3, the third (1992) as Cycle 4, the fourth (1997) as Cycle 5, and the fifth (2002) as Cycle 6. Mortality and reproductive studies are reported independent of morbidity follow-ups. Figure 2-1 illustrates the time line of the study and the period of exposure to herbicides for the subjects.

Cohort Enumeration

Cohort enumeration involved the utilization of all governmental assets available to the USAF, including the Social Security Administration, the Internal Revenue Service, and the VA. Location of subjects was determined using existing military records archived at the National Personnel Records Center, St. Louis, Missouri, and the USAF Human Resources Laboratory, Brooks AFB, Texas (AFHS, 1983). For both the mortality and morbidity branches of the study, the exposed population was defined as Ranch Hand personnel ($n \approx 1{,}269$)[29] who had served among the C-123 crews—pilot, copilot, navigator, and one spray operator—and the ground support crews—typically enlisted flight-line support personnel—between 1962 and 1971 (AFHS, 1984a). AFHS investigators repeated their awareness of the inherent limitations resulting from the small size of the study population in the baseline report, an issue that had been raised by protocol

[29] AFHS reports are not reliable accounts of the absolute number of "exposed" (Ranch Hand) and "unexposed" (comparison) subjects. These numbers change between reports and over time as further study leads to the reclassification of study subjects.

review committees and other involved groups.[30] After they reevaluated the feasibility of including personnel from other branches of service in the AFHS, USAF investigators believed it was sound to limit the exposed cohort to Ranch Hands. They asserted "the Ranch Hand group had a much higher level of exposure that was sustained over a prolonged period of time . . . [implying] that Ranch Hand personnel would be more likely to develop more acute and chronic symptoms . . . and would manifest them sooner than the other exposed military personnel" (AFHS, 1984a).

The initial eligible comparison group of 23,978 was limited to C-130 crews, each comprising three officers and two enlisted persons. Comparison subjects were generally characterized as nonrisk taking, nonvolunteer, and nonherbicide exposed (AFHS, 1982). They had served in the USAF between 1962 and 1971,[31] but had flown cargo, and not defoliant missions, in SEA. They were assumed to be similar to Ranch Hand subjects regarding lifestyle, training profiles, and socioeconomic factors. Comparison subjects were matched to Ranch Hand subjects on age, race,[32] and military occupation at a ratio as high as 1:10.[33] Military occupation was divided into five categories: officer/pilot, officer/navigator, officer/other, enlisted/flight engineer, and enlisted/other (AFHS, 1984a).

Individual-level pools of comparison subjects remained assigned to each Ranch Hand for the duration of the study. For the mortality component of the study, Ranch Hand subjects were matched to 5 (of the possible maximum of 10) randomly selected comparison subjects (AFHS, 1983). Subjects for which the cause of death was determined to be combat related were excluded from mortality analyses.[34] For the morbidity component, previous health status or history was ascertained for all exposed subjects and comparison subjects. Ranch Hand sub-

---

[30]The General Accounting Office reported in 1999 that due to the limited statistical power of the AFHS, the "minimum relative risk that would be likely to be detected" for the cohort was 45, 7.5, and 1.7 for liver cancer, prostate cancer, and all-sites cancer, respectively, in 1982. Those minimum detectable relative risks were projected to decrease to 11, 2.0, and 1.37 for liver cancer, prostate cancer, and all-sites cancer, respectively, for 1992 (GAO, 1999).

[31]For the purposes of Agent Orange-related disability compensation, the VA applies an exposure window of "service on active duty in the Republic of Vietnam during the period beginning on January 9, 1962, and ending on May 7, 1975" (VA, 2003).

[32]Ranch Hands were predominately non-Black—98 percent of officers and 92 percent of enlisted (AFHS, 1984a).

[33]Manual review of personnel records in 1981 (after matching had been conducted) revealed that 18 percent (n = 2,208) of the comparison group did not meet study inclusion criteria (AFHS, 1984a). This effectively reduced the matched ratio of Ranch Hand subjects to comparison subjects from 1:10 to 1:8. Investigators reported that the ineligible comparison subjects were "randomly distributed among the matched sets" and were thus removed from the study without the conduct of a random reassignment of matched sets, and replacement comparison subjects were shifted within subsets (AFHS, 1984a).

[34]The health status prior to combat-related death was determined through review of medical records (AFHS, 1984a).

TABLE 2-2 AFHS Matching Scheme

Study Component	Subject to Comparison Ratio for Analysis	Comparison Selection, Replacement, and Study Duration
Mortality	1:5	Combat deaths excluded; random selection from maximum pool of 10; vital status ascertained periodically for 20 years
Retrospective Morbidity	1:1	Random selection from subset of 5 of maximum pool of 10; living non-compliant comparisons replaced from remaining pool; replacements not health-matched; deceased comparisons not replaced; cross-sectional survey
Prospective Morbidity	1:1	Random selection from subset of 5 of maximum pool of 10; living non-compliant comparisons replaced from remaining pool; replacements "health-matched;" deceased comparisons replaced; 20 years of observation including family health questionnaires (reproductive outcomes)

SOURCE: Adapted from AFHS, 1982.

jects were matched to the first living and compliant comparison randomly selected from the individual-level mortality pool of five (AFHS, 1984a). If the first selected comparison subject was living, but noncompliant, then another subject was randomly selected from the remaining eligible comparison pool. Retrospective health data were collected for deceased (noncombat related) Ranch Hand subjects and comparison subjects through first-order next-of-kin interviews. Original comparison subjects for the prospective morbidity study were those selected for the retrospective morbidity study, with the addition of replacements for deceased comparison subjects (AFHS, 1982). The impact on study power resulting from loss to follow-up (noncompliant or unlocatable) of original prospective morbidity component comparison subjects was addressed through the replacement of unaccountable or noncompliant comparison subjects with the next eligible comparison[35] from the remaining pool of up to 10 (AFHS, 1982). According to the study protocol (AFHS, 1982), replacement comparison subjects were also to be matched on self-reported health perception to original comparison subjects that refused to participate. In the initial (1982) physical examination, replacement comparison subjects were the first willing randomly selected subjects from the available pool (AFHS, 1984a). In the follow-up evaluations, replacement comparison subjects were matched on self-perceived health when possible to refusal or unaccounted-for comparison subjects (AFHS, 2000). The matching schemes for the various components of the study are summarized in Table 2-2,

[35]Eligibility in any cycle reflects eligibility in a previous cycle and not compliance in a previous cycle (AFHS, 2005).

and AFHS population dynamics for the entire morbidity study are presented in Figure 3-2 of Chapter 3.

Reconstruction of Exposure

While Ranch Hand subjects were considered to be exposed as a group, an exposure index was created to categorize degree of potential exposure to Agent Orange among Ranch Hand subjects. Each Ranch Hand subject was assigned to an exposure category (low, medium, or high) based on a composite exposure score (E_i) defined as the quotient of the number of gallons of herbicides sprayed during a subject's tour and the number of airmen with the subject's duties during his tour scaled by a temporally-based TCDD weighting factor (AFHS, 1984a).[36]

$$E_i = (\text{TCDD wt. factor}) \times \frac{\text{gal. herbicides sprayed during subject's (i}^{\text{th}}\text{) tour}}{\text{number of airmen w/ subject's duties during i}^{\text{th}}\text{ tour}}$$

The TCDD weighting factor equaled 1 for post–July 1, 1965 duty and 24 for pre–July 1, 1965 duty. The rationale for it was that the herbicides used in the earlier time period (Agents Pink, Green, Purple, and early batches of Agent Orange) were more heavily contaminated with TCDD than those used thereafter. The derivation of weighting factor is detailed in the baseline morbidity report's *Exposure Index Development* chapter (AFHS, 1984a).

Investigators acknowledged the inability of the exposure classification scheme to directly assess exposure at the individual level or any differences in exposure related to variation in or deviation from typical job duties, but adopted it as a working model (AFHS, 1984a). Exposure scores (E_i) were applied differentially to occupational categories to reflect differences in exposure opportunity associated with the performance of *typical* duties characteristic of each occupational group (Table 2-3) (IOM, 1994).

---

[36]The TCDD weighting factor equaled 1 for post-1965 duty and 24 for pre-1965 duty. The rationale for the weighting factor was that earlier herbicide formulas (Agents Pink, Green, and Purple) were found to be more heavily contaminated with TCDD (NAS, 1974). The volume distribution of herbicides in Vietnam, on which the exposure model was based, was derived from data contained in the HERBS computer tapes (AFHS, 1984a). The HERBS tapes are computer tapes that contain information on location and time of 9,495 fixed-wing spray missions conducted between 1965 and 1971 (Bullman et al., 1994). The exposure index used in Cycles 1–3 was a modified version of the model in the original protocol as investigators discovered that the data needed for the original exposure index did not exist. Investigators later admitted (ca. 2000) that the assumption that more service personnel in the area would reduce individual exposure was probably not valid and that more individuals in a contaminated area likely meant that more individuals were exposed (RHAC, 2000).

TABLE 2-3 Calculated Exposure Index

Occupational Group	Exposure Category	Corresponding Gallons of Herbicides (E_i)
Officer	Low	< 35,000
	Medium	35,000–70,000
	High	> 70,000
Enlisted Flyer	Low	< 50,000
	Medium	50,000–80,000
	High	> 80,000
Enlisted Ground	Low	< 20,000
	Medium	20,000–27,000
	High	> 27,000

SOURCE: AFHS, 1984a.

The calculated exposure index developed for Cycle 1 was implemented in both the first (1985) and second (1987) morbidity follow-ups. In the Cycle 3 report investigators noted that, as structured, the calculated exposure index "[could] be regarded as only fair" (AFHS, 1987) in its ability to characterize actual exposure to herbicides as they had knowledge of preliminary results from the serum TCDD pilot study.

Assessment of exposure was drastically altered with the advent of a serum TCDD assay developed by the CDC in 1987 (Patterson et al., 1987).[37] The assay had a detection limit of 1.25 parts-per-quadrillion (ppq = femtogram or 1×10^{-15}) for a 200-g sample (Patterson et al., 1987) and was strongly correlated with adipose tissue TCDD levels. It was weakly correlated with the original calculated exposure index, indicating the potential for the misclassification of exposure using the index (assuming the assay was the better proxy) (AFHS, 1991b). The new assay eliminated the need for the painful surgical extraction of adipose tissue to determine TCDD body burden.[38] When "serum dioxin" is referred to in AFHS

[37]CDC and AFHS investigators met in 1986 to discuss the serum TCDD assay pilot study (Michalek, 2000; RHAC, 2000). Eventually, sera samples were collected from 150 Ranch Hand subjects and 50 comparison subjects independent of the 1987 Cycle 3 follow-up physical exam; sera were collected at Red Cross Centers in Atlanta, Cleveland, Los Angeles, and Tulsa (CDC, 1988). Forty-seven AFHS participants had had their serum assayed for the pilot and the Cycle 3 follow-up. These serial measures were used to assess test reliability (RHAC, 2000). The assay is congener specific for 2,3,7,8-tetrachlorodibenzo-*p*-dioxin and therefore, when TCDD body burden or dioxin are referred to in AFHS reports the reference is to 2,3,7,8-TCDD burden, and not to toxic equivalents.

[38]TCDD can also be measured from lipids in breast milk (Patterson et al., 1987).

publications, it is actually serum lipid-weight concentration in parts-per-trillion (ppt) and is equal to measured serum TCDD in ppq, which has been corrected for total lipid weight and serum density[39] (AFHS, 1991b). When a "current" level is referred to in reports later than the *Serum Dioxin Analysis of 1987 Examination Results* report (AFHS, 1991b), the value has been extrapolated back to 1987 values based on contemporaneously accepted (by AFHS investigators) TCDD half-life values (AFHS, 1995).[40] When "initial" dioxin is referred to in the AFHS, it is based on TCDD levels as determined by assay measurements extrapolated back to a subject's end of term of service in Vietnam using contemporaneously accepted TCDD half-life estimates (AFHS, 1991b). For the exam cycles that took place after the development of the assay (Cycles 4–6), earlier exposure proxies were replaced with both cohort status (Ranch Hand vs. Comparison) and serum TCDD level—initial or current values.

Data Collection

Data from both the questionnaires and the physical examinations were collected by contracted personnel[41] who were blinded to participant exposure status (AFHS, 1982, 1984a, 2005). Data collected during physical examinations comprised indices of health status that encompassed general health, endocrine, pulmonary, immunologic, neurologic, renal, hepatic, hematologic, dermatologic, psychiatric, cancer, and cardiovascular endpoints. Reproductive data pertained to aspects of lineage, gestation, date of birth, birth defect status, maternal/paternal risk factors, birth outcome, birth weight, and offspring health through age 18 (AFHS, 1982). Questionnaire data included information relating to "demographics, education, occupation, medical history, study compliance, toxic exposures, and reproductive history" (AFHS, 2005). Additional data sources include birth certificates and military personnel and medical (civilian and military) records (AFHS, 1984a). Comprehensive reproductive histories were also ascertained through interviews of current and former wives or partners (AFHS, 1984a). Permission forms for the release of medical data (subject, spouse, and

---

[39]TCDD (ppt) = $\frac{\text{ppq} \times 102.6}{\text{w}}$, where 102.6 is a correction factor for serum density and *w* is equal to the total lipid weight of the sample (AFHS, 1991b).

[40]Original TCDD half-life estimates were based on data from the 1976 Seveso, Italy, industrial accident (AFHS, 1990).

[41]Louis Harris and Associates, Inc. administered questionnaires and Kelsey-Seybold Clinic, P.A., conducted the physical examinations for the baseline study (AFHS, 1984a). The questionnaire was developed by the National Opinion Research Center, but Louis Harris and Associates, Inc. was awarded the contract for administration of the baseline questionnaire (AFHS, 1984a). Under contract with Science Applications International Corporation, the National Opinion Research Center and Scripps Clinic and Research Foundation, administered all follow-up questionnaires and physical examinations, respectively, for the morbidity study (AFHS, 1987).

offspring) were administered during or following questionnaire administration (AFHS, 1984a).

All study participants who had completed the questionnaire were invited to participate in the physical examination (AFHS, 1984a). Endpoints measured during the $2^1/_2$-day physical examination were derived from scientific literature reviews of subject areas (toxicology, chemistry, case reports, and epidemiologic studies) related to chlorophenoxy herbicides and dioxin. The final choice of outcome measures was also influenced by practicality (complexity and length) as well as invasiveness of procedures (AFHS, 1984a).[42] The battery of laboratory tests performed at each physical examination changed over time reflecting changes in science and technology (Appendix B). Biospecimens from study participants—serum (all cycles), urine (Cycles 1–3), whole blood (Cycle 6), semen (Cycle 1), and adipose tissue (Cycle 5)—were banked for future analysis (AFHS, 1984a, 1987, 1990, 1991b, 1995, 2000, 2005). It took approximately 10 months to conduct physical exams for all participants; the cost of the exams was estimated as $16 million in 2000 (RHAC, 2000).

Questionnaires were administered by trained professionals in the subjects' homes for the Cycle 1 evaluation.[43] If a subject was new to the study in any of the follow-up cycles, then he and his spouse received the same questionnaire that was administered at the Cycle 1 evaluation. In-home interview administration for subjects new to the study continued through part of Cycle 3 (AFHS, 2005). Beginning in 1987, administration of the baseline questionnaire for new subjects took place at the physical examination site (Scripps Clinic, La Jolla, California). An interval questionnaire was developed for all returning subjects attending follow-up examinations to capture new information and to update existing data. All interval questionnaires were administered at the physical examination site. Beginning with the Cycle 3 examination, computer assisted personal interview (CAPI) systems facilitated the administration of the interval questionnaire as well as any newly administered baseline questionnaires (AFHS, 2005). Questions were added to the interval questionnaire over time to better address pertinent research questions. When a new question appeared on the questionnaire for a particular follow-up cycle, it was included in subsequent questionnaires to establish a longitudinal record for the item (AFHS, 2005). In cases where new questions were not subject to changes over time, only those subjects who had not previously answered the

[42]AFHS researcher Joel Michalek stated in 2000 that Cycle 1 outcomes were based on a list of veteran complaints compiled by the VA (RHAC, 2000).

[43]Any replacement comparison subjects—there were 346 replacement comparison subjects (23 percent of the comparison population) who completed questionnaires at the baseline—contacted after November 1982 (n = 30), were not interviewed by a Lewis Harris and Associates employee (AFHS, 1984a). Baseline questionnaires were administered to these replacement comparison subjects by USAF personnel at the physical examination site (AFHS, 1984a).

question were queried. A dietary assessment included in the Cycle 4 examination was a one-time query of dynamic variables (AFHS, 2005).[44]

Mortality data collected (VA,[45] SSA,[46] IRS,[47] and USAF[48]) throughout the study include date of death and underlying cause of death (primary and secondary) (AFHS, 1983). According to the protocol, all participants were to be encouraged at the first follow-up examination to consent to a government-funded autopsy in the event of their death (AFHS, 1982).[49] The overwhelming majority of data and biologic samples collected during the course of the study are archived at the AFHS research facility at Brooks City-Base, San Antonio, Texas.

The primary data sources for the elements of the study are listed in Figure 2-2.

Data Analysis

Morbidity Analyses

Subjective (self-reported) and objective (clinically verified) data were gathered through the questionnaires and during the physical examinations (AFHS, 1987). Analytical tests performed reflected a variety of data types (dichotomous, polytomous, and continuous) and numerous research questions that evolved over time—many in later cycles were generated by the results of previous cycles (AFHS, 1984a). Generally, earlier analyses performed sought to identify differences between Ranch Hand subjects and comparison subjects relating to both subjective and objective endpoints by group and exposure opportunity (AFHS, 1987). For the Cycle 1 evaluation, 190 dependent variables were evaluated for associations with self-reported symptoms, medical signs, and vital status (AFHS, 1984a). The majority of analyses performed on data collected for the Cycle 1 evaluation focused on differences by occupational group and exposure category

---

[44]An SEA service-based occupational survey was administered to enlisted Ranch Hand subjects only in 1989 (independent of cycle-specific activities) to evaluate the accuracy of the calculated exposure index as judged by the degree of correlation with the serum TCDD assay (Wolfe et al., 1995b).

[45]The VA's Beneficiary Identification and Record Locator Subsystem (BIRLS) served to locate subjects for whom death benefits had been awarded (AFHS, 1983).

[46]If the Social Security Administration's Office of Remuneration and Earnings had employer-reported earnings data for a previous calendar year, then a subject was presumed to be living (AFHS, 1983).

[47]The National Institute for Occupational Safety and Health facilitated retrieval of Internal Revenue Service mortality-related data (e.g., living if filing tax return and deceased if listed as such on joint tax return) for AFHS (AFHS, 1983).

[48]USAF personnel, finance, and medical records were used to locate subjects and ascertain vital status (AFHS, 1983).

[49]Tissue samples were to be analyzed at the Armed Forces Institute of Pathology (AFHS, 1982).

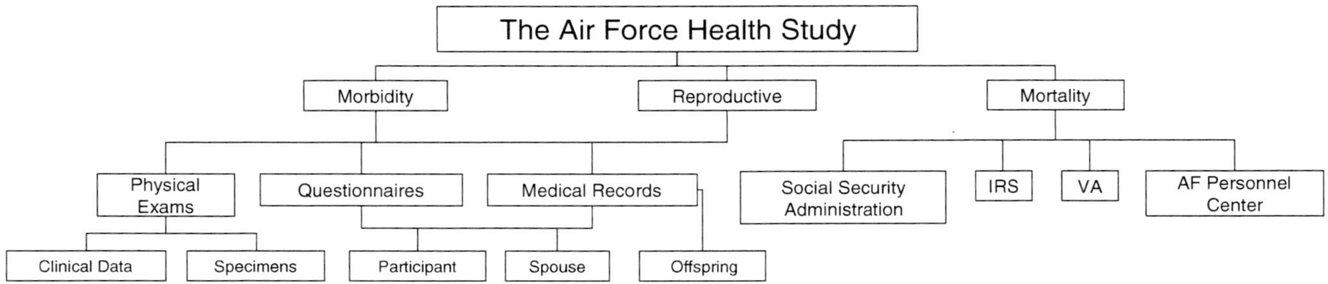

FIGURE 2-2 Data sources for AFHS morbidity study subjects.
SOURCE: M. Yeager, Science Applications International Corporation (SAIC), personal communication, July 13, 2005.

(AFHS, 1984a). In the 1985 Cycle 2 follow-up examination, results reported in all major clinical chapters were for differences in subjective and objective outcomes between the Ranch Hand and comparison groups (AFHS, 1987). For purposes of longitudinal comparison, additional analyses of Ranch Hand subjects versus original comparison subjects (Cycle 1) are included in tabulated form in chapter appendixes in the Cycle 2 follow-up report (AFHS, 1987). Cycle 3 analyses reflected the methodology of the previous cycle—characterization of variation in morbidity by group, occupational category, and exposure index ranking (AFHS, 1990). Separate analyses based on the serum TCDD assay (pilot study and Cycle 3 serum collections) data were published in a stand-alone report—*Serum Dioxin Analysis of 1987 Examination Results* (AFHS, 1991b). In the Cycle 3 follow-up report's executive summary, readers were cautioned to interpret Cycle 3 results carefully as early indications of assay analyses indicated that the qualitative exposure index was "not a good measure of actual dioxin exposure" (AFHS, 1991b).

Three statistical models were created to evaluate the relationship between dioxin body burden and morbidity (over 300 dependent variables) for the 1987 serum dioxin analyses. In two of the models dioxin body burden among Ranch Hand subjects only was considered. Model 1 was based on *initial* dioxin values or the estimated body burden ($t_{1/2}$ = 7.1 years) at the time a Ranch Hand left Vietnam. Model 2 was based on *current* TCDD body burden. Model 2 analyses mainly involved differences in morbidity outcomes (subjective and objective) by temporal strata (relative to time of service) (AFHS, 1991b). Models 1 and 2 were both conducted under what investigators referred to as the "minimal" (Ranch Hand subjects with less than 10 ppt TCDD body burden [n = 345] were excluded as they were considered not to have been exposed to TCDD in Vietnam) and "maximal" (Ranch Hand subjects with less than 5 ppt TCDD body burden [n = 124] were excluded as they were considered not to have been exposed to TCDD in Vietnam) assumptions (AFHS, 1991b). Under Model 3, differences in health status between Ranch Hand subjects and comparison subjects according to current dioxin levels were evaluated (Table 2-4). The 5 ppt spread between the "un-

TABLE 2-4 Model 3 (Serum Dioxin Analysis of 1987 Examination Results)

Category	Current TCDD Body Burden
Ranch Hand Subjects	
Unknown	≤ 10 ppt
Low	15 ppt < TCDD ≤ 33.3 ppt
High	> 33.3 ppt
Comparison Subjects	≤ 10 ppt

SOURCE: AFHS, 1991b.

TABLE 2-5 Model 3 (Cycle 5)

Category	Lipid-adjusted Initial TCDD Body Burden
Ranch Hand Subjects	
Unknown	≤ 10 ppt
Low	15 ppt < TCDD ≤ 94 ppt
High	> 94 ppt
Comparison Subjects	≤ 10 ppt

SOURCE: AFHS, 2000.

known" and "low" Ranch Hand categories was established to ensure clear delineation between the subgroups (AFHS, 1991b).

Six analytical models were used in Cycle 4 (AFHS, 1995). Model 1 contrasted indices of health status between Ranch Hand subjects and comparison subjects. The second model applied to Ranch Hand subjects only and evaluated variation in indices of morbidity according to initial dioxin levels. Model 3 contrasted morbidity of Ranch Hand subjects and comparison subjects by both current and initial TCDD levels. Models 4–6 applied to Ranch Hand health status only and were each based on current TCDD values (Model 4: lipid-adjusted current TCDD; Model 5: whole-weight current TCDD; and Model 6: whole-weight current TCDD adjusted for total lipids) (AFHS, 1995). Changes in percentage of body fat and percentage of body fat at time of duty were treated as covariates in Models 2 and 3 to compensate for the influence of these factors on TCDD half-life value (AFHS, 1995).

The estimated TCDD half-life on which statistical models were based in Cycle 5 changed from the Cycle 4 value of 7.1 years to 8.7 years in Cycle 5 based on then-recent research (Michalek et al., 1996). In the 1992 follow-up, 266 health variables were evaluated using four analytical models (AFHS, 2000). In Model 1, health status was assessed for Ranch Hand subjects and comparison subjects at the group level independent of TCDD body burden. Initial TCDD body burden was the basis for Model 2 and body fat percentage[50] was considered a covariate. In Model 3, variation in health outcomes were evaluated for both Ranch Hand subjects and comparison subjects by lipid-adjusted initial TCDD body burden[51] category (Table 2-5).

[50]Body fat percentage was calculated using inputs of height and weight. Discrepancies in the database were identified in the 1992 follow-up (Cycle 4) resulting from changes in height over time—a decrease in height of > 5 cm was found to have occurred for more than 85 participants (AFHS, 1995).

[51]"[E]xtrapolated initial dose, assume[s] first-order elimination, $I = 4 + (C - 4) \times \exp(\log(2) \times t/h)$, where 4 ppt is considered the median background level of lipid-adjusted dioxin" (AFHS, 2000). The background level of 4 ppt was derived from the results of the Agent Orange Validation Study.

TABLE 2-6 Model 3 (Cycle 6)

Category	Lipid-adjusted Initial TCDD Body Burden
Ranch Hand Subjects	
Background	≤ 10 ppt
Low	15 ppt < TCDD ≤ 118 ppt
High	> 118 ppt
Comparison Subjects	≤ 10 ppt

SOURCE: AFHS, 2005.

Model 4 was based on 1987 serum TCDD values or values from 1992 or 1997 measures extrapolated back to 1987. If a 1992 serum TCDD value was less than 10 ppt, then the measure was not extrapolated back to 1987 levels. Body fat percentage was not a covariate in Model 4.

Analytical models used for Cycle 5 (1997) were applied to Cycle 6 (2002) data analyses with few modifications. The derived initial and 1987 TCDD levels were based on an estimated TCDD half-life of 7.6 years in Cycle 6—this was a change from the half-life estimate of 8.7 years used in the previous cycle—again based on updated research.[52] Model 2 in Cycle 6 varied from Model 2 in Cycle 5 in that body mass index was a covariate in Cycle 6 (AFHS, 2005).[53] The Model 3 lipid-adjusted initial TCDD low to high cutoff point changed from 94 ppt in Cycle 5 to 118 ppt in Cycle 6 (Table 2-6).

Body mass index also replaced body fat percentage as a covariate in Model 3. The singular change in Model 4 for Cycle 6 was the use of the 7.6-year TCDD half-life value to extrapolate to 1987 serum TCDD levels (AFHS, 2005).

Reproductive Outcomes Analyses

Analyses of reproductive outcomes were focused on potential male-mediated effects and only addressed the offspring of participants for whom serum dioxin measures had been made by 1990 (AFHS, 1992).[54] Maternal data (collected from partners) included alcohol, drug, and cigarette use and maternal family histories. Three models were used in the reproductive analyses (AFHS, 1992).[55] For the first two models it was assumed that all "Ranch Hands received

[52]TCDD elimination was found to exhibit an inverse relationship with body fat and was also thought to possibly vary by other related factors (Michalek and Tripathi, 1999).

[53]In Cycle 5, body fat (a covariate) was calculated from body mass index (AFHS, 2000).

[54]Reproductive outcomes were reported in the Cycle 1 technical report (AFHS, 1984a). This discussion refers to analytical models used in the stand-alone technical report of reproductive outcomes (AFHS, 1992).

[55]Subjects were limited to one reproductive outcome (Schwartz, 2000).

TABLE 2-7 Model 3 (Reproductive Outcomes, 1992)

Category	Current TCDD Body Burden
Background	Comparison with ≤ 10 ppt
Unknown	Ranch Hand with ≤ 10 ppt
Low	15 ppt < Ranch Hand with TCDD ≤ 33.3 ppt
High	Ranch Hand with > 33.3 ppt

SOURCE: AFHS, 1992.

a single dioxin dose in Vietnam and only background thereafter" (AFHS, 1992). Model 1 was based on extrapolated initial TCDD level using a half-life of 7.1 years. Model 2 was based on current dioxin levels using the same half-life estimate, and Model 2 also included a "time-by-current dioxin" interaction term (AFHS, 1992). Ranch Hand subjects with current TCDD levels less than or equal 10 ppt (n = 347) were excluded from one set of analyses (using both Models 1 and 2) of reproductive outcomes, and a separate set of analyses (using both Models 1 and 2) were carried out excluding Ranch Hand subjects with less than or equal to 5 ppt (n = 125) (AFHS, 1992). Investigators cited that the "intent of these two analyses was to 'trap' the true dioxin versus reproductive outcome relationship between them" (AFHS, 1992). Models 1 and 2 applied only to Ranch Hand reproductive and offspring experience. Model 3 applied to the reproductive outcomes of both Ranch Hand subjects and comparison subjects based on current TCDD ranking (Table 2-7) (AFHS, 1992).

Mortality Analyses

Cycle 1 mortality analyses evaluated all-cause and cause-specific mortality at the group level as well as dose–response trends based on the qualitative exposure index (AFHS, 1983). Ranch Hand mortality was contrasted with that of the study comparison group and three additional external comparison populations: the 1978 U.S. White Male Mortality Experience,[56] the DOD Nondisability Retired Life Table, and the West Point Class of 1956. These external comparisons were made to evaluate the "healthy worker effect"[57] as well as to identify any

[56]The source of these data was US Department of Health and Human Services: *Vital Statistics of the United States 1978* (AFHS, 1983).

[57]The healthy worker effect (confounding) results from the exclusion or out-migration of ill persons from the occupational setting. In the case of the AFHS, this phenomenon could be considered the "healthy soldier effect" whereby AFHS subjects by the nature of the military selection/retention physical examination criteria, would be healthier than the general population.

differences in group mortality experience between Vietnam veterans and other military members (AFHS, 1983). In the first update to this analysis (AFHS, 1984b), Ranch Hand mortality was compared to that of the internal comparison group, active duty USAF personnel, and to the active U.S. Civil Service population (male) in addition to the three external groups used in the Cycle 1. The 1985 update again contrasted Ranch Hand mortality experience with the internal comparison group, the 1978 U.S. White Male Mortality Experience population, the DOD Nondisability Retired Life Table population, the West Point Class of 1956, and U.S. Civil Service population (male) (AFHS, 1985). The 1986 update provided summary counts and death rates for Ranch Hand subjects and comparison subjects stratified by race and military occupation (AFHS, 1986). For the 1989 mortality update, Ranch Hand mortality was compared to that of the matched subsets of five and to the entire internal comparison population (n = 19,101). External comparison populations were not included (AFHS, 1989).

In all mortality analyses conducted prior to 1991, dose–response was evaluated using the Cycle 1 quantified exposure index. This changed when serum TCDD analyses indicated that the index was a poor proxy for Agent Orange exposure (Wolfe, 1989; AFHS, 1991a). However, AFHS investigators chose not to conduct analyses based on TCDD measurements for the 1991 mortality update because they lacked assay data for 91 deceased Ranch Hand subjects and 238 living Ranch Hand subjects (26 percent of the cohort). Instead, military rank and occupation in SEA were considered the most viable surrogates of exposure (AFHS, 1991a). Ranch Hand mortality was contrasted with that of the total comparison population in the 1991 update. The 1993 mortality update included a dose–response assessment based on TCDD measurements on the subset of participants for which this information was available, along with analyses of the entire Ranch Hand and comparison groups stratified by rank and occupation (AFHS, 1993). The methods used in the 1994 and 1996 updates did not deviate appreciably from the analytical methods of the 1993 report (AFHS, 1994, 1996).

Generally, survival curve estimates and standard mortality ratios adjusted for rank (officer versus enlisted), occupation (flyer versus nonflyer), age, birth year, and TCDD level beginning in 1991 are reported in AFHS mortality reports (AFHS, 1991a, 1993, 1994, 1996).

Data analyses are discussed at length in AFHS technical reports. The above summary discussion of AFHS analyses presents only the most basic details of AFHS analyses—major changes made to analytical models over time and changes in TCDD half-life estimates—which along with the discussion of exposure assessment, provide referential context for the discussion of AFHS results. Results and conclusions presented below are the findings of the AFHS and not the conclusions or findings of this committee.

Results

Dissemination of the results of the AFHS has taken place through two primary channels: reports and papers in peer-reviewed journals. Multi-volume reports detailing study methodology and the findings of the clinical assessments have been issued for all six physical examination cycles and for the mortality and reproductive outcomes investigations. These are both posted on the AFHS website (http://www.brooks.af.mil/AFRL/HED/hedb/afhs/reports.html) and available through the National Technical Information Service of the US Department of Commerce (www.ntis.gov). Papers related to study topics have been published in journals covering epidemiologic, medical, toxicological, exposure assessment, and statistical methodology topics since 1980.[58]

This section briefly summarizes some of the results presented in the AFHS reports. Selected papers produced by the investigators are addressed in the section entitled *AFHS Research and the Institute of Medicine's* Veterans and Agent Orange *Reports*.

Morbidity and Mortality Study Results

Participation in the Cycle 1 evaluation was on a volunteer basis even for personnel on active duty—15 percent of both Ranch Hand subjects and matched comparison subjects were on active duty[59] at the time the Cycle 1 study was implemented, and 17 percent of Ranch Hand subjects and 19 percent of matched comparison subjects held Federal Aviation Administration Certificates indicating active participation in the aviation sector (AFHS, 1984a). During protocol development it was estimated that 39 percent of Ranch Hand subjects would participate in the physical examination (AFHS, 1984a). In actuality, 97 percent of Ranch Hand subjects and 93 percent of comparison subjects completed the questionnaire, and 87 percent of Ranch Hand subjects and 76 percent of comparison subjects underwent physical examination (AFHS, 1984a). Flight status,[60] age, race,

---

[58]A list of these papers is provided on the AFHS web site: http://www.brooks.af.mil/AFRL/HED/hedb/afhs/articles.html.

[59]Retired USAF nurse and Yale researcher Linda Spoonster Schwartz testified before the National Security, Veterans Affairs, and Intergovernmental Relations Subcommittee of U.S. House of Representatives that only limited confidentiality was granted to AFHS study participants on active duty (Schwartz, 2000). In November of 1981, study participants received introductory letters in which the issue of confidentiality of medical findings was discussed. In cases where "serious medical findings which impact public health and safety" were discovered during the morbidity study, a committee comprising a specialist physician, a physician of the subject's choice, a flight surgeon, a legal representative, and a representative from the subject's professional field would make the final determination as the degree of threat any identified medical condition posed to the public's health and safety (AFHS, 1984a).

[60]Even minor abnormalities discovered in the course of a physical examination can adversely impact flight status in both the military and civilian sectors (AFHS, 1984a).

and military status were said to have influenced participation rates. Questionnaires were administered to noncompliant persons by telephone (AFHS, 1984a) and trends among nonresponders were analyzed (AFHS, 1984a). Higher than expected participation rates resulted in many tasks cited as "undone"[61] by the time the Cycle 1 results were reported in 1984, and investigators estimated that the Cycle 1 report represented "100 man-years of in-house work" and the accomplishment of thousands of statistical tests (AFHS, 1984a).

Cycle 1 analyses indicated that at the group level Ranch Hand subjects were found to differ significantly on such outcomes as nonmelanomic skin cancer,[62] self-reported neuroses, liver enzymes, and peripheral leg pulses, although many of these differences were not evident after adjusting for age and smoking history (AFHS, 1984a). Inconsistent with what would be expected with TCDD exposure (Cook et al., 1980), no cases of chloracne or evidence of previous occurrence of chloracne was documented. Like chloracne, other diseases associated with TCDD exposure (soft-tissue sarcoma[63] and porphyria cutanea tarda) were also not observed to be more prevalent among Ranch Hand subjects. Many of the differences observed between Ranch Hand subjects and comparison subjects were based on self-reported measures (e.g., more Ranch Hand subjects perceived their health to be poor), and those differences that were based on clinical measures were within normal ranges and did not correlate with exposure indices. Investigators concluded as of Cycle 1 that Ranch Hand subjects were not experiencing increased rates of or early onset of diseases under study relative to the comparison population. Ranch Hand mortality was found not to vary by frequency, cause, or age relative to comparison subjects. Minor birth defects (such as birthmarks), neonatal deaths, and physical handicaps were significantly higher among Ranch Hand subject offspring versus comparison offspring. Reproductive results were characterized as "mixed" in the Cycle 1 report (AFHS, 1984a) and were considered "preliminary" as they were subject to verification of records.[64]

Cycle 2 analyses indicated that cancer, kidney disease, general cardiovascular health, pulmonary disease and function, and hematologic measures did not

---

[61]Investigators identified five areas as needing further development: database refinement, tailor follow-up examination requirements based on Cycle 1 results, refine exposure index (aerodynamic study of flight conditions), conduct additional statistical analyses and power estimates, and collaborate with other groups with research activities related to herbicides and/or dioxin exposure (AFHS, 1984a).

[62]The influence of sun exposure (UV radiation) could not be evaluated during Cycle 1 analyses, but was slated for evaluation in the Cycle 2 skin cancer evaluation (AFHS, 1984a).

[63]One case of soft-tissue sarcoma was reported among comparison subjects, but diagnosis had not been confirmed at the time of the baseline evaluation, and this case was not included in analyses (AFHS, 1984a).

[64]Reproductive results became a source of controversy, and AFHS investigators were later criticized for the delayed publication (AFHS, 1992) of early reproductive results (GAO, 1999).

vary significantly by group. The differences in peripheral pulse measures observed in the Cycle 1 evaluation were no longer evident, a change investigators attributed to the requirement of pretest smoking abstinence for the Cycle 2 physical examination. Endpoints for which a significant group difference was observed included lower percentages of body fat among Ranch Hand personnel and a higher proportion of erythrocyte sedimentation rate (ESR)[65] abnormalities among Ranch Hand subjects. Rates of self-reported fair or poor health were higher for enlisted Ranch Hand subjects. Ranch Hand subjects had higher rates of basal cell carcinoma as well as higher rates of verified heart disease. Ranch Hand subjects were more likely to self-report abnormalities related to hysteria and social introversion. As was the case in the Cycle 1 evaluation, Ranch Hand personnel were not found to be at increased risk for development of chloracne, soft-tissue sarcoma, or porphyria cutanea tarda. No dose-response pattern was observed based on the calculated exposure index for the included dependent variables. Of the 19 endpoints evaluated in longitudinal analyses, erythrocyte sedimentation rate, Babinski reflex, depression, platelet count, and manual all-pulse index[66] indicated changes over time. Changes in ESR were attributed to differences in laboratory procedures between the Cycle 1 and Cycle 2 evaluations.[67] Results of psychological tests were mixed: Ranch Hand subjects experienced more psychological abnormalities according to the results of the Cornell Medical Index, but comparison subjects experienced more psychological maladies according to the results of the Halstead-Reitan Neuropsychological Test Battery (AFHS, 1987). Overall, there were slight decreases in group differences between Cycle 1 and Cycle 2.

Mortality analyses from the 1984 update failed to detect statistically significant differences in the mortality experience of Ranch Hand personnel relative to the comparison population or as compared to mortality trends among white males in the U.S. population and DOD retired officers (AFHS, 1984b). Trends in mortality were associated with age: Ranch Hand officers born between 1905 and 1935 were found to have a better mortality experience than comparison subjects and a worse mortality experience than comparison subjects for those Ranch Hand subjects born after 1935 (AFHS, 1984b). Overall, the mortality experience of Ranch Hand ground personnel was less favorable than that of the comparison group, but the difference was not statistically significant.

---

[65]Erythrocyte sedimentation rate is used to screen for inflammatory or malignant disease. It is not a definitive diagnostic test (Stevens and Mylecraine, 1994).

[66]Both manual palpitation and Doppler technique were used to evaluate pulse (femoral, popliteal, dorsalis pedis, posterior tibial, and radial) quality in Cycle 2 (AFHS, 1987). A longitudinal trend was observed for the manual technique.

[67]The laboratory portions of the baseline examination were conducted by Kelsey-Seybold Clinic, Houston, Texas. For the follow-up examination Scripps Clinic in La Jolla, California, through SAIC conducted lab analyses (AFHS, 1984a, 1987).

At the time of the 1987 morbidity follow-up evaluation, USAF investigators concluded that the differences in health outcomes between Ranch Hand subjects and comparison subjects were insufficient to attribute trends in adverse health outcomes among Ranch Hand subjects to herbicide exposure (AFHS, 1990). The difference between Ranch Hand subjects and comparison subjects in self-perceived health status was not statistically significant. Recurrent findings were cited in the follow-up. Erythrocyte sedimentation rates continued to be higher for Ranch Hand subjects as a group. Skin cancer incidence remained higher for Ranch Hand subjects. Ranch Hand subjects were more likely to have developed coordination and balance difficulties as well as some psychological disorders. Ranch Hand subjects had more pulse abnormalities—a result observed at the Cycle 1 evaluation, but not at the Cycle 2. At the time the Cycle 2 results were published (1987), one case of soft-tissue sarcoma among Ranch Hand subjects and one case of soft-tissue sarcoma among comparison subjects[68] were reported. Additionally, one case of non-Hodgkin's lymphoma among Ranch Hand subjects had been reported, but not verified (Wolfe, 1989). These cases of soft-tissue sarcoma and non-Hodgkin's lymphoma were verified and included in the report of Cycle 3 results (AFHS, 1990). Ranch Hand subjects had higher rates (statistically significant) of verified and suspected neoplasms. Ranch Hand subjects were found to be experiencing more coordination abnormalities than comparison subjects, and after controlling for insecticide exposure, a significant increasing trend was observed for coordination abnormalities among enlisted Ranch Hand subjects. Statistically significant trends were observed for sleep disorders, verified psychological disorders, and in scores on two psychological batteries[69] (indicators of psychological distress and/or dysfunction). Investigators again noted the lack of chloracne and porphyria cutanea tarda occurrence among Ranch Hand subjects. In summary, investigators stated that as of Cycle 3 there was no evidence of an association between herbicide exposure and increased morbidity among Ranch Hand subjects (AFHS, 1990).

Reevaluation of Cycle 3 data based on TCDD body burden revealed several statistically significant associations for lipid-related abnormalities (cholesterol, high-density lipoprotein [HDL], and cholesterol to HDL ratio) (AFHS, 1991b). Two-hour postprandial glucose, ESR, immunoglobulin A, white blood cell and platelet counts, spirometric indices, benign systemic neoplasms, and decreased testicular size were also directly associated with TCDD body burden. AFHS investigators stated, in summary, that their findings "reveal[ed] a consistent relationship between dioxin [body burden] and body fat," which they believed begged

[68]The single case of soft-tissue sarcoma was mentioned in the baseline report (AFHS, 1984a). There is some variation in reporting of these cases of soft-tissue sarcoma and non-Hodgkin's lymphoma among AFHS reports and publications.

[69]The Symptom Checklist-90-Revised and the Millon Clinical Multiaxial Inventory were used as part of the psychological evaluation during the Cycle 3 follow-up (Appendix B) (AFHS, 1990).

two separate hypotheses: (1) that dioxin causes an increase in body fat, and (2) that body fat modulates TCDD elimination rates (AFHS, 1991b).

As of Cycle 3 (1987), median Ranch Hand (n = 866) serum TCDD level was 12.7 ppt and ranged from no detection to 617.8 ppt. Median comparison (n = 804) serum TCDD was 4.2 ppt and ranged from no detection to 54.8 ppt (AFHS, 1991b). The 1987 TCDD value was considered by AFHS investigators to be the most informative. Subject sera were assayed in Cycles 4–6, but those assays were primarily intended to capture serum TCDD data for subjects whose sera had not previously been assayed. By Cycle 6 TCDD assays were performed for only 12 Ranch Hand subjects (2 percent of Ranch Hand participants) and 94 comparison subjects (8 percent of comparison participants). Table 4-2 recounts the number of assays performed by cycle in Chapter 4.

Cycle 4 analyses indicated that Ranch Hand subjects perceived their health status to be poorer than that of comparison subjects. Investigators noted that this result may have been biased as subjects were aware of TCDD body burden results and thus those with higher levels (Ranch Hand subjects) may have "consciously or subconsciously perceived their health to be poorer than their comparison subjects" (AFHS, 1995). Statistically significant associations were observed between TCDD body burden and percentage of body fat and ESR. Ranch Hand subjects had only a "slightly higher" prevalence of skin neoplasms (both benign and malignant) relative to comparison subjects, which had been found previously to be significant. Risk of neoplastic disease was determined to be similar for both groups. Members of Ranch Hand groundcrews were more likely than members of comparison groundcrews to develop cranial nerve index abnormalities. For the neurological assessment overall, no significant differences were observed between Ranch Hand subjects and comparison subjects, and no exposure-effect trend was evident (AFHS, 1995). TCDD body burden was found to be associated with glucose intolerance. The association was observed in both diabetic and nondiabetic subjects and was also found to exhibit a dose–effect trend. The association was evident longitudinally. While diabetes prevalence did not differ significantly between Ranch Hand subjects and comparison subjects, current dioxin was significantly associated with diabetes onset (AFHS, 1992). Using both the current and initial TCDD body burden models, a statistically significant direct association was observed between TCDD body burden and cholesterol, triglycerides, and the cholesterol-to-HDL ratio as well as for some hepatic enzyme levels (AST, ALT, and GGT)[70] among Ranch Hand subjects. TCDD body burden was not found to be associated with any clinical maladies. No statistically significant group differences were found for neoplastic disease and most of the site-specific cancer evaluations found lower relative risks in the cohort subjects in the high

[70]AST: aspartate aminotransferase; ALT: alanine aminotrasferase; GGT: gamma glutamyltransferase (AFHS, 2000).

dioxin category than those in the background and low dioxin categories (AFHS, 1995). Deaths due to cardiovascular and digestive disease were significantly increased among Ranch Hand groundcrews (AFHS, 1994). This finding was consistent with the previous three mortality follow-up evaluations (AFHS, 1989, 1991a, 1993). The AFHS cited cardiovascular disease, glucose intolerance, and serum lipid abnormalities as the most highly relevant findings in the Cycle 4 follow-up (AFHS, 1995).

Ranch Hand subjects, and specifically enlisted Ranch Hand groundcrew personnel, continued to report their health as fair to poor with significantly greater frequency than comparison subjects in Cycle 5 (AFHS, 2000). Body fat was found to be directly correlated with TCDD body burden, and the pharmacokinetics of TCDD appeared to differ by body fat percentage (AFHS, 2000). Significant differences in ESR were not observed at the group level, but ESR did correlate with TCDD body burden. Longitudinal analysis indicated that Ranch Hand subjects experienced more ESR abnormalities than comparison subjects over time, and this trend was strongest for enlisted Ranch Hand subjects (AFHS, 2000). Ranch Hand subjects were not at increased risk for malignant neoplastic disease development after 15 years of follow-up, and longitudinal analyses did not suggest a difference in the development of malignancies over time by group status. Enlisted Ranch Hand groundcrews had lower rates of neoplastic disease than comparison subjects. A dose–effect trend between TCDD body burden and neuropathy was observed for peripheral nerve disorders, as verified by medical records review. An increase in prevalence of several neuroses was observed for enlisted Ranch Hand groundcrews. Many significant associations were observed between hepatic enzymes (AST, ALT, and GGT) and serum lipid indices (cholesterol, triglycerides, and HDL) and current TCDD body burden (AFHS, 2000). A history of essential hypertension was found to be directly associated with current serum TCDD values among Ranch Hand subjects, and initial serum TCDD body burden was found to be associated with evidence of myocardial infarction. These findings, along with increased frequency of circulatory-related deaths among nonflying enlisted Ranch Hand subjects, indicated that further evaluation of the relationship between TCDD body burden and heart disease was warranted (AFHS, 2000). Enlisted Ranch Hand groundcrews were found to have a significant increased risk of elevated levels of thyroid stimulating hormone (TSH). Type 2 diabetes prevalence was significantly associated with TCDD body burden. Ranch Hand subjects were also more likely than comparison subjects to require insulin control of their diabetes. Time to diabetes onset was directly associated with current serum TCDD levels among Ranch Hand subjects. Fasting glucose and α-1-C hemoglobin levels were directly associated with current and initial serum TCDD levels, and fasting urinary glucose trended with current TCDD levels. Investigators concluded that there was evidence of an association of either Ranch Hand group/subgroup status or serum TCDD levels (current and/or initial) with diabetes, cardiovascular abnormalities, peripheral polyneuropathy, serum lipid abnormalities, and elevation of hepatic enzyme levels.

Analyses of Cycle 6 data revealed increases among enlisted Ranch Hand subjects of reported post-SEA acne occurrence and of post-SEA acne duration. These increases were correlated with current TCDD levels for those subjects who had not reported occurrence of pre-SEA acne (AFHS, 2005). Cardiovascular results varied by model and subgroup. An increased risk of high diastolic blood pressure was observed among Ranch Hand enlisted flyers and Ranch Hand subjects in the high-exposure category (Model 3/initial TCDD). Ranch Hand subjects were more likely to suffer from heart disease than comparison subjects in the enlisted-flyer stratum. Mean platelet count was higher for Ranch Hand enlisted flyers. Among enlisted Ranch Hand groundcrew personnel (Model 1) and Ranch Hand subjects in the low and high initial TCDD categories (Model 3) an increase in abnormal red blood cell morphology was observed. An increase in mean ESR was observed for Ranch Hand subjects in the low and high categories (Model 3). White blood cell count was inversely associated with current TCDD values (Model 4). Associations for diabetes indices varied by statistical model. Ranch Hand subjects were at significantly higher risk of abnormal 2-hour postprandial urinary glucose levels versus comparison subjects (Model 1). Under Model 2, mean fasting insulin and the probability of requiring insulin to control diabetes were directly correlated with initial TCDD, and the time to onset of diabetes was inversely correlated with initial TCDD. The requirement of insulin management of diabetes was also correlated with initial TCDD under Model 3 for the high category. Current TCDD (Model 4) was directly associated with the need for oral hypoglycemic or insulin control of diabetes and inversely associated with time to diabetes onset. Risk of elevated levels of α-1-C hemoglobin was directly associated with current TCDD (Model 4). Mean TSH was significantly higher for Ranch Hand subjects versus comparison subjects as was luteinizing hormone for Ranch Hand officers only versus comparison subjects (Model 1) (AFHS, 2005). The risk of abnormal antinuclear antibody titer increased (Model 2) with initial TCDD level (AFHS, 2005).

Reproductive Study Results

Although rudimentary reports of reproductive outcomes were published in the 1982 (baseline) morbidity report, it was not until 1996 that a comprehensive report of the reproductive experience of the Ranch Hand subjects was published. Cycle 1 results were considered preliminary and were based on maternal reporting only. Medical data collection/verification began for 9,921 conceptions and 8,100 live births one year after the Cycle 1 report was released (AFHS, 1992). Results did not reflect a dose–effect trend under any of the implemented analytical models. For several outcomes—for example, circulatory system disorders and genital anomalies—rates were greater for children born to Ranch Hand subjects in the low-dioxin categories versus Ranch Hand subjects in the high-dioxin category or the comparison group (AFHS, 1992).

Michalek and colleagues (1998b) evaluated preterm birth, intrauterine growth retardation (IUGR), and infant death in offspring of veterans with quantifiable 1987 or 1992 dioxin measures (Ranch Hand offspring: n = 859; comparison offspring: n = 1,223). Offspring analyses were restricted to singleton live births conceived during or subsequent to the subject's SEA tour. Ranch Hand offspring were categorized by paternal dioxin level. Subject assay measures greater than 10 ppt, were extrapolated to "initial dioxin" level or to the time of conception. Offspring whose father's 1987 or 1992 dioxin level—if both were available the 1987 measure was used—was ≤ 10 ppt were assigned to the background. Initial dioxin levels ≤ 79 ppt but >10 ppt were assigned to low, and those > 79 ppt were assigned to the high categories. Children of fathers in the high and background categories were at increased risk of preterm birth. All offspring of Ranch Hand subjects were at increased risk of infant death. Offspring of any category were not at increased risk of IUGR. Evaluation of sex of offspring indicated that offspring sex was not associated with paternal dioxin levels (Michalek et al., 1998c).

In 1998, a follow-up report of reproductive outcomes documented at Cycle 1 was released (AFHS, 1998). According to the follow-up report, which was based on verified reports of reproductive anomalies, statistically significant odds ratios relating to birth defects and neonatal death with respect to paternal service in SEA (pre- versus post-SEA outcomes) were observed (AFHS, 1998), although more than 6,000 negative responses were not subject to records verification. An elevated rate of neural tube defects[71] among Ranch Hand offspring was reported in the journal *Epidemiology* three years before the updated USAF report was released (Wolfe et al., 1995a).

Additional Mortality Study Results

As already noted, a baseline mortality report (AFHS, 1983) and several updates (AFHS, 1984b, 1985, 1986, 1989, 1991a, 1993, 1996) have been published as part of the study. The mortality investigation has also been the subject of three papers in the peer-reviewed literature.

Michalek and colleagues (1990) analyzed cumulative mortality through December 31, 1987. Ranch Hand subjects were similar to comparison subjects with respect to all-cause mortality. Results for unadjusted cause-specific analyses indicated that Ranch Hand subjects did not differ significantly from comparison subjects. After adjusting for rank and military occupation—there were too few non-Caucasian subjects to adjust for race—there were still no significant trends

[71]Three of four neural tube defects identified were cases of spina bifida (IOM, 1996).

in mortality. When analyses were adjusted for time since beginning of SEA tour of duty (≤ 5 years), Ranch Hand subjects had experienced a significantly greater than expected number of deaths from external causes, with the overwhelming majority caused by nonmilitary aviation accidents. Unadjusted analyses indicated that more Ranch Hand subjects than comparison subjects had died from diseases of the digestive tract. However, this finding was not statistically significant and was not suggestive of an herbicide effect—the majority resulted from alcoholic liver disease.

In view of the data collected between 1979 and December of 1993, AFHS investigators concluded that there were no significant differences between Ranch Hand subjects and comparison subjects for overall all-cause mortality, nor were any differences in group mortality (officer/enlisted or flyer/nonflyer) evident. No significant differences were observed for cause-specific mortality, excepting an observed increase in deaths due to diseases of the circulatory system among enlisted groundcrew. This finding was again reported in the 1994 mortality update. Mortality results were also published in the *American Journal of Epidemiology* (Michalek et al., 1998a). This paper reported a greater number of observed Ranch Hand deaths due to digestive disease than expected, but 7 of the 9 observed deaths were due to cirrhosis and hepatic disease. The authors warned that they were not able to control for alcohol consumption in the analysis.

A 20-year update—covering cohort mortality through December 31, 1999—was published in 2005 (Ketchum and Michalek, 2005). That paper reported, for the first time, an elevated relative risk for all-cause mortality among all Ranch Hand veterans. The observed increased risk was driven by outcomes among the enlisted groundcrew (based on 88 deaths in Ranch Hand veterans). When separated by reported cause, death due to circulatory disease in enlisted groundcrew was notable (based on 40 deaths).

Following 20-years' worth of observation and analysis and the generation of more than 20,000 pages of printed material, investigators stated that "diabetes represents the most important health problem seen in the AFHS" (AFHS, 2005; RHAC, 2000).

Costs

AFHS funding is a line item in the DOD annual budget, where it is referred to as the *Ranch Hand II Epidemiology Study*. Budgets from Fiscal Year (FY) 2000 (which provides figures back to FY 1998) onward are available online (DTIC, 1999, 2000, 2001, 2002, 2003, 2004, 2005); the committee obtained earlier information from study staff.[72] Data, shown in Table 2-8, indicate that costs were the highest in the years where physical examinations took place. For most of

[72]M. Blancas, Air Force Health Study, personal communication, November 4, 2005.

TABLE 2-8 AFHS Budget by Fiscal Year and Exam Cycle

Exam Cycle	Fiscal Year	Fiscal Year $(M)
	1981	1.30
1	1982	7.00
	1983	1.00
	1984	1.40
2	1985	8.50
	1986	4.80
3	1987	9.10
	1988	5.50
	1989	3.10
	1990	1.40
	1991	1.50
4	1992	9.70
	1993	8.90
	1994	3.70
	1995	3.20
	1996	3.00
5	1997	8.80
	1998	10.22
	1999	4.12
	2000	4.18
	2001	4.18
6	2002	11.29
	2003	10.07
	2004	4.65
	2005	*4.77*
	2006	*4.19*

NOTE: FY 1998–2004 are final amounts; *2005–2006 are estimates.*

SOURCES: M. Blancas, Air Force Health Study, personal communication, November 4, 2005; DTIC, 2000, 2001, 2002, 2003, 2004, 2005.

the cycles, these costs are spread over two years. All told, approximately $143 million has been spent or allocated for conducting the AFHS. Study funding is thus provided by direct congressional appropriation and is not at the discretion of the USAF.

The yearly budget justifications include breakouts for major categories of work. These indicate that a total of ~$20.8 million[73] was spent or is allocated for

[73]$8.3 million in FY 2002; $7.7 million in FY 2003; $2.3 million in FY 2004; $1.6 million in FY 2005; $0.9 million in FY 2006.

the Cycle 6 physical examinations, questionnaires, and participants' database, of which ~$16.0 million was in the two years where examinations were being conducted (DTIC, 2003, 2004, 2005). Processing and documentation of the database has averaged ~$2.8 million per year over the past five years' budgets.

The AFHS FY 2006 budget (DTIC, 2005) includes allocations to perform documentation and organization of the data assets in anticipation of their future disposition:

> Continue to process and document examination data. Continue archiving previous cycles' examination data and digitize and archive the Cycle 6 data as received. Conduct medical records coding and verification of examination database and Cycles 1 through 6 coding. . . . Prepare for and complete transition or turnover of archives and specimens to designated agencies.

A total of $1,612,000 is assigned to these and other data analysis and support tasks.[74] The documentation and organization activities were apparently planned as a routine part of the study's shutdown and were not related to the *Veterans and Agent Orange*–series report recommendations concerning the AFHS discussed in the Chapter 1. In Chapters 3 and 4, the committee offers several recommendations regarding how the data assets should be documented and organized. It believes that these activities may well fall under the existing budget items listed above.

Study staffing levels have varied over time; personnel comprised two USAF active duty personnel, 10 federal civil service, and 26 contract employees at the beginning of 2005 (Michalek, 2005). There have also been additional outside personnel associated with analysis and data gathering contracts.

COMPENSATION AND BENEFITS FOR VIETNAM VETERANS

The Department of Veterans Affairs and Public Law 102-4

When illness or injury is related to military service, the VA provides medical care, vocational rehabilitation, and a range of other federal benefits as appropriate to those veterans (or their dependents) whose cases have been declared *service connected* (Brown, 2005). For injuries and acute diseases with clearly defined causes or exposures, proof of service connection is relatively straight forward, and if a veteran can provide the VA disability rating specialist with the necessary supporting documentation, then benefits are awarded according to the degree of the severity of the disease or injury. The disability rating scheme is based on a graduated scale ranging from 10 to 100 percent. Compensation grants related to

[74]The other tasks specified in the line item were: support of the annual mortality analysis, conduct of data analysis for journals and reports to Congress, and continued maintenance of study's local area network. An additional $1,677,000 was allocated for data analysis under a separate line item.

environmental or occupational exposures such as Agent Orange represent some of the most difficult disability cases to adjudicate (Brown, 2005). Proof of service connection is far more difficult to establish for longer-latency chronic diseases for which a substantial lapse of time since exposure has occurred. To establish direct service connection the onus is on the veteran to meet minimum VA evidentiary criteria: "evidence of a scientific association," "evidence of military exposure," "evidence of exposure magnitude," and "evidence of temporal plausibility" (Brown, 2005). Claims are decided on an individual basis, and if the evidence indicates that "a veteran's illness or injury is at least as likely as not to have been caused by the environmental or occupational exposure" (Brown, 2005), then the claim is settled in favor of the veteran or his or her dependents.

Excepting the evidentiary requirements listed above, the VA can grant benefits based on what is known as a *presumptive service connection* (Brown, 2005). A condition presumed to be connected to military service generally needs to manifest within a prescribed postservice time frame and must result in at least 10 percent disability. Presumptive connection relieves the veteran of the task of meeting the burden of proof[75] of service connection. Agent Orange claims proved to be problematic for the VA and veterans seeking compensation, as the nature of exposure at the individual level was largely unknown and the toxicokinetics (relationship between dose and transport to site of toxic activity) and toxicodynamics (mechanisms of toxicants at the site of toxic activity and the downstream functional consequences) of 2,4-D and 2,4,5-T as well as that of TCDD have yet to be fully elucidated (Bier, 2003; Brown, 2005). To expedite the compensation awards process in the case of Agent Orange-related claims, in 1991 Congress placed provisions into Pub. L. 102-4, *The Agent Orange Act of 1991*. Pub. L. 102-4 required the VA to contract with the NAS to independently review all available scientific data pertaining to the health effects of herbicides used during the Vietnam War (not limited to Agent Orange) and dioxin exposure.[76] Although respective NAS committees evaluate the strength of the evidence between specific outcomes and herbicide/dioxin exposure, it is the VA that has the ultimate authority regarding compensation policy and dispensation of awards. The VA is not limited to the input of the NAS, and has its own panel of experts that recommends actions to the Secretary of Veterans Affairs regarding the establishment of presumptive service connection for a particular health outcome. NAS reports consti-

---

[75]When many veterans separate from service they often retain only the minimum documentation of their service experience—their ETS (end of term of service) orders and their DD214/DD13. They may not possess a complete copy of their medical record. Recovering these documents and reconstructing service experience years and even decades after separation from service can be an onerous task, and veterans may not have access to germane documentation.

[76]Pub. L. 102-4 also called for the IOM to conduct biennial reviews of related material for a follow-up period of 10 years (IOM, 1999). In 2001, Pub. L. 107-103 extended IOM biennial reviews through 2014 (IOM, 2005).

tute an important input to this process, but the VA can and has made decisions on other bases.

AFHS Research and the Institute of Medicine's "Veterans and Agent Orange" Reports

In accordance with Pub. L. 102-4, the VA asked the NAS to form a series of committees to "determine (to the extent that available scientific data permit meaningful determinations)" the following regarding associations between specific health outcomes and exposure to TCDD and other chemical compounds in herbicides:

- whether a statistical association with herbicide exposure exists, taking into account the strength of the scientific evidence and the appropriateness of the statistical and epidemiologic methods used to detect the association;
- the increased risk of the disease among those exposed to herbicides during service in the Republic of Vietnam during the Vietnam era; and
- whether there exists a plausible biological mechanism or other evidence of a causal relationship between herbicide exposure and the disease.

In fulfillment of its charge, the first committee given this task assembled a list of health outcomes to evaluate based on an exhaustive literature survey that included more than 6,000 abstracts and articles, 230 of which were epidemiologic investigations. Fourteen of the 230 studies were related to the Air Force Health Study. Thirty-two outcomes or categories of outcomes were identified.

Veterans and Agent Orange: Health Effects of Herbicides Used in Vietnam (*VAO*) (IOM, 1994), was the first comprehensive evaluation published under the congressional mandate.

Determinations of health risks related to veterans were based on the appropriateness and strength of statistical association reported in the scientific literature as well as biologic plausibility and mechanistic evidence of or inference to causality[77] (IOM, 1994). The strength of the scientific evidence is characterized by a qualitative scale based on criteria first established by the International Agency for Research on Cancer (IARC, 1977):

- sufficient evidence of an association,
- limited or suggestive evidence of an association,

[77]While evidence of causality is considered, diseases are classified on the basis of "statistical association, not on causality" (IOM, 1994).

- inadequate or insufficient evidence to determine whether an association exists, and
- limited or suggestive evidence of no association.[78]

AFHS mortality and morbidity results were reviewed in great detail with respect to all major disease categories and contributed with varying degrees of influence to the overall knowledge foundation on which the original report of the Veterans and Agent Orange (VAO) series was based. A total of 13 reports and papers were cited (IOM, 1994). Application and interpretation of AFHS results by the committee was limited by the statistical methods and results presentation employed by investigators. The committee noted specifically that inclusion of more Cycle 1 data,[79] statement of a priori hypotheses, and greater "exploration of an overall effect" would have improved the clarity and generalizability of AFHS outcomes (IOM, 1994).

Two then-new AFHS publications (AFHS, 1995; Wolfe et al., 1995a) were reviewed in *VAO Update 1996* (IOM, 1996). The AFHS 1995 mortality update was one of three studies of "high quality" that led to the addition of spina bifida to the disease category of limited or suggestive evidence of an association. The previously reviewed (IOM, 1994) AFHS 1990 report of increased risk of non-melanomic skin cancer among Ranch Hand subjects contributed to the category change of skin cancer from limited or suggestive evidence of no association to inadequate or insufficient evidence to determine whether an association exists.

In *VAO Update 1998* (IOM, 1999), urinary bladder cancer was upgraded from a condition for which there was limited or suggestive evidence of no association to an outcome for which there was inadequate or insufficient evidence to determine whether an association exists. AFHS findings did not contribute to this change.

---

[78]Sufficient evidence of an association is declared when "a positive association has been observed between herbicides and the outcome in studies in which chance, bias, and confounding could be ruled out with reasonable confidence." Limited or suggestive evidence of an association refers to conditions for which "evidence is suggestive of an association between herbicides and the outcome but is limited because chance, bias, and confounding could not be ruled out with confidence." Inadequate or insufficient evidence to determine whether an association exists is the determination made when "the available studies are of insufficient quality, consistency, or statistical power to permit a conclusion regarding the presence or absence of an association." Limited or suggestive evidence of no association describes outcomes for which "several adequate studies, covering the full range of levels of exposure that human beings are known to encounter, are mutually consistent in not showing a positive association between exposure to herbicides and the outcome at any level of exposure" (IOM, 1994).

[79]The committee concluded that—using Models 1 and 2—the "most relevant baseline data" had been excluded from most analyses of the reproductive data and that the committee's critique of methods used in reproductive analyses could be generally applied to the AFHS (IOM, 1994).

In 1999, the VA commissioned an evaluation of type 2 diabetes risk by the IOM independent of the biennial VAO updates. The IOM released *Veterans and Agent Orange: Herbicide/Dioxin Exposure and Type 2 Diabetes* in 2000. The results of the AFHS Cycle 5 morbidity analyses (AFHS, 2000) related to diabetes and the contents of a paper on the cohort (Longnecker and Michalek, 2000) were reviewed in great detail. Endpoints measured included type 2 diabetes incidence, time to disease onset, severity of disease, and a battery of related laboratory tests. These metrics were analyzed using four different exposure models that were run adjusted and unadjusted for the age, race, military occupation, personality type, body fat, and family history (IOM, 2000). Further analyses carried out at the request of the IOM committee served to strengthen the importance of AFHS results (Personal communication, J.E. Michalek, Air Force Health Study, July 28, 2000). These indicated an increased prevalence of and a decreased time to onset of type 2 diabetes was associated with dioxin exposure among Ranch Hand subjects. Previously VAO-reviewed AFHS material (Henriksen et al., 1997) was also considered in the committee's conclusion that there was limited or suggestive evidence of an association between herbicide or dioxin exposure and type 2 diabetes (IOM, 2000). Two AFHS papers were cited in the report's discussion of the biologic plausibility of an association between diabetes and dioxin exposure: Michalek and Tripathi (1999), reporting a compensatory metabolic relation between dioxin and insulin regulation in study participants; and Longnecker and Michalek (2000), finding an apparent association between serum dioxin levels and fasting glucose levels among nondiabetic AFHS comparison group members with less than 10 ppt serum dioxin.

Nine then-new AFHS reports and papers (including those addressed in the type 2 diabetes report) were reviewed in *Veterans and Agent Orange: Update 2000* (IOM, 2001). Other than the type 2 diabetes decision, there were no changes to the categorizations of health outcomes from the previous update as the new literature supported existing conclusions.

No new major AFHS reports had been released at the time the next two update reports were published.[80] However, a number of journal articles related to AFHS (Barrett et al., 2001; Michalek et al., 2001a,b,c; Steenland et al., 2001) were reviewed in both *VAO Update 2002* (IOM, 2003a) and *VAO Update 2004* (IOM, 2005; Akhtar et al., 2004; Barrett et al., 2003; Michalek et al., 2003; Pavuk et al., 2003). No changes were made in the strength of evidence categories by either of the IOM committees because, again, new evidence supported existing conclusions.[81]

A table adapted from *VAO Update 2004* (IOM, 2005) is included as Appendix C. It provides, as part of a comprehensive list of the Vietnam veterans'

---

[80]The Cycle 6 follow-up examination results were not released until July of 2005.

[81]A new health outcome—chronic lymphocytic leukemia—was added in 2002 (IOM, 2003a).

health outcomes literature, summary information on AFHS publications and indicates in which volume of the VAO report series a review may be found. The table includes information on the type of study, a summary description of the topics addressed, and the size of the study population. Additional information on, and reviews of, the AFHS reports and papers may be found in the text of the Veterans and Agent Orange reports referenced in the Appendix.

In the period since the Agent Orange Act of 1991 was passed, the AFHS has contributed to the establishment of a presumptive service connection[82] for type 2 diabetes in Vietnam veterans and for spina bifida in their offspring. As of September 2004, 191,649 Vietnam-era veterans were receiving compensation for diabetes mellitus (VA, 2005), and 1,187 children of Vietnam veterans were receiving compensation for spina bifida as of September 2005, the majority of which are presumptively connected to Vietnam service (G. Peters, Veterans Benefits Administration, personal communication, September 2, 2005). The Veterans Benefits Administration of the VA does not have complete documentation on the number of Vietnam veterans who have received compensation for conditions recognized as service connected due to their association with herbicide or dioxin exposure.

REFERENCES

AFHS (Air Force Health Study). 1982. *An Epidemiologic Investigation of Health Effects in Air Force Personnel Following Exposure to Herbicides: Study Protocol, Initial Report.* Brooks AFB, TX: USAF School of Aerospace Medicine. SAM-TR-82-44.

AFHS. 1983. *An Epidemiologic Investigation of Health Effects in Air Force Personnel Following Exposure to Herbicides. Baseline Mortality Study Results.* Brooks AFB, TX: USAF School of Aerospace Medicine. NTIS AD-A130 793.

AFHS. 1984a. *An Epidemiologic Investigation of Health Effects in Air Force Personnel Following Exposure to Herbicides. Baseline Morbidity Study Results.* Brooks AFB, TX: USAF School of Aerospace Medicine. NTIS AD-A-138-340.

AFHS. 1984b. *An Epidemiologic Investigation of Health Effects in Air Force Personnel Following Exposure to Herbicides. Mortality Update: 1984.* Brooks AFB, TX: USAF School of Aerospace Medicine. NTIS-AD-A-162-687.

AFHS. 1985. *An Epidemiologic Investigation of Health Effects in Air Force Personnel Following Exposure to Herbicides. Mortality Update: 1985.* Brooks AFB, TX: USAF School of Aerospace Medicine. NTIS-AD-A-163-237.

[82]As of March 3, 2005, the VA recognized the following diseases as presumptively connected to Vietnam service: chloracne, Hodgkin's disease, multiple myeloma, non-Hodgkin's lymphoma, porphyria cutanea tarda, respiratory cancers (lung, bronchus, larynx, and trachea), soft-tissue sarcoma, acute and subacute peripheral neuropathy, prostate cancer, and spina bifida in offspring of veterans (VA, 2003).

AFHS. 1986. *An Epidemiologic Investigation of Health Effects in Air Force Personnel Following Exposure to Herbicides. Mortality Update: 1986.* Brooks AFB, TX: USAF School of Aerospace Medicine. USAFSAM-TR-86-43.

AFHS. 1987. *An Epidemiologic Investigation of Health Effects in Air Force Personnel Following Exposure to Herbicides. First Follow-up Examination Results.* 2 vols. Brooks AFB, TX: USAF School of Aerospace Medicine. USAFSAM-TR-87-27.

AFHS. 1989. *An Epidemiologic Investigation of Health Effects in Air Force Personnel Following Exposure to Herbicides. Mortality Update: 1989.* Brooks AFB, TX: USAF School of Aerospace Medicine. USAFSAM-TR-89-9.

AFHS. 1990. *An Epidemiologic Investigation of Health Effects in Air Force Personnel Following Exposure to Herbicides.* 2 vols. Brooks AFB, TX: USAF School of Aerospace Medicine. USAFSAM-TR-90-2.

AFHS. 1991a. *An Epidemiologic Investigation of Health Effects in Air Force Personnel Following Exposure to Herbicides. Mortality Update: 1992.* Brooks AFB, TX: Armstrong Laboratory. AL-TR-1991-0132.

AFHS. 1991b. *An Epidemiologic Investigation of Health Effects in Air Force Personnel Following Exposure to Herbicides. Serum Dioxin Analysis of 1987 Examination Results.* 9 vols. Brooks, AFB, TX: USAF School of Aerospace Medicine. AL-TR-91-0009.

AFHS. 1992. *An Epidemiologic Investigation of Health Effects in Air Force Personnel Following Exposure to Herbicides. Reproductive Outcomes.* Brooks AFB, TX: Armstrong Laboratory. AL-TR-1992-0090.

AFHS. 1993. *An Epidemiologic Investigation of Health Effects in Air Force Personnel Following Exposure to Herbicides. Mortality Update: 1993.* Brooks AFB, TX: Armstrong Laboratory. AL/AO-TR-1993-0161.

AFHS. 1994. *An Epidemiologic Investigation of Health Effects in Air Force Personnel Following Exposure to Herbicides. Mortality Update: 1994.* Brooks AFB, TX: Armstrong Laboratory. AL/AO-TR-1994-0128.

AFHS. 1995. *An Epidemiologic Investigation of Health Effects in Air Force Personnel Following Exposure to Herbicides. 1992 Followup Examination Results.* Brooks AFB, TX: Epidemiologic Research Division. Armstrong Laboratory. AL-TR-920107.

AFHS. 1996. *An Epidemiologic Investigation of Health Effects in Air Force Personnel Following Exposure to Herbicides. Mortality Update 1996.* Brooks AFB, TX: Epidemiologic Research Division. Armstrong Laboratory. AL/AO-TR-1996-0068.

AFHS. 1998. *An Epidemiologic Investigation of Health Effects in Air Force Personnel Following Exposure to Herbicides. Reproductive Outcome Update.* Brooks AFB, TX: Epidemiologic Research Division. Armstrong Laboratory. AFRL-HE-BR-TR-1998-0073.

AFHS. 2000. *An Epidemiologic Investigation of Health Effects in Air Force Personnel Following Exposure to Herbicides. 1997 Follow-up Examination Results.* Brooks AFB, TX: Human Systems Program Office. Armstrong Laboratory. AFRL-HE-BR-TR-2000-02.

AFHS. 2005. *An Epidemiologic Investigation of Health Effects in Air Force Personnel Following Exposure to Herbicides. 2002 Followup Examination Results.* Brooks AFB, TX: Epidemiologic Research Division. Armstrong Laboratory. AFRL-HE-BR-SR-2005-0003.

Akhtar FZ, Garabrant DH, Ketchum NS, Michalek JE. 2004. Cancer in US Air Force veterans of the Vietnam War. *Journal of Occupational and Environmental Medicine* 46(2):123–136.

Alcott EB. 1995. *A History of the Ranch Hand Epidemiologic Investigation.* Brooks AFB, TX: Office of History, Human Systems Center.

Barrett DH, Morris RD, Akhtar FZ, Michalek JE. 2001. Serum dioxin and cognitive functioning among veterans of Operation Ranch Hand. *Neurotoxicology* 22:491–502.

Barrett DH, Morris RD, Jackson WG Jr, Michalek JE. 2003. Serum dioxin and psychological functioning in US Air Force veterans of the Vietnam War. *Military Medicine* 168(2):153–159.

Bier D. 2003. Amino acid pharmacokinetics and safety assessment. *Journal of Nutrition* 133(6 Suppl. 1):2034S–2039S.

Boyne WJ. 2000. Ranch Hand: Even then, the defoliation missions over Vietnam were controversial. *Air Force Magazine* 83(8):84–89. [Online]. Available: http://www.afa.org/magazine/Aug2000/0800ranch.asp [accessed April 7, 2005].

Brown M. 2005. The role of science in the Department of Veterans Affairs disability compensation policies for environmental and occupational illnesses and injuries. *Journal of Law and Policy* 13(2):593–612.

Buckingham WA. 1982. *Operation Ranch Hand: The Air Force and Herbicides in Southeast Asia, 1961–1971.* Washington, DC: Office of Air Force History.

Buckingham WA. 1997. *Operation Ranch Hand: Herbicides in Southeast Asia, 1961–1971.* [Online]. Available: http://www.cpcug.org/user/billb/ranchhand/ranchhand.html [accessed May 12, 2005].

Bullman TA, Watanabe KK, Kang HK. 1994. Risk of testicular cancer associated with surrogate measures of Agent Orange exposure among Vietnam veterans on the Agent Orange Registry. *Annals of Epidemiology* 4:11–16.

Butler DA. 2005. Connections: the early history of scientific and medical research on "Agent Orange." *Journal of Law and Policy* 13(2):527–552.

CDC (The Centers for Disease Control Veterans Health Studies). 1988. Serum 2,3,7,8-tetrachlorodibenzo-*p*-dioxin levels in US Army Vietnam-era veterans. *Journal of the American Medical Association* 260:1249–1254.

Cecil PF. 1986. *Herbicidal Warfare: The Ranch Hand Project in Vietnam.* New York: Praeger.

Cook RR, Townsend JC, Ott MG, Silverstein LG. 1980. Mortality experience of employees exposed to 2,3,7,8-teterachlorodibenzo-*p*-dioxin (TCDD). *Journal of Occupational Medicine* 22:530–532.

de Sola D. 2004. Vietnamese sue over Agent Orange *(CNN Law Center).* [Online]. Available: http://www.cnn.com/2004/LAW/08/15/agent.orange.suit/index.html [accessed October 10, 2005].

DTIC (Defense Technical Information Center). February 1999. *RDT&E Budget Item Justification Sheet, Ranch Hand II Epidemiology Study, PE number: 0605306F.* [Online]. Available: http://www.dtic.mil/descriptivesum/Y2000/AirForce/0605306f.pdf [accessed August 31, 2005].

DTIC. February 2000. *RDT&E Budget Item Justification Sheet, Ranch Hand II Epidemiology Study, PE number: 0605306F.* [Online]. Available: http://www.dtic.mil/descriptivesum/Y2001/AirForce/0605306f.pdf [accessed August 31, 2005].

DTIC. June 2001. *RDT&E Budget Item Justification Sheet, Ranch Hand II Epidemiology Study, PE number: 0605306F.* [Online]. Available: http://www.dtic.mil/descriptivesum/Y2002/AirForce/0605306f.pdf [accessed August 31, 2005].

DTIC. February 2002. *RDT&E Budget Item Justification Sheet, Ranch Hand II Epidemiology Study, PE number: 0605306F.* [Online]. Available: http://www.dtic.mil/descriptivesum/Y2003/AirForce/0605306f.pdf [accessed August 31, 2005].

DTIC. February 2003. *RDT&E Budget Item Justification Sheet, Ranch Hand II Epidemiology Study, PE number: 0605306F.* [Online]. Available: http://www.dtic.mil/descriptivesum/Y2004/AirForce/0605306f.pdf [accessed August 31, 2005].

DTIC. February 2004. *RDT&E Budget Item Justification Sheet, Ranch Hand II Epidemiology Study, PE number: 0605306F.* [Online]. Available: http://www.dtic.mil/descriptivesum/Y2005/AirForce/0605306f.pdf [accessed August 31, 2005].

DTIC. February 2005. *RDT&E Budget Item Justification Sheet, Ranch Hand II Epidemiology Study, PE number: 0605306F.* [Online]. Available: //www.dtic.mil/descriptivesum/Y2006/AirForce/0605306f.pdf [accessed August 31, 2005].

500 vets claim herbicide effects. 1978, October 12. *The Washington Post.* [Online]. Available: http://pqasb.pqarchiver.com/washingtonpost_historical/results.html?st=basic&uid=&MAC=50a23aa1f3f5c6104e90e36051420d61&QryTxt=500+vets+claim+herbicide+effects&sortby=REVERSE_CHRON&restrict=articles [accessed February 7, 2005].

Galston AW. 2001. Falling leaves and ethical dilemmas: Agent Orange in Vietnam. In: Galston AW, Shurr EG, eds., *New Dimensions in Bioethics*. Dordrecht, The Netherlands: Kluwer Academic Publishers. [Online]. Available: http://www.yale.edu/isps/journal/volume2/galston.html [accessed May 3, 2005].

GAO (General Accounting Office). 1999. Agent Orange: Actions Needed to Improve Communications of Air Force Ranch Hand Study Data and Results. GAO/NSIAD-00-31. Washington, DC: GAO. [Online]. Available: http://www.gao.gov/new.items/ns00031.pdf [accessed May 6, 2005].

Gough M. 1986. *Dioxin, Agent Orange: The Facts*. New York: Plenum Press.

Henriksen GL, Ketchum NS, Michalek JE, Swaby JA. 1997. Serum dioxin and diabetes mellitus in veterans of Operation Ranch Hand. *Epidemiology* 8(3):252–258.

Herbicide victim study urged. 1979, June 5. *The Washington Post*. [Online]. Available: http://pqasb.pqarchiver.com/washingtonpost_historical/access/170786222.html?dids=170786222:170786222&FMT=ABS&FMTS=ABS:AI&fmac=&date=Apr+10%2C+1979&author=&desc=Herbicide+Victim+Study+Urged [accessed February 7, 2005].

IARC (International Agency for Research on Cancer). 1977. Some fumigants, the herbicides 2,4-D and 2,4,5-T, chlorinated dibenzodioxins and miscellaneous industrial chemicals. *IARC Monographs on the Evaluation of the Carcinogenic Risk of Chemicals to Man, Vol. 15*. Lyon, France: IARC.

IOM (Institute of Medicine). 1994. *Veterans and Agent Orange: Health Effects of Herbicides Used in Vietnam*. Washington, DC: National Academy Press.

IOM. 1996. *Veterans and Agent Orange: Update 1996*. Washington, DC: National Academy Press.

IOM. 1999. *Veterans and Agent Orange: Update 1998*. Washington, DC: National Academy Press.

IOM. 2000. *Veterans and Agent Orange: Herbicide/Dioxin Exposure and Type 2 Diabetes*. Washington, DC: National Academy Press.

IOM. 2001. *Veterans and Agent Orange: Update 2000*. Washington, DC: National Academy Press.

IOM. 2003a. *Veterans and Agent Orange: Update 2002*. Washington, DC: The National Academies Press.

IOM. 2003b. *Characterizing Exposure of Veterans to Agent Orange and Other Herbicides Used in Vietnam: Final Report*. Washington, DC: The National Academies Press.

IOM. 2005. *Veterans and Agent Orange: Update 2004*. Washington, DC. The National Academies Press.

Ketchum NS, Michalek JE. 2005. Postservice mortality of Air Force veterans occupationally exposed to herbicides during the Vietnam War: 20-year follow-up results. *Military Medicine* 170(5): 406–413.

Lathrop GD. 1980. Response to the NAS Report Re: The Air Force study of personnel exposed to herbicide orange. [Memorandum June 6, 1980]. The Alvin L. Young Collection of Agent Orange at the National Agricultural Library. Brooks AFB, TX: USAF School of Aerospace Medicine. [Online]. Available: http://www.nal.usda.gov/speccoll/findaids/agentorange/container.htm [accessed April 4, 2005].

Lavy TL. 1987. *Human Exposure to Phenoxy Herbicides* (Veterans Administration Monograph). Washington, DC: U.S. Government Printing Office, pp. 1–17.

Longnecker MP, Michalek JE. 2000. Serum dioxin level in relation to diabetes mellitus among Air Force veterans with background levels of exposure. *Epidemiology* 11(1):44–48.

McConnell AF. 1970. Mission: Ranch Hand. *Air University Review* 21(2):89–94.

Meek SL. 1981. An estimate of the relative exposure of US Air Force crewmembers to Agent Orange. Thesis (M.S. Public Health). University of Washington School of Public Health, Department of Environmental and Occupational Health Sciences. The Alvin L. Young Collection on Agent Orange at the National Agricultural Library. [Online]. Available: http://www.nal.usda.gov/speccoll/findaids/agentorange/container.htm [accessed April 4, 2005].

Michalek JE. 2000. Department of Defense News Briefing: Dr. Joel Michalek Briefs on Agent Orange Study [March 29, 2000, Transcript]. DefenseLINK News. [Online]. Available: http://www.defense.gov/transcripts/2000/t03292000_t0329afa.html [accessed July 5, 2005].

Michalek JE. 2005 (January 5). *The Air Force Health Study: An Overview and Update.* PowerPoint presentation before the Committee on the Disposition of the Air Force Health Study, Washington, DC.

Michalek JE, Tripathi RC. 1999. Pharmacokinetics of TCDD in veterans of Operation Ranch Hand: 15-year follow-up. *Journal of Toxicology and Environmental Health* 57:369–378.

Michalek JE, Wolfe WH, Miner JC. 1990. Health status of Air Force veterans occupationally exposed to herbicides in Vietnam II. Mortality. *Journal of the American Medical Association* 264(14): 1832–1836.

Michalek JE, Pirkle JL, Caudill SP, Tripathi RC, Patterson DG, Needham LL. 1996. Pharmacokinetics of TCDD in veterans of Operation Ranch Hand: 10-year follow-up. *Journal of Toxicology and Environmental Health* 47:209–220.

Michalek JE, Ketchum NS, Akhtar FZ. 1998a. Post-service mortality of Air Force veterans occupationally exposed to herbicides in Vietnam: 15 year follow-up. *American Journal of Epidemiology* 148(8):786–792.

Michalek JE, Rahe AJ, Boyle CA. 1998b. Paternal dioxin, preterm birth, intrauterine growth retardation, and infant death. *Epidemiology* 9(2):161–167.

Michalek JE, Rahe AJ, Boyle CA. 1998c. Paternal dioxin and the sex of children fathered by veterans of Operation Ranch Hand [Letter to the Editor]. *Epidemiology* 9(4):474–475.

Michalek JE, Ketchum N, Longnecker MP. 2001a. Serum dioxin and hepatic abnormalities in veterans of Operation Ranch Hand. *Annals of Epidemiology* 11(5):304–311.

Michalek JE, Akhtar FZ, Arezzo JC, Garabrant DH, Albers JW. 2001b. Serum dioxin and peripheral neuropathy in veterans of Operation Ranch Hand. *Neurotoxicology* 22:479–490.

Michalek JE, Akhtar FZ, Longnecker MP, Burton JE. 2001c. Relation of serum 2,3,7,8-tetrachlorodibenzo-*p*-dioxin (TCDD) level to hematological examination results in veterans of Operation Ranch Hand. *Archives of Environmental Health* 56(5):396–405.

Michalek JE, Ketchum NS, Tripathi RC. 2003. Diabetes mellitus and 2,3,7,8-tetrachlorodibenzo-*p*-dioxin elimination in veterans of Operation Ranch Hand. *Journal of Toxicology and Environmental Health, Part A* 66(3):211–221.

Midwest Research Institute (MRI). 1967. Assessment of Ecological Effects of Extensive or Repeated Use of Herbicides. MRI Project No. 3103-B. Kansas City, MO: MRI. NTIS AD-824-314.

Minarik CE. 1964 (January). Crops Division Defoliation Program. In: Mattie VZ, ed. *Proceedings of the First Defoliation Conference, 29–30 July, 1963.* Fort Detrick, MD: U.S. Army Biological Laboratories, pp. 21–24.

NAS (National Academy of Sciences). National Research Council, Assembly of Life Sciences. 1974. *The Effects of Herbicides in South Vietnam.* Washington, DC: National Academy of Sciences.

NRC (National Research Council), Assembly of Life Sciences. 1980. *Review of US Air Force Protocol: Epidemiological Investigation of Health Effects in Air Force Personnel Following Exposure to Herbicide Orange.* Washington, DC: National Academy of Sciences.

OTA (Office of Technology Assessment, U.S. Congress). 1983. *OTA Review of Centers for Disease Control Protocols for Epidemiologic Studies of the Health of Vietnam Veterans.* Washington, DC: OTA.

Patterson DG, Hampton L, Lapeza CR, Besler WT, Green V, Alexander LR, Needham LL. 1987. High-resolution gas chromatography/high-resolution mass spectrometric analysis of human serum on a whole-weight and lipid basis for 2,3,7,8-tetrachlorodibenzo-*p*-dioxin. *Analytical Chemistry* 59:2000–2005.

Pavuk M, Schecter AJ, Akhtar FZ, Michalek JE. 2003. Serum 2,3,7,8-tetrachlorodibenzo-*p*-dioxin (TCDD) levels and thyroid function in Air Force veterans of the Vietnam War. *Annals of Epidemiology* 13(5):335–343.

RHAC (Ranch Hand Advisory Committee). 2000 (October 19–20). Meeting minutes. [Online]. Available: http://www.fda.gov/ohrms/dockets/ac/00/transcripts/3654t1.pdf [accessed August 15, 2005].

Schuck PH. 1987. *Agent Orange on Trial: Mass Toxic Disasters in the Court.* Cambridge, MA: Belknap Press of Harvard University Press.

Schwartz LS. 2000. *Agent Orange—Actions Needed to Improve Communications of Air Force Ranch Hand Study Data and Results* (GAO/NSIAD-00-31). Statement at the March 15, 2000, hearing of the United States House of Representatives' Subcommittee on National Security, Veterans Affairs, and Intergovernmental Relations, Subcommittee, United States House of Representatives. regarding GAO's December 1999 report: Agent Orange—Actions Needed to Improve Communications of Air Force Ranch Hand Study Data and Results (GAO/NSIAD-00-31) March 15, 2000. [Online] Available: http://www.vva.org/legiss/31500tes.htm [accessed January 4, 2006].

Steenland K, Calvert G, Ketchum N, Michalek J. 2001. Dioxin and diabetes mellitus: an analysis of the combined NIOSH and Ranch Hand data. *Occupational and Environmental Medicine* 58:641–648.

Stellman JM, Stellman SD, Christian R, Weber T, Tomasallo C. 2003. The extent and patterns of usage of Agent Orange and other herbicides in Vietnam. *Nature* 422(6933):681–687.

Stevens KR, Mylecraine L. 1994. Issues in Chronic Toxicology. In: Hayes W, ed. *Principles and Methods of Toxicology.* 3rd Ed. New York: Raven Press, pp. 663–697.

VA (Department of Veterans Affairs). 2003. Agent Orange brief: Agent Orange—general information. [Online]. Available: http://www1.va.gov/agentorange/docs/a1brief2003.doc [accessed May 6, 2005].

VA. 2005. Veterans Benefits Administration: Annual benefits report fiscal year 2004. [Online]. Available: http://www.vietnam.ttu.edu/star/images/252/2520308007A.pdf and http://www.vietnam.ttu.edu/star/images/252/2520308007Bvba.va.gov/bln/dmo/reports/fy2004/2004_abr.pdf [accessed August 15, 2005].

Warren WF. 1968. A review of the herbicide program in South Vietnam. Working Paper No. 10-68. NTIS AD 779–797. San Francisco: Scientific Advisory Group.

Wilcox FA. 1989. *Waiting for an Army to Die: The Tragedy of Agent Orange.* Cabin John, MD: Seven Locks Press.

Wolfe WH, Principal Investigator, Air Force Health Study. 1989. *Air Force Health Study.* Statement at the July 10, 1989 hearing of the Committee on Veterans' Affairs Subcommittee on Hospitals and Health Care, U.S. House of Representatives.

Wolfe WH, Michalek JE, Miner JC, Rahe AJ, Moore CA, Needham LL, Patterson DG. 1995a. Paternal serum dioxin and reproductive outcomes among veterans of Operation Ranch Hand. *Epidemiology* 6:17–22.

Wolfe WH, Michalek JE, Miner JC, Papa TM. 1995b. Self-reported herbicide exposure in veterans of Operation Ranch Hand. Unpublished paper. Corresponding author: Joel E. Michalek, Ph.D.

Young AL, Reggiani GM, eds. 1988. *Agent Orange and Its Associated Dioxin: Assessment of a Controversy.* Amsterdam: Elsevier.

3

The Air Force Health Study Database

This chapter addresses matters concerning the medical records and other study data collected as part of the Air Force Health Study (AFHS). It details the number of study subjects in the Ranch Hand and comparison cohorts and how those figures have changed over the course of the study. The chapter also catalogs the electronic and hard copy information collected and addresses the question of whether obstacles exist to retaining and maintaining these data.

Some of the content in this chapter was previously presented in the committee's interim letter report (IOM, 2005).

DATA COLLECTION AND DATABASE CHARACTERISTICS

Collection

Chapter 2 provides in-depth information on the collection of AFHS data over the course of the study. The information in that chapter related to medical records and other study data is summarized here, and some additional details on changes in the study population over time are presented.

The original cohort of Ranch Hand personnel totaled 1,242[1] subjects who had served in the C-123 crews in Operation Ranch Hand herbicide spray missions and included pilots, copilots, navigators, spray operators, and ground support crews. This study was designed as a matched cohort study; it used a complex

[1]Twenty-two Ranch Hands had been killed in action (AFHS, 1984a).

strategy to enroll comparison subjects. Specifically, a pool of 23,978 subjects comprising C-130 crewmembers who had served in the Southeast Asia theater but who were not involved in spray missions were identified and deemed to be an appropriate comparison group. The exposure period for the Ranch Hand subjects spanned from 1962 to 1971, and the pool subjects served during the same period. From the comparison pool, 1,241 subjects were chosen to be part of the original comparison group. Comparison subjects were matched to Ranch Hand subjects by age, race, and military occupation.

Most of the AFHS research is focused on the morbidity component of the study, where exceptionally detailed data gathering took place. The initial physical examination and surveying of these AFHS subjects (Cycle 1) was conducted in 1982 and subsequent cycles were conducted in 1985, 1987, 1992, 1997, and 2002.

The AFHS uses a rather complex terminology in its reports to designate the status of its subjects. Comparison subjects enrolled in the study at the beginning of Cycle 1 evaluations are referred to as *original* comparison subjects. Because some of the original comparison subjects were deemed to be ineligible subsequent to enrollment (when more detailed investigation showed that they did not meet the selection criteria),[2] a second category of comparison subjects was established to indicate those comparison subjects that were *shifted* from the pool to replace ineligible subjects during Cycle 1. A third category is called *replacement* comparison subjects. Replacement comparison subjects are those subjects available for study inclusion from the individual-level pools of up to 10 comparison subjects. This replacement strategy was implemented to reduce the effect on study power of loss to follow-up on comparison subjects. If an original comparison subject did not participate in a particular cycle visit but participated in a later cycle, he was still designated as an original comparison. Cohort enumeration is discussed in detail in Chapter 2.

Subjects who participated in Cycle 1 were termed either *partially* or *fully compliant*, depending on whether they completed only the questionnaire[3] required of all subjects or both the questionnaire and physical exam. Cycle 1 questionnaires were administered by Louis Harris and Associates, Inc. The National Opinion Research Center (NORC), under contract with Science Applications International Corporation (SAIC), administered questionnaires during Cycles 2–6. The physical examination was conducted by the Kelsey-Seybold Clinic in Houston,

---

[2]During Cycle 1 it was discovered that 18 percent of the comparison population was ineligible for study inclusion (AFHS, 1984a).

[3]A short telephone questionnaire was offered to those subjects that refused to participate in the questionnaire. Refusal subjects who completed this short telephone survey are another "compliance" class reported in the Cycle 1 report (AFHS, 1984a). If a Ranch Hand survived the war but died prior to Cycle 1, next of kin were contacted and—if they consented—were administered a proxy version of the participants' baseline questionnaire.

TABLE 3-1 Participation in Physical Examinations by Cycle

	Ranch Hand Subjects		Comparison Subjects*	
Examination	Eligible	Participated	Eligible	Participated
Cycle 1—1982	1,209	1,046 (87%)	1,666	1,223 (73%)
Cycle 2—1985	1,199	1,017 (85%)	1,713	1,292 (75%)
Cycle 3—1987	1,188	996 (84%)	1,730	1,298 (75%)
Cycle 4—1992	1,149	953 (83%)	1,761	1,280 (73%)
Cycle 5—1997	1,102	870 (79%)	1,920	1,251 (65%)
Cycle 6—2002	1,043	777 (74%)	2,044	1,174 (57%)

NOTE: These numbers reflect corrections made to earlier cycles due to the identification of misclassified study subjects in later cycles and therefore vary slightly from the numbers published in early AFHS reports.

*Totals include original, shifted, and replacement comparison subjects.

SOURCE: Table C-1 (*Compliance of Ranch Hands by Examination Year*) and Table C-2 (*Compliance of All Comparisons by Examination Year*) (AFHS, 2005b).

Texas, in Cycle 1 and at the Scripps Clinic and Research Foundation in La Jolla, California, for Cycles 2–6. Summaries of participation by cycle are presented in Table 3-1[4] and Figure 3-1. Demographic characteristics of the Cycle 6 participants are presented in Table 3-2.

Figure 3-2 details the participation of both Ranch Hand and comparison subjects throughout the study and provides summary counts by cycle for the following subject subclasses: new to the cohort (N),[5] deceased (D), unlocatable (U), refused to take part in the exam or were noncompliant (F), and found to be ineligible (I). The population numbers presented in Figure 3-2 represent the best available information. However, as is sometimes the case with long-term longitudinal studies, there are some inconsistencies in the study population numbers reported by the AFHS at various times, and some data are missing altogether.

Among the 1,241 comparison subjects first identified for participation in the morbidity study, 212 individuals were deemed ineligible (primarily due to the determination that their tour of duty did not occur in the designated territory)

[4]After the first (1982) physical examination cycle, "eligible" subjects include those new to the study and exclude those who died after the conclusion of the previous cycle. Subjects were deemed to have "participated" in a cycle if they were fully compliant with the physical examination. The numbers reported in the table reflect corrections made to earlier cycles due to the identification of misclassified study subjects in later cycles and therefore vary slightly from the numbers published in early AFHS reports and shown in Figure 3-2.

[5]A subject would be classified as *new to the cohort* if his status as a Ranch Hand or comparison subject was being corrected from the initial classification, or if he was moved from the pool of potential comparison subjects to the status of an active study participant.

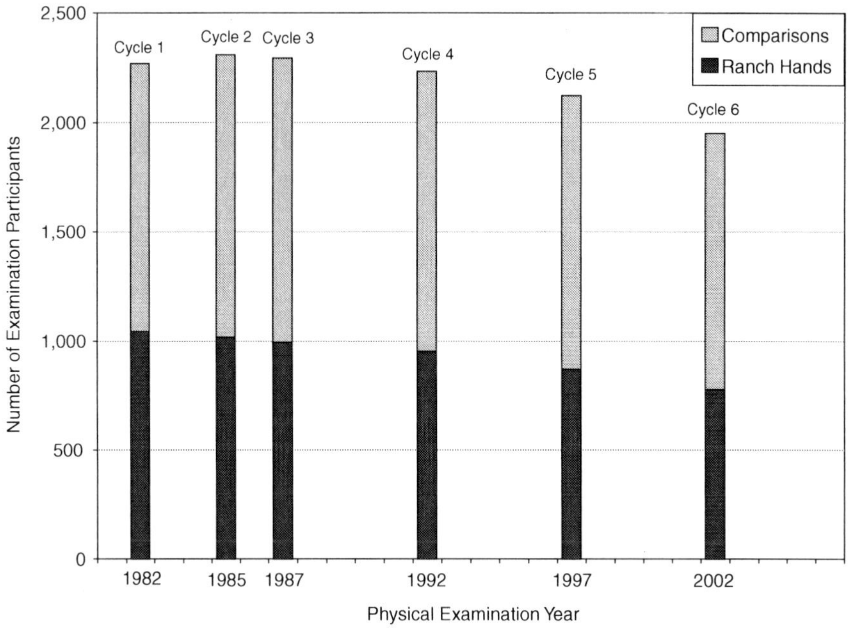

FIGURE 3-1 AFHS physical examination participation by year and cycle.

TABLE 3-2 Selected Demographic Characteristics of Cycle 6 (2002) Participants

	Ranch Hand Subjects	Comparison Subjects
Number of subjects	777	1,174
Mean age	63.1	63.0
Race (%)		
Black	6.3	6.5
Nonblack	93.7	93.5
Military occupation (%)		
Officer	39.5	39.4
Enlisted flyer	17.1	15.8
Enlisted groundcrew	43.4	44.9

SOURCE: Table 8-1. Associations between Matching Demographic Variables (Age, Race, and Military Occupation) and Estimates of Herbicide or Dioxin Exposure (AFHS, 2005b).

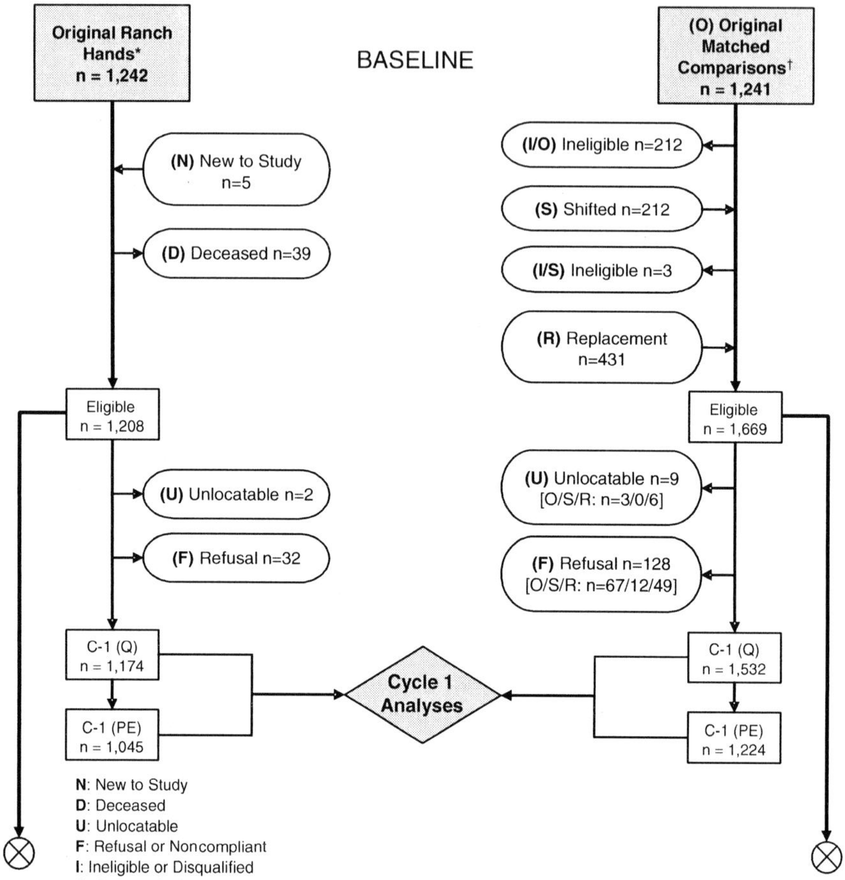

* Total does not reflect the 22 Ranch Hands known at the Baseline to have been killed in action.
† One Ranch Hand (Black officer) remained unmatched to a comparison.
‡ Numbers of eligible and participating Ranch Hands reflect AFHS reports (AFHS, 2000 & 2005b) and not the numbers that would be expected—Cycle 5, PE: n=869; Cycle 6, Eligible n=1,042, PE: n=776—from reported changes in the study population recorded in AFHS reports.

NOTE: Flowchart numbers reflect what was known to AFHS investigators at any given cycle according to AFHS reports and do not reflect corrections made to earlier cycles due to the identification of misclassified subjects in later cycles. Identical study population counts vary on occasion within and across cycle reports. Thus, this reconstruction should be considered a general overview of AFHS population dynamics. Eligibility in any cycle reflects eligibility in a previous cycle, and not compliance in a previous cycle, corrected for between-cycle newly identified or deceased subjects.

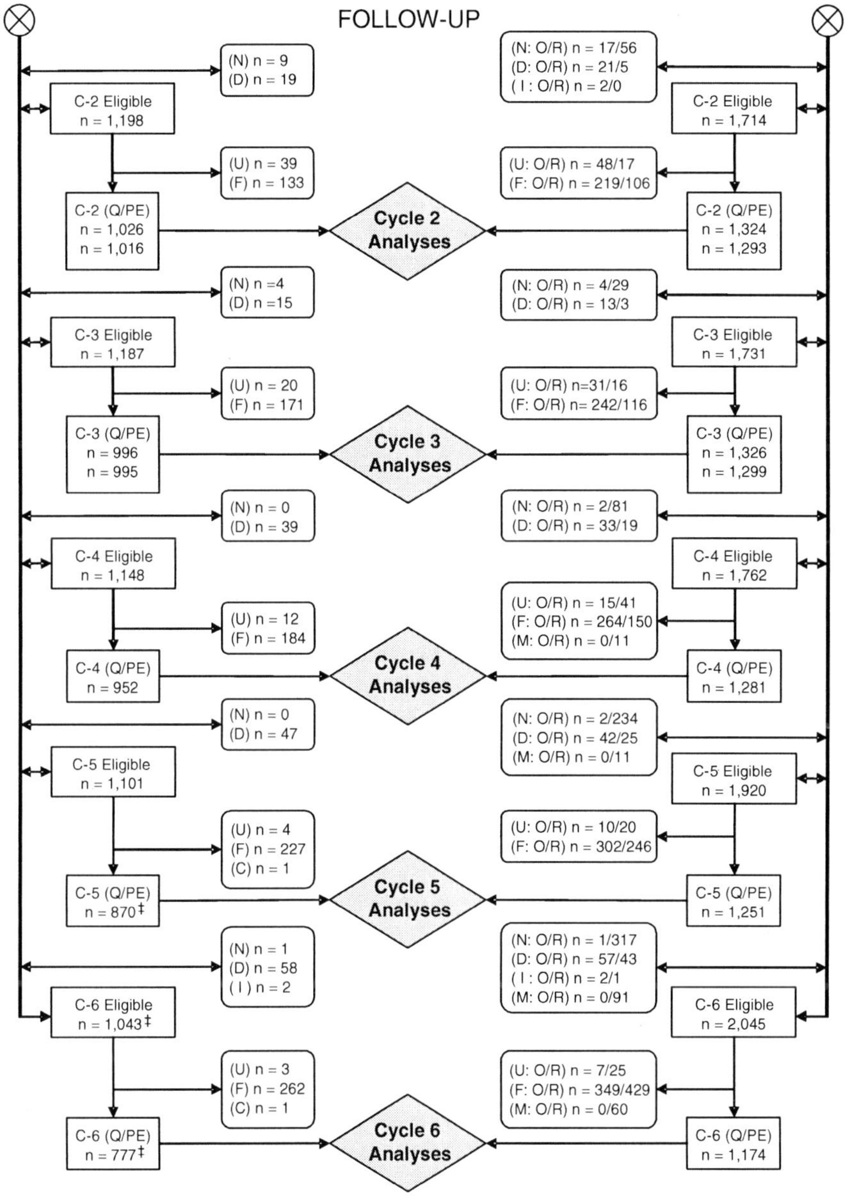

FIGURE 3-2 AFHS-Morbidity Study Population.
SOURCE: AFHS, 1984a, 1987, 1990, 1995, 2000, 2005c.

during the Cycle 1 examinations and were removed, resulting in 1,029 original comparison subjects. Subsequently, 212 new comparison subjects were added or shifted[6] into the original comparison group. In addition, five new Ranch Hand subjects were identified toward the end of the Cycle 1 assessment and enrolled. Additional, or new (N), Ranch Hand subjects were added at subsequent cycles as well when further investigation revealed that they met the criteria for Ranch Hand designation. Between Cycles 1 and 2, four additional Ranch Hand subjects were identified in this manner.

Original comparison subjects who did not participate in an earlier cycle but did participate in a later cycle are designated in Figure 3-2 with an "N:O" or as *new original* comparisons.

An intricate strategy was used to add new subjects to the comparison group from the individually matched pools of up to 10 potential comparison subjects for each Ranch Hand subject. These additional comparison subjects are identified in Figure 3-2 as replacement comparison subjects (R). Because the investigators expected greater non-compliance from comparison subjects than from Ranch Hand subjects, 431 subjects were added as replacements before Cycle 1. Between Cycles 4 and 5, 234 replacement subjects were added. Replacements were already matched at the individual pool level on age, race, and military occupation; in Cycles 2–6, they were also matched on the (self-reported) perception of overall health of the Ranch Hand subject. Where an exact health perception match was not available, the closest match was made. The rationale for the actual number of replacements added at each cycle—which exceeded the 1:1 matched ratio of the original study design—was not provided in AFHS documentation.

Data on the factors influencing study participation were collected, analyzed, and the results presented in the *Study Selection and Participation* chapters[7] of the final reports for each of the cycle examinations. Some potential participants gave investigators specific reasons why they chose not to be a part of the data gathering exercises (lack of interest or time, or job commitments, for example) while others did not respond to contacts, failed to honor appointments, or communicated a desire not to have any contact with or from the AFHS under any circumstances. Among potential participants for whom data were available, veterans who refused to participate were more likely to self-report fair or poor health than those who were fully compliant. The Cycle 6 report noted that "[t]his pattern of . . . reporting poorer health has been observed since the baseline examination" (AFHS, 2005b).

Comprehensive information was collected on the reproductive history of current and former spouse(s) and partner(s) of subjects in Cycles 1–4. This was done via a questionnaire that was administered to that person either onsite (if the per-

---

[6]Distinctions are not made between original and shifted comparison subjects in reports after Cycle 1; both are referred to as original comparison subjects.

[7]These chapters are called *Study Selection and Participation Bias* in Cycles 1 and 2.

son accompanied the subject to the cycle exam), over the phone, or by postal questionnaire. Information was collected in private to facilitate obtaining independent histories. Consent was obtained for medical records review to verify some data. Information on fertility, miscarriages, stillbirths, induced abortions, intrauterine growth retardation, and live births (pre- and full-term) were collected and coded. For live births, birth defects data were obtained along with general information on the health and well-being of the child through age 18.[8]

For the first five mortality studies (AFHS, 1983, 1984b, 1985, 1986, 1989) the original matched cohort of one Ranch Hand to five comparison subjects was used for internal comparisons as well as several external comparison populations, as detailed in Chapter 2. The entire comparison pool population was used for additional analyses in the 1989 mortality follow-up. These numbered 20,340 veterans at the 20-year follow-up: 1,262 Ranch Hand subjects and 19,078 comparison subjects (Ketchum and Michalek, 2005). Date of death was obtained using U.S. Air Force (USAF) Military Personnel Center records, the Department of Veterans Affairs Death Beneficiary Identification and Record Location System, and the Internal Revenue Service database of active Social Security numbers (SSNs). Death certificates provided information on the underlying cause(s) of death (Michalek et al., 1990). These data were verified and coded and are a part of the electronic database. They were combined with basic demographic information (age, race, military occupation, and the like) for all-subject analyses and with the data collected in the cycle exams for more detailed examinations with the smaller cohort of morbidity study participants.

Database Characteristics

The AFHS database is vast. It comprises electronically stored data and programs and a number of materials originally collected in hard copy form, which also exist as PDFs.

Electronically Stored Data and Programs

The AFHS's electronically stored data consists of information collected from subjects during the six cycles of in-person physical examinations and in computer-aided telephone interviewing, computer-assisted personal interviewing, and machine and hand coding of questionnaires and other data intake instruments. In addition, the SAS and Fortran programs and Excel spreadsheets used to analyze these data have been retained.

The AFHS investigators maintain what are referred to in this report as *master* data files for each of the cycles. These master data files are used as the starting

[8]The most recent paper on this component of the study was published in 1998 (Michalek et al., 1998a). It contains a citation to the study's earlier reproductive outcomes work.

TABLE 3-3 AFHS Electronically Stored Data Assets

Type	Description	Number
*.dat	Flat files	11,140
*.sd2, *.sas7bdat	SAS databases	5,694
*.sas	SAS programs	35,444
*.for	Fortran programs	8,844
*.xls	Excel spreadsheets	2,184

SOURCE: Michalek, 2005.

point for all analyses.[9] Within a cycle, there are separate master files for various components of the cycle's data gathering effort: responses to questionnaires, results of particular physical exams, and so on. Data in these files are stored by the subject's study identification number, which the AFHS refers to as a *case number*. The separate files relate case numbers to participant names, military records, and other information that does not vary between cycles. Working files are created from these master files and used for specific analyses. Raw and working files are saved for potential future reference (for example, if it was necessary to verify a seemingly anomalous value or reexamine the steps that led to a particular result) but are not otherwise used.

Table 3-3 lists the number of files contained in the database. The database presently resides on two servers—an IBM 580 (Kiowa) and a Compaq ProLiant ML370—housed in the AFHS research facility at Brooks City-Base, San Antonio, Texas. The data[10] take up ~525 GB of space on the machines, including operating system and backup files (J. Robinson, Air Force Health Study, personal communication, September 21, 2005).

The committee does not have a comprehensive listing of all of the data collected during the course of the AFHS. However, it has compiled lists of the general classes of endpoints analyzed in the six cycle examinations as cited in AFHS technical reports. These are presented in 16 tables contained in Appendix B. The tables are organized to parallel the manner in which the data are addressed in AFHS technical reports. Their contents are indexed in Table 3-4 below.

The tables in Appendix B indicate that not all questionnaire components, physical examination parameters, or other information gathered was analyzed during the cycle in which it was collected. Most standard physical examination assessments and laboratory tests were performed at all cycles. However, other

[9]The original form in which data are delivered to the AFHS is referred to as a *raw* data file. A raw data file is quality-control checked against paper copy or other alternative documentation and corrected where necessary before a master data file is created. Summary variables derived from collected information—such as body mass index—are also incorporated into master data files.

[10]This includes PDFs of the hard copy materials (discussed below).

TABLE 3-4 Index of Appendix B Tables

Table	Category
B-1	General health assessment
B-2	Neoplasia assessment
B-3	Neurologic assessment
B-4	Psychological assessment
B-5	Gastrointestinal assessment
B-6	Dermatologic assessment
B-7	Cardiovascular assessment
B-8	Hematologic assessment
B-9	Renal assessment
B-10	Endocrine assessment
B-11	Immunologic assessment
B-12	Pulmonary assessment
B-13	Reproductive assessment
B-14	Laboratory data
B-15	Covariable data
B-16	Questionnaire data

tests were deleted or added as the investigators had the opportunity to consider early results and form new hypotheses, or take account of changes in technology or standards of practice. Some variables—such as information on sleeping difficulties and dietary habits—were only assessed at one cycle as part of a focused investigation. Although these tables are not a comprehensive or definitive list of the information contained in the AFHS database(s), they illustrate the scope of material stored.

The committee's interim letter report (IOM, 2005) offered recommendations for several database documentation activities that will—if carried out—produce authoritative lists of what variables were collected and when. These recommendations are also listed at the end of this chapter.

For a time in the early 2000s, deidentified[11] data from Cycles 2–5 were available to the public through the AFHS website and the Government Printing Office (AFRL, 2000a,b,c; 2001). The data were in both SAS and flat file formats and comprised the clinical datasets for the various component of the physical exam: general health, dermatology, cancer, heart disease, diabetes, endocrinology, and

[11]Deidentification is the process of removing or altering data in a record that could be used to identify a subject. Under the HIPAA Privacy Rule (45 CFR §164.514 (a–c)), data are considered to be deidentified if either a qualified expert determines that the risk that it could be used to identify a subject is "very small" or if they do not include any of eighteen specified potentially identifying pieces of information.

the like (RHAC, 2000). Laboratory, reproductive outcomes, and mortality datasets were also available. These data were made accessible, at least in part, in response to a 1999 General Accounting Office[12] report that criticized the lack of public access and recommended that AFHS "establish and publicize a timetable for the release of all study data and provisions to release the data in a format (such as compact disc or the Internet) that is easily accessible to the general public" (GAO, 1999).[13] However, AFHS later withdrew the data from their website, owing to questions over whether the study subjects had given consent for the posting (RHAC, 2003).

Nonelectronic Materials

The AFHS data collection also comprises a number of materials originally collected in hard copy or other nonelectronic form. These include paper originals of cycle physical exam reports and completed questionnaires; medical records from the subjects' physicians, dentists, and other health providers; X rays and other diagnostic imagery; lists of medications taken; military administrative records such as duty station orders, flight records, performance reports, awards and decorations, and discharge documents; vital status records such as birth and death certificates; limited information on the subjects' spouse(s) and children; research reference materials; and the study's reports and papers. These materials are currently stored in a secure building at the study's Brooks City-Base facility in Texas. They take up ~5,350 cubic feet of records storage systems space (J. Robinson, Air Force Health Study, personal communication, September 21, 2005). All have been scanned and the images stored in electronic files in Portable Document Format (PDF). The PDF files containing a particular subject's materials are cataloged in a directory labeled with the subject's name and case number. There are over 8.8 million such PDF files (Michalek, 2005).

Electrocardiogram (ECG) strips, X rays, and Super-VHS video tapes collected during the cycle exams are also stored at the AFHS facilities. Twelve-lead scalar resting ECGs were obtained from subjects during all six exam cycles. The ECGs were evaluated and information regarding various parameters were coded and placed into the electronic database, along with variables characterizing any prior heart problems in the subject.[14] The X-ray films—primarily, chest X rays—were taken during Cycles 2–6 and fill ~50 linear feet of storage space.[15]

---

[12]Now called the Government Accountability Office.

[13]A follow-up publication of the study director's testimony before a congressional committee reiterated the criticisms and recommendation (Kwai-Cheung, 2000).

[14]Depending on the cycle, these parameters included ST-T, P, U, and Q-wave morphology; QRS and QT interval; axis deviation; and evidence of bradycardia, tachycardia, arrhythmia, abnormal sinus rhythm, and myocardial infarction.

[15]Source: J. Robinson, Air Force Health Study, personal communication, September 21, 2005.

TABLE 3-5 AFHS Hard Copy Data Assets

Type	Description	Number
Files		
*.pdf	Image files†	8,812,945
Hard copy materials		
ECGs	Paper tracings	[not enumerated]
X ray films	Images on film	15,390
SVHS tapes	Dental videos (1994)	1,166
	Dental videos (1997)	1,908

†Text in these files is not searchable.
SOURCE: Michalek, 2005.

The SVHS format video tapes in the data collection store high-resolution images of subjects' teeth taken during the Cycle 4 and 5 exams. The tapes were made as part of a National Institute of Dental and Craniofacial Research (NIDCR) adjunct to the study examining the association between exposure to elemental mercury via dental amalgams and measures of neurologic function (Kingman et al., 2005). They were used to document the examinations, supply images of subjects' dental restorations, and provide a means of resolving postexam discrepancies in collected data. NIDCR funded the examination and conducted the data analysis; collected data were given to the AFHS for integration into the database. A separate consent was obtained from the subjects who participated in the project. The tapes take up ~160 linear feet of storage space.[16]

Table 3-5 shows the quantities of these materials.

OBSTACLES AND LIMITATIONS TO FURTHER USE OF AFHS DATA

The committee considered three primary categories of obstacles and limitations to further use of the AFHS medical records and other study data: those related to the design and execution of the study; logistical—that is, those relating to the management and analysis of the data; and procedural—those addressing how personal information on study subjects is handled. These are discussed below.

[16]Source: J. Robinson, Air Force Health Study, personal communication, September 21, 2005.

Limitations Related to the Design and Execution of the Study

The AFHS—like all epidemiologic studies—suffers from limitations related to factors intrinsic to its design and resulting from implementation decisions made by the investigators. Many of these are specific to the study of the health effects of wartime exposure to herbicides and would carry into future research on this topic, although some of the limitations can be addressed by making different assumptions in analyses. However, the limitations would not necessarily extend to more general studies using the data assets.

Study limitations were a central topic of the 1999 GAO report on the AFHS (GAO, 1999). The GAO study director, Kwai-Cheung Chan (2000), summarized that report's findings as follows:

> The [AFHS] has two major limitations: it has difficulty in detecting low to moderate increases in risks of rare diseases because of the relatively small size of the Ranch Hand population, and its findings cannot be generalized to all Vietnam veterans because Ranch Hands and ground troops were exposed to different levels of herbicides in different ways. Blood measurements of dioxin . . . suggest that the Ranch Hands' exposure levels were significantly higher than those of many ground troops. But ground troops may have been exposed in ways (such as through contaminated food and water) that Ranch Hands were not, and little is known about the potential effects of such differences.

GAO asserted that "the Air Force has not clearly or effectively communicated these limitations to the public" (GAO, 1999) and suggested that lack of knowledge of these issues was leading to misunderstanding of the study's results.

In congressional testimony concerning the GAO report in 2000, Dr. Linda Spoonster Schwartz—a Yale University researcher and retired Major USAF nurse—offered additional observations (Schwartz, 2000). Among her comments were that the AFHS protocol (AFHS, 1982) stated that data collected from active duty personnel[17] were not confidential because information that indicated a risk to "public safety or national defense" would be made known to the USAF. The fact that a subject's information could affect his career could, she said, have had an influence on the subject's responses and willingness to submit to certain tests. Dr. Schwartz also indicated that, since all of the AFHS participants were in Vietnam at one time, it could not be assumed that the comparison subjects had no significant exposure to herbicides,[18] and that this called into question the validity of the comparison group for studies of the health effects of herbicides.

---

[17]At the time of the Cycle 1 exam,185 Ranch Hands and 184 comparison subjects were on active duty; in addition, 210 Ranch Hand subjects and 234 comparison subjects held current military or civilian flying certificates, which have rigorous physical and mental fitness requirements (AFHS, 1984a).

[18]Serum dioxin levels in study subjects are not a reliable proxy for exposure because these levels decrease over time in the absence of exposure, blood draws were not taken until several years after the end of US military involvement in Vietnam, and not all herbicides were contaminated with dioxin.

Dr. Joel Michalek, then principal investigator of the AFHS, spoke in a January 2005 presentation before the committee about how the study had dealt with obstacles (Michalek, 2005). He noted four limitations of the study related to herbicide health effects research: the inherently small size of the cohort; lack of any biomarkers of herbicide exposure other than dioxin; little information on participants' locations in the theater of operations; and unavailability of a detailed exposure history. Michalek also indicated that AFHS investigators had confronted several exposure-related design and analysis issues. Lack of a good herbicide exposure metric led to concerns over exposure misclassification and bias that were recognized in the study's original protocol (AFHS, 1982).[19] After CDC developed an assay for measuring serum TCDD levels in the late 1980s that AFHS adopted as a proxy, more issues arose. One of these was the effect of measurement error in the estimation of TCDD half-life, an issue because this value was used to estimate a common baseline serum dioxin level for each study participant. Papers by Caudill et al. (1992) and Michalek et al. (1992) discuss this in greater detail. Later papers addressed the validity of dioxin body burden as an exposure index (Michalek et al., 1995), reliability of the dioxin assay (Michalek et al., 1996), and the correction of bias in half-life calculations (Michalek et al., 1998b). The AFHS web site notes a weakness specific to the examination of questions outside of the study's stated mission to evaluate the health effects of wartime exposure to herbicides: "[b]ecause all of our study subjects served in Vietnam or Southeast Asia, contrasting Ranch Hands with comparisons may not fully reveal health differences associated with service in Vietnam" (AFHS, 2005a).

An additional obstacle identified by this committee is related to study design. As described above, the design allowed the addition of replacement comparisons at each cycle. The integration of replacements in statistical analyses cannot be handled using standard statistical techniques.

Subjects who were found to have been misclassified (designated as a comparison subject when in fact they were a Ranch Hand subject and vice versa) were in turn reassigned to the other group and followed under this new group assignment. Such a design, coupled with the usual issues of missing data and losses to follow-up, complicates the reanalysis of results presented in AFHS reports and papers.

Logistical Limitations

Logistical limitations are those related to documentation and organization of the data assets. These issues were the focus of the committee's interim letter report (IOM, 2005).

[19]The protocol also addresses a number of other recognized study difficulties and planned correction measures.

As noted in that report, the amount, detail, and quality of documentation of the data vary by the cycle in which the data were collected. Data from the most recent cycle (Cycle 6, collected in 2002) appear to be well documented, and the data dictionary for this cycle (SAIC, 2003) contains many desirable features: it exists as a searchable PDF, and it contains thorough descriptions of the variables and how information gathering changed from Cycle 5. Documentation for earlier cycles is less complete and is not necessarily in printed or electronically stored form. For example, committee members noted that investigators referred to hand-written annotations in their data dictionary to determine the meaning of coded responses to a questionnaire item during a May 2005 visit to the AFHS research facility.

AFHS reports and papers focus on analyses of a particular cycle's data; little longitudinal (across cycles) analysis has been done to date. Data from early cycles are in different file formats than later data, requiring the analyst to be familiar with this fact and be able to write code that accommodates it. The data location for a particular piece of information—for example, the questionnaire or the master data file where a variable can be found—may change between cycles. Variable names for the same piece of information sometimes change between cycles. Data formatting—whether responses are coded as a numeric value versus an alphanumeric character—are not always consistent between cycles. Differences sometimes exist in how data are coded in identically labeled variables: for example, the year of the subject's birth (DOBYY) is given as the last two digits of the year in the Cycle 4 database, but it is given by all four digits in the Cycle 6 database. Technology (sensitivity or limit of detection or quantitation in laboratory tests, for example) has changed over time; it is therefore possible that an observation coded as below the limit in one cycle may have a value associated with it in a later cycle. And, missing data codes, error codes, and codes for specific outcomes are not uniformly documented or necessarily consistent between cycles.

Because the data may vary in so many and subtle ways, it is necessary to carefully consult the variable name and data dictionaries for each cycle where such documents exist—and to know where such information may be found in their absence—in order to carry out analyses.

The interim letter report offered several specific recommendations intended to create a more complete and uniform accounting of the AFHS medical records and other study data. The final section of this chapter recapitulates these recommendations.

The other electronically stored materials—the SAS and Fortran programs and Excel spreadsheets used to analyze these data—are not necessarily documented in a form that would allow them to be easily understood. This is not an obstacle to retaining and maintaining these files, but it might present a challenge to someone who wishes to review the steps taken to generate the results of an analysis published by the AFHS investigators. However, any future need to access these thousands of programs is uncertain at best.

The study's hard copy materials present an obstacle unrelated to their documentation and organization. As already noted, the AFHS currently is storing ECG strips, X-ray films, SVHS tapes, and large volumes of paper records. There are costs to store and maintain these assets in a manner that minimizes the risk that the subjects' privacy and confidentiality may be unintentionally compromised.

The AFHS has been in existence for approximately 25 years. The committee found that data and specimens have been maintained at a level typical of most long-term epidemiologic research. Over the course of the study, the best practices in epidemiologic investigations and specimen storage have changed, and the technology for managing and analyzing data and samples has advanced. The AFHS has evolved in response to these advances. Study personnel were not tasked with updating and harmonizing the system over time or rendering it accessible to outside researchers, and there was no particular incentive to expend time and funds on efforts to do so. Thus, the observations offered here on the state of the data should therefore not be viewed as a criticism of the work of the AFHS staff.

Procedural Limitations: Confidentiality and Other Ethical, Legal, and Social Issues (ELSI)

The medical records and other AFHS study data have features that present challenges to the preservation of the privacy of the study subjects and the confidentiality of their personal information. Two prominent features related to the electronic records files and materials originally collected in hard copy but not digitized are discussed below.

Data in AFHS electronic records files are stored by case number. However, such coding does not guarantee the privacy of study subjects. The subjects, the Ranch Hands in particular, are not a randomly chosen cohort, picked from a vast, anonymous population. They are a relatively small and well-defined group, many of whom are either known or can be found through publicly available sources. With names as a starting point, other information on the subjects (service rank, tours of duty, and the like) could be gathered and hypothetically, matched against variables in the electronic database to determine which person was designated by which case number. The exceptionally large amount of data available on each subject makes this task easier than would be the case in a less extensive epidemiologic study. And, were such an effort successful, great amounts of personal information would be revealed.

A second feature relates to the nature of certain supporting documentation in the study's collection. Some data assets such as medical records from subjects' health providers, military administrative records, and vital status records were collected in hard copy form. Information varies from subject to subject, and the majority of it has not been coded and placed in electronic records files. Instead, it has served as a supplemental information source that could be consulted when uncertainties or inconsistencies arose in the interpretation of the electronic records. All of these materials have been scanned into PDF image files. The privacy and confidentiality concern with both the hard copy and PDF materials is that almost all contain personal information (names, addresses, SSNs), and it is not practical to redact or otherwise deidentify them. Although destroying these materials is an option, that step would impair the ability of any future investigators to check and correct data.

Issues such as these are inherent to large-scale epidemiologic studies. The committee does not believe that the AFHS data assets present any extraordinary or insurmountable issues. The AFHS has successfully managed these in the past, as have investigators on other epidemiologic studies.

Additional ELSI, including consent, are discussed in Chapter 6.

FINDINGS, CONCLUSIONS, AND RECOMMENDATIONS

On the basis of its review of AFHS reports, its site visit to the study facility, the scientific literature, and other information presented in this chapter, the committee has reached the following findings regarding the medical records and other study data collected in the course of the Air Force Health Study. As noted in the interim letter report, the committee finds that:

> The medical records and other study data collected in the course of the AFHS have been properly maintained. However, they are not currently organized and documented in a manner that allows them to be easily understood, evaluated, managed, or analyzed by persons outside of the AFHS.

The committee also finds that:

> Obstacles, including privacy concerns, exist to retaining and maintaining the medical records and other study data.

A database as large and complex as AFHS's requires proper documentation in order to maximize its effective use, especially when the data represent information accumulated over decades of time. Without such documentation, accessing and analyzing even the most basic information could prove to be a tedious undertaking. Such documentation is necessary whether the database is only to be used by a dedicated staff or is made available to a wider audience.

The committee thus believes that there is merit in creating a more complete and uniform accounting of the AFHS medical records and other study data whatever policy decision may be taken in response to its recommendations. The data assets may be subject to records retention statutes or regulations and may therefore need to be appraised for possible preservation. It thus makes sense that they be in a form that is comprehensible to people who are not already familiar with them so that reasoned decisions can be made. Any future uses of the data—should such options be pursued—would be facilitated by having them documented completely and in a uniform manner.

Much of the knowledge of these data files is currently stored within the collective minds and personal notes of the AFHS staff charged with maintaining it. Unless the salient information for future access and analysis is documented, it will inevitably be lost. The committee recognizes that resources are required to produce such documentation but believe the investment is necessary and, in the end, worth the effort.

The committee's interim letter report offered several recommendations for addressing the obstacles to retaining and maintaining the AFHS medical records and other study data related to the organization and documentation of these materials. These are reiterated below.

Approaches to addressing the other obstacles identified here are presented in Chapter 6 in the context of the committee's recommendations for further study.

Recommendations Contained in the Interim Letter Report

The interim letter report (IOM, 2005) describes the committee's conclusion that the present state of the documentation and organization of AFHS medical records and other study data was an obstacle to retaining and maintaining these materials after the currently scheduled termination date of the study. The committee therefore recommended that:

> **Action should be taken prior to the currently scheduled termination date of the AFHS to reorganize and document the study's medical records and other study data in a form and format that allows them to be easily understood, evaluated, managed, or analyzed by persons outside of the AFHS.**

The following actions were recommended:

- Create a comprehensive inventory of master data files, organized by examination cycle. This inventory should include the file name and type (flat file,[20] SAS database, and so on); a brief description of its contents; and the name, column location, and length; variable type (character or numeric); data codes; and description of each variable stored in the file. The *Variable Name Dictionary for the Air Force Health Study, 1992 Questionnaire and Analyses* (Michalek, 2000c) is an example of such a document.[21]

---

[20]A flat file contains records that are stored without structured relationships or formatting. This simplified form allows data to be used by a variety of applications and minimizes the possibility of data loss due to software obsolescence.

[21]Variable name dictionaries also exist for the Cycle 2 (Michalek, 2000a) and Cycle 3 (Michalek, 2000b) physical exams.

• Create a comprehensive inventory of the variables contained in the master data files, organized by examination cycle and by questionnaire, physical examination report, or other data intake instrument. The *Data Dictionary for Physical and Psychological Examination and Laboratory Data, Air Force Health Study, Cycle 6* (SAIC, 2003) is an example of such a document.[22] The contents of this Cycle 6 data dictionary include

1. an annotated version of the data collection forms, comprising the variables and codes used in the associated database,
2. a synopsis of the variable names and their descriptions,
3. the summary variables created and codes used,
4. the number of study subjects examined for each test,
5. changes in the database structure from the previous examination, and
6. notes on data comparability between cycles.

In addition, the laboratory results section of the dictionary contains descriptions of assays, units of measurement and normal ranges, and data codes.

The committee recommends that such information be compiled for all variables in all examination cycles and that it include notation of whether any attributes of a variable have changed over the course of the study.

• Create a master data codebook containing the name of every data variable represented anywhere in the AFHS database—that is, at any examination cycle—along with a brief description of the variable, the master data file(s) in which it was stored, and its pertinent attributes. This codebook would be derived from the documents outlined above and would constitute a comprehensive distillation of database contents. It should make clear during which examination cycles a particular piece of information was gathered and the variable name(s) associated with that information over the course of the study. A master identification table with rows containing variable descriptions, columns representing each of the six exam cycles, and the intersections listing the variable name used in that cycle, would be a useful adjunct to this effort.

• Create a document/database describing the contents, format, and location of the AFHS collection of materials that have been scanned into PDF image files—subjects' medical records, diagnostic imagery, military and vital status records, and the like—and explaining the collection's organizational structure. This document/database will serve as a directory to these data.

---

[22]There is a separate data dictionary for the Cycle 6 Health Interval and 1982 baseline questionnaires (NORC, 2003).

The committee recommended that these documents/databases be in a form and format that facilitates easy access to their contents; searchable electronic files with paper backup for archival purposes would accomplish this.

In addition, the committee recommended that an overall plan be developed and implemented for archiving the medical records and other study data of the AFHS.[23] Ease of accessibility to the data should be a primary consideration in this effort. The committee noted that federal regulations addressing the preparation of electronic records for transmittal to the National Archives (36 C.F.R. § 1228.270) contain specific information about file formats and media that are appropriate for long-term storage.

The committee believes that it is incumbent on the USAF, as the custodian of the AFHS research materials, to ensure their proper documentation and organization. It therefore recommends that:

> **If available AFHS program funds are not sufficient to accomplish the actions elucidated above, supplemental funding should be provided to carry out such work in a complete and timely manner.**

REFERENCES

AFHS (Air Force Health Study). 1982. *An Epidemiologic Investigation of Health Effects in Air Force Personnel Following Exposure to Herbicides: Study Protocol, Initial Report.* Brooks AFB, TX: USAF School of Aerospace Medicine. SAM-TR-82-44.

AFHS. 1983. *An Epidemiologic Investigation of Health Effects in Air Force Personnel Following Exposure to Herbicides. Baseline Mortality Study Results.* Brooks AFB, TX: USAF School of Aerospace Medicine. NTIS AD-A130 793.

AFHS. 1984a. *Air Force Health Study (Project Ranch Hand II). An Epidemiologic Investigation of Health Effects in Air Force Personnel Following Exposure to Herbicides. Baseline Morbidity Study Results.* Brooks AFB, TX: USAF School of Aerospace Medicine. NTIS AD-A138-340.

AFHS. 1984b. *An Epidemiologic Investigation of Health Effects in Air Force Personnel Following Exposure to Herbicides. Mortality Update: 1984.* Brooks AFB, TX: USAF School of Aerospace Medicine. NTIS-AD-A-162-687.

AFHS. 1985. *An Epidemiologic Investigation of Health Effects in Air Force Personnel Following Exposure to Herbicides. Mortality Update: 1985.* Brooks AFB, TX: USAF School of Aerospace Medicine. NTIS-AD-A-163-237.

AFHS. 1986. *An Epidemiologic Investigation of Health Effects in Air Force Personnel Following Exposure to Herbicides. Mortality Update: 1986.* Brooks AFB, TX: USAF School of Aerospace Medicine. USAFSAM-TR-86-43.

AFHS. 1987. *An Epidemiologic Investigation of Health Effects in Air Force Personnel Following Exposure to Herbicides. First Follow-up Examination Results.* 2 vols. Brooks AFB, TX: USAF School of Aerospace Medicine. USAFSAM-TR-87-27.

AFHS. 1989. *An Epidemiologic Investigation of Health Effects in Air Force Personnel Following Exposure to Herbicides. Mortality Update: 1989.* Brooks AFB, TX: USAF School of Aerospace Medicine. USAFSAM-TR-89-9.

---

[23]The committee's recommendations constitute elements of such a plan.

AFHS. 1990. *An Epidemiologic Investigation of Health Effects in Air Force Personnel Following Exposure to Herbicides.* 2 vols. Brooks AFB, TX: USAF School of Aerospace Medicine. USAFSAM-TR-90-2.

AFHS. 1995. *An Epidemiologic Investigation of Health Effects in Air Force Personnel Following Exposure to Herbicides. 1992 Follow-up Examination Results.* Brooks AFB, TX: Epidemiologic Research Division, Armstrong Laboratory. AL-TR-920107.

AFHS. 2000. *An Epidemiologic Investigation of Health Effects in Air Force Personnel Following Exposure to Herbicides. 1997 Follow-up Examination Results.* Brooks AFB, TX: Epidemiologic Research Division, Armstrong Laboratory. AFRL-HE-BR-TR-2000-02.

AFHS. 2005a. Frequently Asked Questions. [Online]. Available: www.brooks.af.mil/AFRL/HED/hedb/afhs/FAQ.html [accessed October 30, 2005].

AFHS. 2005b. *An Epidemiologic Investigation of Health Effects in Air Force Personnel Following Exposure to Herbicides. 2002 Follow-up Examination Results.* Brooks AFB, TX: Epidemiologic Research Division, Armstrong Laboratory. AFRL-HE-BR-SR-2005-0003.

AFRL (Air Force Research Laboratory). 2000a. Air Force Health Study 1987 Follow-up, Cycle 3. Project Ranch Hand II. [computer files]. Washington, DC: Air Force Research Laboratory and Government Printing Office (GPO).

AFRL. 2000b. Air Force Health Study 1992 Follow-up, Cycle 4. Project Ranch Hand II. [computer files]. Washington, DC: AFRL and GPO.

AFRL. 2000c. Air Force Health Study 1997 Follow-up, Cycle 5. Project Ranch Hand II. [computer files]. Washington, DC: AFRL and GPO.

AFRL. 2001. Air Force Health Study 1985 Follow-up, Cycle 2. Project Ranch Hand II. [computer files]. Washington, DC: AFRL and GPO.

Caudill SP, Pirkle JL, Michalek JE. 1992. Effects of measurement error on estimating biological half-life. *Journal of Exposure Analysis and Environmental Epidemiology* 2(4):463–476.

GAO (General Accounting Office). 1999, December 17. *Agent Orange—Actions Needed to Improve Communications of Air Force Ranch Hand Study Data and Results.* GAO/NSIAD-00-31. Washington, DC: GAO.

IOM (Institute of Medicine). 2005. *Disposition of the Air Force Health Study—Interim Letter Report.* Washington, DC: The National Academies Press. [Online]. Available: http://www.nap.edu/catalog/11483.html [accessed December 1, 2005].

Ketchum NS, Michalek JE. 2005. Postservice mortality of Air Force veterans occupationally exposed to herbicides during the Vietnam War: 20-year follow-up results. *Military Medicine* 170(5):406–413.

Kingman A, Albers JW, Arezzo JC, Garabrant DH, Michalek JE. 2005. Amalgam exposure and neurological function. *Neurotoxicology* 26(2):241–255.

Kwai-Cheung Chan, Director, Special Studies and Evaluations, National Security and International Affairs Division, GAO. 2000. *Persisting Problems With Communication of Ranch Hand Study Data and Results.* Statement at the March 15, 2000, hearing of the Subcommittee on National Security, Veterans Affairs, and International Relations, Committee on Government Reform, House of Representatives. GAO/T-NSIAD-00-117.

Michalek JE. 2000a. *Variable Name Dictionary for the Air Force Health Study. 1985 Physical Exam Questionnaire and Analyses.* Brooks AFB, TX: Air Force Research Laboratory. AFRL-HE-BR-SR-2001-0003. [Online]. Available: http://handle.dtic.mil/100.2/ADA387644 [accessed October 30, 2005].

Michalek JE. 2000b. *Variable Name Dictionary for the Air Force Health Study. 1987 Analyses Data Sets for 1987 Report and Dioxin Report.* Brooks AFB, TX: Air Force Research Laboratory. AFRL-HE-BR-SR-2000-0003. [Online]. Available: http://handle.dtic.mil/100.2/ADA380762 [accessed October 30, 2005].

Michalek JE. 2000c. *Variable Name Dictionary for the Air Force Health Study. 1992 Questionnaire and Analyses.* Brooks AFB, TX: Human Effectiveness Directorate, Human Systems Wing. AFRL-HE-BR-SR-2000-0008. [Online]. Available: http://handle.dtic.mil/100.2/ADA387728 [accessed August 31, 2005].

Michalek, JE. 2005 (January 5). *The Air Force Health Study: An Overview and Update.* Washington, DC. [PowerPoint presentation] The Committee on the Disposition of the Air Force Health Study.

Michalek JE, Wolfe WH, Miner JC. 1990. Health status of Air Force veterans occupationally exposed to herbicides in Vietnam. II. Mortality. *Journal of the American Medical Association* 264(14): 1832–1836.

Michalek JE, Tripathi RC, Caudill SP, Pirkle JL. 1992. Investigation of TCDD half-life heterogeneity in veterans of Operation Ranch Hand. *Journal of Toxicology and Environmental Health* 35(1):29–38. Erratum in: *Journal of Toxicology and Environmental Health* 36(4):431.

Michalek JE, Wolfe WH, Miner JC, Papa TM, Pirkle JL. 1995. Indices of TCDD exposure and TCDD body burden in veterans of Operation Ranch Hand. *Journal of Exposure Analysis and Environmental Epidemiology* 5(2):209–223.

Michalek JE, Tripathi RC, Kulkarni PM, Pirkle JL. 1996. The reliability of the serum dioxin measurement in veterans of Operation Ranch Hand. *Journal of Exposure Analysis and Environmental Epidemiology* 6(3):327–338.

Michalek JE, Rahe AJ, Boyle CA. 1998a. Paternal dioxin, preterm birth, intrauterine growth retardation, and infant death. *Epidemiology* 9(2):161–167.

Michalek JE, Tripathi RC, Kulkarni PM, Gupta PL, Selvavel K. 1998b. Correction for bias introduced by truncation in pharmacokinetic studies of environmental contaminants. *Environmetrics* 9(2):165–174.

NORC (National Opinion Research Center). 2003. *Air Force Health Study 2002–2003 Follow-Up Examinations. Data Dictionary: Health Interval Questionnaire; 1982 Baseline Questionnaire.* Chicago, IL: NORC, University of Chicago.

RHAC (Ranch Hand Advisory Committee). 2000. Transcript: Ranch Hand Advisory Committee Meeting, October 19–20, 2000, Day One. [Online]. Available: www.fda.gov/ohrms/dockets/ac/00/transcripts/3654t1.pdf [accessed October 17, 2005].

RHAC. 2003. Transcript: Ranch Hand Advisory Committee Meeting, March 13, 2003. [Online]. Available: http://www.fda.gov/ohrms/dockets/ac/03/transcripts/3937T1.doc [accessed October 17, 2005].

SAIC (Science Applications International Corporation). 2003. *Data Dictionary for Physical and Psychological Examination and Laboratory Data Air Force Health Study, Cycle 6.* Brooks AFB, TX: Human Systems Wing/YASP. USAF contract: F41624-01-C-1012. SAIC project: 01-0813-04-2273.

Schwartz LS. 2000. *Agent Orange—Actions Needed to Improve Communications of Air Force Ranch Hand Study Data and Results* (GAO/NSIAD-00-31). Statement at the March 15, 2000, hearing of the United States House of Representatives' Subcommittee on National Security, Veterans Affairs, and Intergovernmental Relations, Subcommittee, United States House of Representatives. Regarding GAO's December 1999 report: Agent Orange—Actions Needed to Improve Communications of Air Force Ranch Hand Study Data and Results (GAO/NSIAD-00-31). March 15, 2000. [Online]. Available: http://www.vva.org/legiss/31500tes.htm [accessed January 4, 2006].

4

The Air Force Health Study Specimens Repository

This chapter describes the laboratory specimens collected during the course of the Air Force Health Study (AFHS). It enumerates what type of specimens were collected, the size of the samples, when they were obtained from the study subjects, how they are currently stored, and the ease with which they can be accessed for research. This information is used to draw conclusions concerning whether obstacles exist to retaining and maintaining the materials.

Some of the content in this chapter was previously presented in the committee's interim letter report (IOM, 2005).

SPECIMEN COLLECTION AND SHIPMENT

Specimen collection was performed as part of the multiday physical examination in each of six cycles carried out by the AFHS during the period 1982–2002.[1] These activities were conducted at the Kelsey-Seybold Clinic in Houston, Texas, in Cycle 1 and at the Scripps Clinic in La Jolla, California, by Science Applications International Corporation (SAIC) Inc., a contract service provider to the AFHS, in later cycles. The protocols for collection, shipment, assay, and storage of various biological specimens are documented in respective biomedical

[1]Sera were also collected at American Red Cross Centers in conjunction with the 1987 TCDD assay pilot study, and insulin-sensitivity testing of 60 Cycle 5 participants was performed at the General Clinical Research Center at the University of Arkansas for Medical Sciences/Central Arkansas Veterans HealthCare (Patterson et al., 1987; Kern et al., 2004).

TABLE 4-1 Number and Type of Specimens Collected from AFHS Subjects by Year and Cycle

Year Exam Cycle	1982 1	1985 2	1987 3	1992 4	1997 5	2002 6	Total # of samples
Blood serum							
# of samples	15,883	6,927	4,588	8,932	8,484	5,853	50,667
# of vials	5–10	3	2	4	4	3	
Volume (ml)	2	5	10	7	10	10	
Whole blood							
# of samples						19,510	19,510
# of vials						10	
Volume (ml)						1	
Urine							
# of samples	2,269	2,309	2,294				6,872
# of vials	1	1	1				
Volume (ml)	50	50	10				
Semen							
# of samples	8,845						8,845
# of vials	1–10						
Volume (ml)	1						
Adipose tissue*							
# of samples					313		313
Weight (g)					10		

*A sample of approximately 10 g was extracted by liposuction (AFHS, 2000).

SOURCE: J. Robinson, Air Force Health Study, personal communication, September 21, 2005.

test plans—created by SAIC—for Cycles 2–6.[2] A detailed protocol is not available for Cycle 1. Cycle 1 laboratory methods are discussed in the original protocol (AFHS, 1982); they are also briefly described in the Cycle 2 biomedical test plan (SAIC, 1985) where shift in laboratory techniques or methods between Cycles 1 and 2 is discussed.

Table 4-1 provides summary counts of the types and quantities of biological specimens collected in each cycle. Sera were stored in all six cycles and aliquot volumes varied by cycle ranging from 2 to 10 ml per aliquot. The number of aliquots per subject also varied ranging from 1 to 10 vials in Cycle 1, 3 vials in Cycles 2 and 6, 2 vials in Cycle 3, and 4 vials in Cycles 4 and 5. In Cycle 6, ten 1-ml aliquots of whole blood were also stored with ethylenediaminetetraacetic acid (EDTA) as an anticoagulant. There was no separation of white blood cells.

[2]These documents are now in the public domain (https://www.formrouter.net/forms@NAS/Public_Access_Form.html).

One aliquot of urine was stored from participants during Cycles 1–3 (1982, 1985, and 1987). Urine aliquot volumes were 50 ml in Cycles 1 and 2 and 10 ml in Cycle 3. The Cycle 1 semen specimens were stored in 1-ml vials with 1–10 aliquots per subject.

A separate blood draw was performed to obtain samples for a 2,3,7,8-tetrachlorodibenzo-*p*-dioxin (dioxin) assay carried out by the Centers for Disease Control (CDC). Table 4-2 delineates the number of assays conducted by exam cycle. Multiple samples were drawn for a subset of the population for use in dioxin half-life studies. The methodology and results of these analyses is presented in Chapter 2 of the Cycle 6 examination report (AFHS, 2005).

Most subjects also underwent a glucose tolerance test with bloods and urines collected two hours after the first blood draw. Suspicious skin lesions were biopsied and their pathology determined in all cycles. These samples were not stored in the repository.

Specimen aliquots were packaged on dry ice and shipped overnight to the AFHS facilities at Brooks City-Base in San Antonio, Texas, where they have been maintained in –70°C freezers (J. Robinson, Air Force Health Study, personal communication, September 21, 2005). No samples were lost during shipment for any of the six cycles.

The current AFHS specimen collection includes portions of frozen whole blood collected originally for dioxin analysis, which were returned to AFHS from CDC. With this exception, no other samples have been returned to the AFHS repository subsequent to distribution to third-party investigators. Of the latter, relatively few have accessed AFHS specimens and, of those who have, some arranged for collection of samples specifically for their own purposes. As an example, adipose tissues were collected in 1997 (Cycle 5) and are held at UC

TABLE 4-2 Number of Dioxin Assays Performed on AFHS Subjects by Year and Cycle

Year[s]	Cycle[s]	Ranch Hand	Comparison	Total
1987 only*	3	277	771	1,048
1992 only	4	76	179	255
1997 only	5	18	95	113
2002 only	6	12	94	106
1987 and 1992	3, 4	30	35	65
1987 and 1997	3, 5	146	0	146
1987, 1992, and 1997	3, 4, 5	218	0	218
Total	777	1,174	1,951	

*Includes assays for 150 Ranch Hands and 50 comparisons conducted for pilot study (Patterson et al., 1987).

SOURCE: AFHS, 2005.

Davis (as indicated in Table 4-1). According to documentation provided to the committee (J. Robinson, Air Force Health Study, personal communication, September 21, 2005), past uses of AFHS specimens that have resulted in removal of samples from the collection include

- 200 samples of sera from the Cycle 1 collection provided for infectious disease antibody testing at the University of Cincinnati in 1984,
- 626 samples of sera from Cycle 1 used for dioxin half-life studies by AFHS and CDC in 1987,
- 4 samples of sera from Cycle 4 from individuals with consistently low immunoglobulin A levels provided to Duke University in 1993,
- 4 samples of sera from Cycle 4 provided to the University of Virginia in 1993, and
- 100 samples of sera (cycle not specified; described as "late 1980s") used by CDC to test for *Legionella* antibodies.

OBSTACLES AND LIMITATIONS TO FURTHER USE OF AFHS SPECIMENS

Limitations Inherent to the Nature of Specimens Collected and Their Subsequent Storage and Preservation

As indicated in Table 4-1, the type and quantity of specimens collected varied by cycle, with some specimen types being collected only once or for only a subset of study participants. Limitations in specimen volumes and the number of aliquots archived would necessitate the prudent restriction of future uses of AFHS specimen assets with appreciable biomaterial requirements.

Although the stored specimens are suitable for many current assays and potentially for new assays as yet unidentified, there are clearly some analytes (such as volatile organic compounds in blood) that require different methods of handling and preservation than those employed in the AFHS in order to ensure analytic viability. There also exist other analyte classes for which the adequacy of the storage conditions over the duration of storage is generally not well established. It is clear that some analytes will not be measurable as special precautions that are sometimes instituted for specific studies were not taken with the specimens. For example, some blood processing protocols require specimen protection from light to prevent degradation of carotenoids. The addition of metaphosphoric acid is a standard practice for serum ascorbic acid measurement (Paoli, 2005). Other analyses require the addition of antioxidants to protect certain chemical species. Ascorbic acid—an antioxidant—is sometimes added to urine specimens as an analyte preservative.

Although whole blood has been stored, it was not done in the presence of a dimethyl sulfoxide containing freezing medium. Thus, the white blood cells

(WBC) are not viable. Additionally, without intact cells it is currently not feasible to assay for gene expression in WBCs. However, emerging technologies may make these types of studies possible.

Thus, it is not possible for the committee to make an exhaustive prediction of what assays could be run in the future, especially given the rapid development of instrument technologies and assay methods with improved analytical sensitivity and specificity. However, it is reasonable for the committee to conclude that there will be an appreciable demand for these specimens given the accompanying physical exam and laboratory data collected over the 20-year course of the AFHS. The National Health and Nutrition Examination Survey (NHANES)[3] repository provides a practical example for determining the utility of AFHS specimens for any specific future study. The committee feels that researchers should bear the burden of demonstrating the suitability of specimens for their particular studies, and these data must be provided before specimens are released.

Logistical Limitations

Logistical limitations to the future use of AFHS specimens include deficiencies in or absence of documentation regarding the methods of collection and processing of specimens,[4] the need to reaccomplish inventory controls through the reorganization of specimens, the improvement of documentation of specimen locations, and, where feasible, the annotation of specimen history. More importantly, preserving the specimens for future uses will require continued support of a specialized facility.

The working group responsible for issues regarding specimens during the committee's May 2005 site visit (Drs. Hankinson and Kalman) interviewed program staff and conducted exercises to evaluate access to and preservation of specimen whole blood, serum, urine, and semen. Their findings are presented in the committee's interim letter report (IOM, 2005) and recapitulated here.

Storage

Specimens are stored at –70°C in a total of 21 freezers in a single room in a building that also houses other AFHS functions. This storage temperature was the accepted state of the art in the 1980s.[5] A few smaller collections of AFHS

[3]Information on NHANES can be found at http://www.cdc.gov/nchs/nhanes.htm.

[4]Variability in laboratory procedures notwithstanding, the ability to detect true variation in selected laboratory endpoints is predicated on the elimination or control of variation in specimen collection and processing.

[5]The practice in 2005 is to store biologic samples at least to –80°C; liquid nitrogen storage—which maintains samples at still lower temperatures (below –130°C)—is used in some studies (Paoli, 2005).

biospecimens have been dispersed to collaborating investigators and would need to be recombined, destroyed, or be handled by some other custodial arrangement prior to the termination of the AFHS.

Specimen Access

Specimens have been maintained in lots, reflecting the manner in which they were received; in some cases several vials from multiple individuals were in zipper-sealed plastic bags, and in other cases several vials were held together with rubber bands. Labels on stored samples are not uniform but in general contain the subject's case number, last and first name, and middle initial. Some aliquots also indicate the subject's age, the sample type (e.g., SER3), collection time, and date.

Multiple steps were required to locate particular specimens. First, the subject's case number and the first four letters of his last name are keyed into a master (computer-based) database that identifies the box in which the sample is stored and the freezer in which that box is located. However, boxes have been moved over time, and locations stored in this database have not been updated and are thus not reliable. The AFHS investigators recently completed a physical inventory of all boxes in the repository and were able to locate all boxes listed in the database. To locate a particular box, one must refer to the hard copy list generated in the physical inventory to determine the current freezer and shelf location of a particular specimen. For example, the database may indicate that a subject's serum specimen from Cycle 2 is located in freezer 19, drawer 2, box 4, but the inventory hard copy might indicate that the actual location of the specimen is freezer 14, drawer 2, box 4.[6] Despite the intricacy of the inventory records, staff was able to locate specimens requested by the working group with little difficulty.

Neither the existing database nor the hard copy reinventory provide data regarding the number of aliquots or volumes stored. It appears that these data were not recorded consistently. For those cycles that had quantities recorded, the current volumes in the record reflect the original quantities received. These have not been updated to indicate removal from the original amounts received.

Specimen Integrity and Condition

No documentation exists for the thermal history of the specimens. However, the physical condition of the freezers appears to be adequate. All had external labels indicating that they had been inspected at 6-month intervals for at least the past three years. The freezers have been monitored for failure throughout the course of the study—in earlier years by physical inspection and later through

[6]The working group was told that drawer and box numbers were maintained in moves.

electronic monitoring and alarm systems. Three people are on call at all times to move samples in case of a freezer failure. Empty freezers maintained at –70°C are available for immediate transfer of samples in case of freezer breakdown. In the earlier years of the study, there was one instance where specimens were compromised by an equipment failure. This occurred in 1986 when 656 urine samples were lost because of a freezer outage.

Thus, the biorepository has been well preserved and certainly appears comparable in quality to repositories housed by other large epidemiologic studies (e.g., the Physicians' Health Study[7] and the NYU Women's Health Study[8]).

Retrieval and inspection of three specimens from randomly selected subjects showed no signs of leakage or major thaws. The appearance of one urine specimen examined by the working group was open to interpretation: the position of the fluid in the vial was consistent with either minor thawing and refreezing, or the initial freezing of the specimen occurring in two phases.

Some residuals from serum samples sent to CDC for dioxin analysis were returned to the AFHS repository. These samples are kept separate from the others, and they are marked as returns in an inventory document. With this exception, all samples in the repository appear to have remained frozen since collection. As noted above, specimens have been sent to Duke University, the University of Cincinnati, and the University of Virginia for various analyses over the course of the study. None of these were returned to the inventory. During the Cycle 5 physical examination, 313 adipose tissue samples were collected; they are being held by a collaborating investigator at the University of California-Davis. The committee does not have any information on the condition and storage circumstances of these samples.

During the committee's first meeting, the AFHS investigators mentioned that they planned to conduct a reassay experiment to evaluate the analytical viability of the specimens. The plan called for analyzing specimens from a small sample of subjects over the six study cycles. These samples will be assayed for endpoints for which historical values are available. Results are expected to generally indicate the current condition of preserved specimens, although their interpretation is not straightforward, and the suitability of these samples for specific analytes will need to be determined in some cases.

A major reinventory and physical reorganization of the specimens is planned for the final year of the study and was recommended in the Committee's letter report (IOM, 2005). This effort will reconcile the inventories and create a new

---

[7]The Physicians' Health Study is a randomized trial. Phase I began in 1982 and Phase II is scheduled for termination in 2007. Over 26,000 blood specimens were collected during Phase I, and more than 11,000 blood specimens have been collected in Phase II (http://phs.bwh.harvard.edu/).

[8]The New York University Women's Health Study is an observational study in which blood samples from more than 17,000 participants have been collected. Specimens are stored in –80°C freezers (http://mcrcr4.med.nyu.edu/womenshealthstudy).

database that would not only provide the actual current location of all specimens but would also indicate the volumes and types of biological material in storage for each individual.

Based on the specimen storage method employed in the NIOSH/FAA Working Women's Health Study, the planned AFHS reorganization will collect all specimens for an individual in one or more sequential boxes. Currently, AFHS specimens are stored in freezers by cycle and specimen type, not by individual. This effort will greatly decrease the effort associated with the retrieval of specimens. However, if the request is for a single type of specimen (e.g., urine), many more boxes will have to be pulled than if the inventory were organized by biospecimen type. Organization by subject will, however, facilitate the withdrawal of a subject's entire specimen archive should he not consent to research in the future.[9] Combining of the specimens from various cycles will necessitate very careful pulling of requested specimens in the future so that not only the correct specimen type but also the correct collection time period for an individual is selected. It is not clear that each vial has the cycle number or date of collection on the label. Thus, any vials without this information should have it added during this reorganization.

Many of the specimens are stored in volumes (e.g., 5-ml to 50-ml vials) much larger than what is required for most assays. It would be desirable to realiquot specimens (e.g., 100-µl to 500-µl aliquots) before sending them out for analysis. This would minimize additional freeze–thaw cycles. While the collaborating laboratory may be able to perform the realiquoting, this is not an ideal solution because the repository would lose control over the specimens and their freeze–thaw history. Realiquoting has cost implications—supervision and technician time and processing and freezer space needs—but is a means to help maintain the specimen integrity for future use.

Procedural Limitations: Privacy and Other Ethical, Legal, and Social Issues

Individual specimens are currently labeled by individual name among other identifiers. This requires that managers of the specimen repository be bound by privacy and confidentiality agreements and that specimens provided to any future users either be relabeled[10] and realiquoted or that privacy requirements be otherwise assured. The operation of a future specimen repository would need to have the capability to satisfy such requirements.

Related issues, including informed consent, are discussed in Chapter 6.

---

[9]Specimen control issues are discussed in Chapter 6.

[10]The current state-of-the-art is to use bar codes for specimens held in repositories. It is not known if relabeling with bar codes was planned in the AFHS reorganization of specimens.

FINDINGS, CONCLUSIONS, AND RECOMMENDATIONS

On the basis of its review of AFHS reports, its site visit of the study facility, the scientific literature, and other information presented in this chapter, the committee has reached the following findings regarding the laboratory specimens and other study data collected during the AFHS.

As noted in the interim letter report, the committee finds that:

> The laboratory specimens collected in the course of the AFHS have been properly maintained. However, they are not currently organized and documented in a manner that allows them to be easily understood, evaluated, managed, or analyzed by persons outside of the AFHS.

The committee also finds that:

> Obstacles, including privacy concerns, exist to retaining and maintaining the laboratory specimens.

The letter report noted that there were two primary options for the disposition of the laboratory specimens collected by the AFHS: disposal or maintenance for possible future use. Regardless of what decision is made concerning their disposition, the committee believes that there is value in fully documenting and reorganizing the laboratory specimens prior to the study's presently scheduled termination date. This would be helpful in auditing their proper disposal if that decision were taken and would be vital to facilitating any possible future use.

The committee's interim letter report offered several recommendations for addressing the obstacles to retaining and maintaining the AFHS laboratory specimens that related to the organization and documentation of these materials. These are listed in the following section.

Approaches to addressing the other obstacles identified here are presented in Chapter 6 in the context of the committee's recommendations for the further study.

Recommendations Contained in the Interim Letter Report

The interim letter report (IOM, 2005) explicates the committee's conclusion that the present state of the documentation and organization of AFHS laboratory specimens was an obstacle to retaining and maintaining these materials after the currently scheduled termination date of the study. The committee therefore recommended that:

> **Action should be taken prior to the currently scheduled termination date of the AFHS to reorganize and document the study's laboratory specimens in a form and format that allows them to be easily understood, evaluated, managed, or analyzed by persons outside of the AFHS.**

The following actions were recommended:

- Reinventory all laboratory specimens held by the AFHS, verifying their location and ascertaining the number and volume of aliquots and type of sample. Carry out a visual inspection of specimen condition while performing this activity, and identify any problematic samples.
- Update and create a single specimen database that includes case number, exam cycle, specimen type, and freezer location.
- Compile all information regarding specimen history (receipt, realiquoting, freeze–thaw cycles, dispersal, and the like) into a single reference database. Where data gaps are present, note their existence.
- Compile all protocols regarding receipt, maintenance, dispersal, and return of specimens for all cycles into a single reference document.
- Document the status of all laboratory specimens sent to outside investigators. Ensure that extant specimens are either disposed of using current best practices or reintegrated into the inventory, clearly marked with their history.
- Perform the currently planned reassay to aid in the evaluation of specimen stability and condition.

The interim letter report also noted that the committee was in agreement with a planned reinventory and physical reorganization of their repository that would collect all specimens for a study subject in one or sequential boxes.[11] They were told of the plan in their May 2005 site visit and understand that the effort was subsequently initiated. The committee recommended that—if the planned reorganization was carried out—the exam cycle or date of collection be added to any vials that were not already marked with such information.

As already noted in Chapter 3, the committee believes that it is incumbent on the U.S. Air Force, as the custodian of the AFHS research materials, to ensure their proper documentation and organization for both historic reasons and for possible future use. It therefore recommends that:

If available AFHS program funds are not sufficient to accomplish the actions elucidated above, supplemental funding should be provided to carry out such work in a complete and timely manner.

REFERENCES

AFHS (Air Force Health Study). 1982. *An Epidemiologic Investigation of Health Effects in Air Force Personnel Following Exposure to Herbicides: Study Protocol, Initial Report.* Brooks AFB, TX: USAF School of Aerospace Medicine. SAM-TR-82-44.

[11]Currently, specimens are stored in freezers by cycle and specimen type.

AFHS. 2000. *An Epidemiologic Investigation of Health Effects in Air Force Personnel Following Exposure to Herbicides. 1997 Followup Examination Results.* Brooks AFB, TX: Epidemiologic Research Division. Armstrong Laboratory. AFRL-HE-BR-TR-2000-02.

AFHS. 2005. *An Epidemiologic Investigation of Health Effects in Air Force Personnel Following Exposure to Herbicides. 2002 Followup Examination Results.* Brooks AFB, TX: Epidemiologic Research Division. Armstrong Laboratory. AFRL-HE-BR-SR-2005-0003.

IOM (Institute of Medicine). 2005. *Disposition of the Air Force Health Study—Interim Letter Report.* Washington, DC: The National Academies Press. [Online]. Available: http://www.nap.edu/catalog/11483.html [accessed December 1, 2005].

Kern P, Said S, Jackson W, Michalek J. 2004. Insulin sensitivity and serum TCDD in Air Force veterans occupationally exposed to herbicides during the Vietnam War. *Organohalogen Compounds* 66:3166–3173.

Paoli PD. 2005. Biobanking in microbiology: from sample collection to epidemiology, diagnosis and research. *FEMS Microbiology Reviews* 29:897–910.

Patterson DG, Hampton L, Lapeza CR, Besler WT, Green V, Alexander LR, Needham LL. 1987. High-resolution gas chromatography/high-resolution mass spectrometric analysis of human serum on a whole-weight and lipid basis for 2,3,7,8-tetrachlorodibenzo-*p*-dioxin. *Analytical Chemistry* 59:2000–2005.

SAIC (Science Applications International Corporation). 1985. *Biomedical Test Plan.* Air Force Contract No. F14689-85-D-0010. SAIC Project No. 2-816-04-195.

5

Value of the AFHS Research Assets

The previous three chapters of this report provide a detailed description of the Air Force Health Study (AFHS) (Chapter 2), and address the current state of the study's medical records and other study data (Chapter 3) and specimens (Chapter 4). This chapter summarizes and builds on that foundation to draw conclusions regarding the scientific merit of retaining and maintaining the data assets of the AFHS, and the advisability of further study of such records, data, and specimens. It also addresses privacy and security concerns related to the retention and maintenance of the AFHS data assets.

SCIENTIFIC MERIT OF THE DATA ASSETS

Based on the information contained in Chapters 2–4 and the additional details presented below, the committee has reached the following findings:

The AFHS Data Assets Are Unique: No Other Epidemiologic Dataset on Vietnam Veterans Contains as Detailed Information Over as Long a Time Period

Subjects in the AFHS morbidity study have undergone up to six cycles of detailed physical examinations and questionnaire data collection over a 20-year period. Physical examination data sources include blood draws, urine and semen collections, skin and fat biopsies, stool smears, spirometry, chest X rays, electrocardiograms, dermatology and peripheral vascular examinations, neurological assessments, psychological testing, and myriad other clinical endpoints. Subjects were asked to provide their medical records, as well as those of their children (up to age 17), their present partner, and any previous partner. These hard copy records were duplicated and exist as part of AFHS data assets. In addition, questionnaires were administered eliciting information on education; employment; income; marital and fertility history; child and family health; health habits; recreation, leisure, and physical activities; toxic substances exposure; military experience; and wartime herbicide exposure. In all, 2,758 subjects participated in at least one cycle exam.

In addition, reproductive data were gathered and coded on 9,921 conceptions and 8,100 live births. The mortality component of the study has followed for nearly 25 years more than 20,000 Vietnam War-era veterans who served in Southeast Asia.

More than 86,000 biologic specimens have been collected over the course of the study; approximately half of these are serum. Blood was collected in all six cycles and serum stored; stored semen is available only from Cycle 1 (1982), and urine is available only from Cycles 1–3 (1982, 1985, and 1987). In the last (sixth) cycle, whole blood was also stored. Chapters 3 and 4 detail the data and specimens collected over the course the study.

Participation rates in the morbidity study have been relatively high, particularly among the Ranch Hands. Of the 1,208 Ranch Hands eligible at the time of the baseline examination, 1,045 (87 percent) took part. Although participation has dropped over time—from 85 percent at Cycle 2 to 74 percent at Cycle 6—the relatively high participation rates suggest that there may not be substantial selection biases in the cohort. Selection bias would exist, for example, if subjects with a health outcome differentially dropped out by exposure status. Among refusal subjects at Cycle 6, 5.4 percent of Ranch Hand refusals cited health reasons as their barrier to participation. Among comparison subjects, 5.1 percent of original comparisons and 5.4 percent of replacement comparisons refused to participate due to health reasons (AFHS, 2005). Passive refusal (non-response to invitation) rates were higher for comparison subjects versus Ranch Hands. The committee notes that the rate of attrition over time is high enough to potentially introduce other sources of bias, and that the introduction of such biases could compromise the internal validity of the study. However, it also notes that AFHS participation rates are comparable to those commonly observed in other longitudinal epidemiologic studies.

All told, the AFHS has more data points and a higher rate of follow-up than the Framingham Heart Study, according to a USAF representative (RHAC, 2004). Approximately $143 million has been spent or allocated for collecting, managing, and analyzing these materials.

Although several other epidemiologic studies of Vietnam veterans have been conducted, few have longitudinal data or have collected and analyzed any biologic samples. Two ongoing studies—the VA Normative Aging Study (Bell et al., 1972; Bossé and Spiro, 1995; MAVERIC, 2001) and the Vietnam Era Twin

Registry (Henderson et al., 1990; Goldberg et al., 2002; Seattle ERIC, 2005)—collect similar but less comprehensive data and specimens from U.S. veterans, some of whom had wartime service in Vietnam.[1] It is beyond the scope of the committee's work to synopsize and review the epidemiologic literature on Vietnam veterans. However, *Veterans and Agent Orange: Update 2004* (IOM, 2005a) and earlier reports in the Veterans and Agent Orange (VAO)—series (IOM, 1994, 1996, 1999, 2000, 2001, 2003) provide details on them. A table adapted from *VAO Update 2004* is included as Appendix C. It contains a comprehensive list of the Vietnam veterans' health outcomes literature and indicates in which volume of the VAO report series a review may be found. The table includes information on the type of study, a summary description of the topics addressed, and the size of the study population. It also contains a listing of AFHS publications reporting epidemiologic results through 2004. In brief, the table and VAO supplementary materials indicate that very few prospective morbidity studies with a broad set of health outcomes have been conducted. In addition, in most of these studies only self-reported health outcomes were obtained. The study most similar to the AFHS—an investigation of health outcomes among U.S. Army Chemical Corps[2] specialists—shares many of AFHS' limitations (a relatively small cohort of veterans with atypical exposures) and has much less detailed information on its subjects. Even in studies of particular health outcomes—most typically, forms of cancer—data were not obtained through direct examination of subjects, although physicians' records were sometimes consulted to verify self-reported diagnoses.

It must be noted that the AFHS cohort is a relatively small sample that is not representative of the US male population at large or of Vietnam veterans. This does not preclude its use in studies of issues beyond those involving exposure to the herbicides employed in the Vietnam War. However, it does mean that the results of such studies must be appropriately qualified and their limitations forthrightly discussed. Most "occupational" cohorts have similar limitations and researchers have developed means of dealing with these issues in their work.

The Data Collected by the AFHS Appear to Be of High Quality and the Specimens Appear to Be Well Preserved

The committee did not perform a comprehensive review of all AFHS data and specimens. However, the survey conducted by a subcommittee during a May 2005 site visit to the study's San Antonio, Texas home led it to conclude that

[1]Additional detail on these two studies is provided in Chapter 6.

[2]The US Army Chemical Corps were responsible for the storage, preparation, and spraying of herbicides using hand equipment and H-34-type helicopters (Kang et al., 2001). They conducted spray operations such as defoliation around Special Forces camps; clearance of perimeters surrounding airfields, depots, and other bases; and small-scale crop destruction.

these materials were collected, coded, documented, and stored in a manner consistent with best practices at the time they were obtained.

All information collection and laboratory analysis activities were subjected to rigorous quality control procedures. These procedures are most recently documented in the quality control chapter of the Cycle 6 final report (AFHS, 2005). Earlier reports chronicle the procedures used in analogous chapters. The procedures were intended to ensure that data were properly recorded, coded, and entered into SAS databases. Information was subjected to validity checks, missing and outlying values were investigated and verified, and subjective observations (clinical impressions in medical exams, for example) were reviewed.

The working groups that visited the site found that requested data could be extracted from SAS datasets and that randomly chosen specimens could be retrieved and appeared to have been properly stored. Details of their findings are contained in the interim letter report of the committee (IOM, 2005b) and are also covered in Chapters 3 and 4 of this report. The interim letter report also offered several recommendations for documenting and organizing the data assets in a form and format that would facilitate easy access to their contents.

Analysis of the AFHS Data Assets Has Contributed to the Literature Addressing the Health of Vietnam Veterans

In Spring 2005, Institute of Medicine (IOM) staff undertook a survey of citations to papers produced by AFHS investigators. Science Citation Index was used to determine the number and title of papers that referenced any one of 45 papers published in peer-reviewed scholarly publications addressing the results of analyses of AFHS data assets. A total of 733 citations were found. Of these, 273 (37 percent) were self-citations, that is, a citation in which the citing and the cited paper had at least one author in common.[3] The remaining 460 (63 percent) were from other authors. Seven AFHS papers account for the majority of these citations by other authors (301 of the 460, or 65 percent). They address TCDD half-life/pharmacokinetics (159 citations), diabetes (58), and other health outcomes (84). Table 5-1 provides additional details on these papers. Although this analysis does not yield any information about the quality of the cited paper or the context in which it was cited, it does yield a rough idea of the extent to which AFHS research has attracted the notice of the scientific community.

AFHS data and biospecimens have had a particular influence on scientific understanding of the pharmacokinetics of TCDD and its half-life[4] in humans be-

[3]Given that AFHS is a longitudinal study, it is de rigueur for later publications by the investigators to reference earlier work.

[4]Half-life refers to the amount of time it takes to reduce the original concentration of an analyte by 50 percent within a circumscribed compartment such as serum or plasma.

TABLE 5-1 AFHS Papers with the Greatest Number of Citations by Other Authors

AFHS Paper	Topic	Total Citations	Citations by Other Authors
Pirkle et al., 1989	Serum dioxin half-life	110	80
Wolfe et al., 1990	Veterans' health status	88	56
Michalek et al., 1996	Pharmacokinetics of TCDD	65	44
Henriksen et al., 1997	Serum dioxin and diabetes mellitus	54	37
Wolfe et al., 1994	Serum dioxin half-life	37	35
Wolfe et al., 1995	Paternal serum dioxin and reproductive outcomes	43	28
Longnecker and Michalek, 2000	Serum dioxin and diabetes mellitus	24	21

cause there are so few longitudinal studies that have collected serum from an exposed population. Within two years of the development of a serum TCDD assay, Pirkle and colleagues published estimates of TCDD half-life based on serial measures (collected 1982 and 1987) for 36 Ranch Hand subjects using a first-order kinetics model. Subsequent analyses (Caudill et al., 1992; Wolfe et al., 1992; Michalek et al., 1992; Wolfe et al., 1994; Michalek et al., 1996; Michalak et al., 1998; Michalek and Tripathi, 1999; Michalek et al., 2002; Emond et al., 2005) of AFHS data and the application of earlier AFHS findings (Warner et al., 2005) have served to refine TCDD half-life estimates with respect to elapsed time since exposure as well as the influence of body fat, the handling of nondetects and truncation of extrapolated values. In conjunction with studies of other exposed populations (Piacitelli et al., 2000; Steenland et al., 2001; Aylward et al., 2005), a revised two-compartment open pharmacokinetic model was subsequently developed. While the serial nature of AFHS TCDD data have enabled them to significantly impact half-life estimates, the data are limited by the length of elapsed time between exposure and assay. Additionally, they cannot inform half-life estimates for TCDD-exposed females, for whom longer half-lives have been observed (Aylward et al., 2005).

AFHS reports and papers have also had an influence on the determinations of Institute of Medicine committees charged with evaluating the strength of the scientific evidence regarding exposure to the herbicides used in the Vietnam War and adverse health outcomes. As noted in Chapter 2,[5] AFHS research was cited

[5]Chapter 2 contains the committee's discussion of this topic in the section entitled *AFHS Research and the Institute of Medicine's "Veterans and Agent Orange" Reports*.

as influential in their decisions regarding spina bifida in the children of Vietnam veterans and type 2 diabetes among Vietnam veterans.

The IOM committee responsible for *Veterans and Agent Orange: Update 1996* (IOM, 1996), while acknowledging the limitations imparted by the small population size, cited AFHS as one of three studies of "relatively high quality" that influenced their determination of limited/suggestive evidence of an association between spina bifida and paternal herbicide exposure. Based in part on the committee's finding, spina bifida compensation legislation (Section 421 of Public Law 104-204, Title 38) was proposed in July 1996 and signed in September 1996 (IOM, 1999). This legislation altered the US Code to include dispensation of benefits to offspring of Vietnam veterans born with spina bifida (excluding spina bifida occulta). The VA's subsequent implementation of the legislation in September 1997 (62 FR 51274-96) marked the first time that VA benefits had been extended to affected offspring based on paternal exposure.

An IOM committee assembled in 1999 at the behest of the VA conducted a review of the scientific literature related to type 2 diabetes and herbicide and dioxin exposure. This committee's report, *Veterans and Agent Orange: Herbicide/Dioxin Exposure and Type 2 Diabetes* (IOM, 2000) discusses AFHS research at length and cites it among the information that was influential in its finding that there was limited/suggestive evidence of an association between exposure to herbicides and/or dioxin and type 2 diabetes. The VA subsequently classified type 2 diabetes as a "presumptive condition" for in-country Vietnam veterans, allowing persons with the disease to seek benefits without showing specific proof of a relationship between their service and the condition. No figures are available on the impact of this program, but a 2001 VA press release indicated that the cost of the benefit was projected to be $3.3 billion over the first five years of its availability, based on the assumption that approximately 220,000 veterans would be receiving benefits (VA, 2001).

There has been relatively little collaboration between AFHS and outside investigators. However, some studies have been conducted.

As noted elsewhere in the report, AFHS researchers and a team from the National Institute of Dental and Craniofacial Research collaborated on a study of silver-mercury amalgam fillings and adverse health outcomes, with a specific focus on neurological morbidity (Kingman et al., 2005).

Sleep disturbances among Ranch Hand subjects were evaluated in a collaborative effort between AFHS and Texas Tech University researchers. Questionnaire data from participants of Cycles 3 and 4 were used to evaluate the nature and frequency of reported sleep disorders. Researchers hypothesized that dioxin somehow targets arousal mechanisms and thereby interferes with normal sleep patterns. Results of this research have been submitted for publication; they were presented in draft form in a June 2005 meeting the Ranch Hand Advisory committee (Liu et al., 2005).

Investigators at University of California-Davis conducted a glucose transport study using 313 adipose tissue samples collected in conjunction with the Cycle 5 physical examination. This molecular epidemiology study matched samples from 313 AFHS volunteers to comparisons recruited from outside the cohort. The molecular markers selected included glucose transporter 4 (GLUT4), an adiposity index, an inflammation marker (NFκB), a signal messenger for toxic action of dioxin, and a housekeeping gene used as a normalization standard. The results of this study have not been published, but preliminary findings are available (RHAC, 2005).

Other efforts have involved the provision of AFHS subjects' biospecimens to other institutions for use in various assays. In 1984, 200 sera samples were sent to the University of Cincinnati for *Strongyloides stercoralis* antibody testing. Duke University and the University of Virginia each received 4 AFHS sera specimens in 1993 for an immunology related study. Nearly 700 sera specimens have been sent to the CDC, in addition to those sent for the standard AFHS morbidity study TCDD assays, for *Legionella* antibody testing and TCDD half-life studies (addressed above).

The committee also identified an instance where data derived from publicly available AFHS reports were combined with other data and analyzed. Researchers compared the prevalence of chronic disease and behavioral risk factors among AFHS study participants (Cycles 1–5; Ranch Hand and comparison subjects) to a subset of age, race, and education-level comparable participants of the National Health and Nutrition Survey (Pfizer, 2005).

Any future on the AFHS data assets is likely to attract the attention of those involved with veterans' health policy because so few epidemiologic studies have been conducted on Vietnam veterans, and almost none on veterans with quantified TCDD body burden.

FUTURE POTENTIAL OF THE DATA ASSETS

The completion of the Cycle 6 physical examinations marked the end of major data gathering activities planned by the AFHS before the currently scheduled termination date of the study in 2006.[6] However, investigators, contractors, and collaborators continue to analyze data and specimens and publish results. Since the beginning of 2005, the Cycle 6 final report has been released, four papers have been published in peer-reviewed journals (Ketchum and Michalek, 2005; Kingman et al., 2005; Pavuk et al., 2005a,b), and several more are under submission or in preparation. These include a study using longitudinal data being prepared under contract by Science Applications International Corporation (SAIC, 2005).

[6]The study continues to conduct periodic mortality updates.

It is clear that these remaining analyses will only scratch the surface of possible scientific hypotheses that can be investigated. Even in the absence of new health outcome information, the AFHS data assets could be used to examine myriad health questions. The committee does not have specific recommendations regarding the type of hypotheses that should be pursued. Rather, should the assets be made available to the scientific community, it believes that these details are best left to the investigators who propose to carry out the work. The committee offers, below, some possible topics for future work to illustrate the richness of the data and to indicate possible avenues for research.

Researchers Can Reanalyze Outcomes Examined by the AFHS Using Different Assumptions and Approaches Than Have Been Applied to Date

The AFHS was initiated to investigate the possible long-term health effects of wartime exposure to herbicides in Vietnam veterans. The study has, by and large, maintained the analysis protocols and assumptions established at its initiation. These include the use of rather basic means of characterizing herbicide exposure[7] and the application of data from replacement subjects when original matched comparisons were unable or unwilling to participate in later cycle exams. It is outside the scope of this report to provide detailed critical analysis of these assumptions. However, it is axiomatic that different assumptions might yield different results concerning the association between herbicide or dioxin exposures and health outcomes. Advances in both knowledge and technology also allow new and more sophisticated analyses to be conducted.

For example, the research of Stellman and colleagues (Stellman et al., 2003a,b; Stellman and Stellman, 2004) has recently yielded a far more detailed understanding of which herbicides were applied where and when, and how dioxin contamination of the 2,4,5-T-based herbicides changed over time. This information could possibly be used to refine exposure assessment models for dioxin-contaminated herbicides and separately factor exposure to non-dioxin-contaminated herbicides.[8] Preliminary research suggests the calendar period of service in-theater, the number of days that spraying took place during that service, and the time spent in Southeast Asia—all previously unfactored surrogates of dioxin exposure—are effect modifiers in analyses of Ranch Hand veterans' postservice health outcomes (Michalek, 2005).

---

[7]The "Reconstruction of Exposure" section of Chapter 2 describes the various means used to characterize herbicide exposure in the cohort. Most analyses use either an exposure surrogate based on wartime occupation or a categorical variable based on a serum dioxin level measured—at minimum—some 16 years after the last exposure.

[8]Such analyses were proposed in a 2004 AFHS presentation before the Ranch Hand Advisory Committee (RHAC, 2004).

When a Ranch Hand subject's comparison was unavailable for a cycle exam, AFHS study protocol dictated that a new comparison be selected from that person's pool of matched (on age, race, and military occupation) potential comparisons. In Cycles 2–6, when feasible, the *new* replacement comparison was matched to the *unavailable* comparison on self-perceived health status—excellent, good, fair, or poor. The replacement of noncompliant comparison subjects during the course of the 20 years of follow-up introduces major complexities into the survival analyses of the comparison group. AFHS chose to treat replacements as identical to originals for the purpose of analyses. However, there is no reason why this assumption has to be maintained and more complex approaches—taking into account the specific times of entry into the comparison cohort, for example—could be explored. Further studies could be accomplished under novel or modified matching strategies, or by excluding replacement comparison subjects.

The cohort's repeated examinations and questionnaires have introduced time-dependent variables into the dataset, and there are correlations among these measurements. These data offer a valuable opportunity to explore how trends in risk factors influence the development of various diseases. Only in recent years has adequate statistical software become available to handle this situation, creating the opportunity for a number of longitudinal analyses that would have been difficult to perform in earlier years.[9]

New Analyses Can Be Performed on the Existing Medical Records and Other Study Data That Examine Questions That Were Not Addressed in the AFHS

AFHS analyses focused on the influence of herbicide or dioxin exposure on health outcomes. However, data were collected on a wide range of potential influences on disease and health and a number of health outcomes not addressed in the AFHS reports could be studied with these data. Some of these may not be directly related to herbicide exposure but may still be important for furthering knowledge about veterans' health and the natural history and risks of disease.

For example, one could investigate associations between occupational exposures to chemical agents, dusts, and fumes and levels of pulmonary function. At each of the six cycles, subjects were asked about their occupational history.[10]

[9]As of late 2005, a longitudinal analysis of AFHS data was underway.

[10]It should be noted that, in Cycle 1, the coding was contracted to Louis Harris and Associates, Inc.; for Cycles 2–6 occupational and industrial codes were attributed by the NORC. The coders were not trained industrial hygienists, and the reliability of the coding has not been verified. For Cycles 1–4, the 1980 Census Alphabetical Index of Industries and Occupations was used, and for Cycles 5 and 6 the 1990 Census revision was used. These facts would have to be accounted for in any analyses using occupational data.

Subjects were asked about the jobs they held since the last examination, up to a maximum of five jobs. These were coded to the Bureau of the Census' North American Industry Classification System and Occupation Classification System. In addition, self-reported exposure to a number of agents was elicited, including dates and frequency of exposure, the reason for leaving employment, and use of personal protective equipment. Separately, pulmonary function measurements (FEV_1 and FVC) were measured during all physical exams except Cycle 2.[11] To ascertain whether occupation affects pulmonary function, analyses using hierarchical linear models (for example) could be undertaken.

Appendix B lists, in tabular form, endpoints that were analyzed in one or more physical exam cycles. Many of the table entries represent multiple endpoints (e.g., the SCL90 battery is a 90-question psychological test that counts as one entry in Table B-3). With myriad variables collected during at least one exam cycle, the potential for investigating various associations is great. Other forms of study design such as nested case–cohort and case–control studies may be appropriate for such research. And in some of these studies, it may be desirable to limit the study group to only the Ranch Hands or only the comparison group.

Advances in Biospecimen Analysis Technology and Science Can Be Employed to Conduct Studies That Were Not Contemplated in the AFHS Protocol

A report by RAND describes the breadth of tissue banking in the United States, thought to span thousands of collections and over 300 million specimens in 1999 (Eiseman and Haga, 1999). These include several massive collections such as the National Pathology Repository at the Armed Forces Institute of Pathology (AFIP), which holds over 12 million wet tissue specimens from more than 2.8 million subjects (AFIP, 2005) and the Coriell Cell Repositories, which maintain nearly a million vials of cryopreserved cells and over 120,000 cell cultures (Coriell Institute for Medical Research, 2005). Although these and other specimen holdings represent much larger and wider populations, the biological samples collected in the AFHS are a distinctive resource because of the depth of the accompanying detailed information from the physical exams, clinical measurements, and questionnaires. The serial nature of the physical exam data and variety of specimen types from individual subjects (sera, whole blood, urine, and semen) are also strengths. Clinical and biomarker measures include over 210 parameters with over 60 measured at all six cycles (Appendix B, Table B-14).

[11]The Cycle 2 exam report stated that pulmonary function studies were not performed "[b]ecause of the essentially negative pulmonary analyses from the baseline examination" (AFHS, 1987).

Storage conditions maintained by the AFHS are adequate for some future analyses of the specimens.[12] Examples include element analysis, standard blood chemistry, steroid hormones, fatty acids, and lipoproteins. Among the potential future uses of these samples are studies of biomarkers of exposure to environmental agents in the Vietnam theater—as was the study of serum 2,3,7,8-tetrachlorodibenzo-*p*-dioxin as a biomarker of exposure to Agent Orange—or exposures to other environmental hazards (Ryan et al., 2004). Studies of biomarkers of response or susceptibility in relation to health endpoints studied in the AFHS are also possible.

The whole blood collected during Cycle 6 would be an excellent source of DNA for possible genetic studies (Kelly and Woolley, 2005; Sun et al., 2005), including whole genome scans. It is also possible to obtain sufficient DNA from stored serum samples for limited genotype analysis. Thus, although it is unlikely that genetic studies were contemplated at the beginning of the AFHS, they are now feasible.

Other changes in technology (Hirsch et al., 2003; Chou et al., 2005) and the availability of new methods (Shevkoplyas et al., 2005) have made possible uses of the specimens that would not have been feasible—or imagined—when the study protocol was written. For example, serum proteomics was unknown 10 years ago. Studies are now examining specific patterns of proteins detectable in stored sera and their utility in the early diagnosis of disease, and in identifying therapeutic targets and disease response markers (Figeys, 2003; Domon and Broder et al., 2004; Chen et al., 2005; Srivastava et al., 2005). Additional examples of *potential* future analyses are listed below.[13]

- Polychlorinated biphenyl, polychlorinated dibenzofuran, and polychlorinated dibenzo-*p*-dioxin congeners that, like 2,3,7,8-TCDD, bind to the aryl hydrocarbon (Ah) receptor can be measured from sera and evaluated (TEQs) for associations with observed health outcomes (Warner et al., 2005).
- Polymorphisms are known to exist in many of the genes involved in response to dioxin such as cytochrome P4501A1 (Huang et al., 2002) and the Ah receptor (Chan et al., 2004). DNA isolated from stored whole blood or serum and genotyped would allow the investigation of gene–environment interactions in response to dioxin (Landi et al., 2005).

---

[12]Chapter 4's discussion of obstacles to retaining and maintaining the specimens indicates that there are some analytes that require different methods of handling and preservation than those employed in the AFHS in order to ensure analytic viability. This precludes conducting certain types of tests in the future.

[13]It should be noted that the committee has not researched in-depth whether these could feasibly be applied to the AFHS specimens.

• There is limited data on oxidative stress biomarkers over time. Sera and urine samples could be used for studies that investigate changes in these biomarkers, polymorphisms in oxidative stress genes, and their relation to disease outcome (Lenaz et al., 1999; Shertzer et al., 2004).
• Sperm samples could be used for analysis of DNA adducts and possible levels of environmental chemicals (Horak et al., 2003).
• Serum inflammatory markers and polymorphisms in inflammation-related genes can be studied in relation to several psychiatric illnesses (Kahl et al., 2006).
• Although highly susceptible to degradation, RNA can be extracted from whole blood and sera stored at –80°C using polymerase chain reaction (PCR) methods (Paoli, 2005) to explore the progression to cancer, diabetes, or other diseases in relation to dioxin and other factors (M.T. Landi, National Cancer Institute, personal communication, April 16, 2005).

Many of these newer technologies have very small sample requirements, making them applicable to the AFHS repository. As biospecimen analysis technology and science are rapidly evolving, more opportunities are likely to become available in the coming years. Additional considerations in the future use of specimens, including consent issues, are discussed in Chapter 6.

Although the AFHS specimen collection may be physically amenable to newly developed analytical technologies, the application of stored specimens to research interests in disciplines such as disease pathology, epidemiology, and genetics is firmly anchored to the existence of and quality of the associated subject records. Therefore, although pertinent aspects concerning the disposition of various AFHS resources are addressed separately in this report, the value of the collective AFHS resource (biomaterial and data holdings) exceeds the value of the sum of its component parts.

The Study's Period of Analysis Can Be Expanded Through Follow-Up of the Cohorts Using Publicly-Available Information

When the AFHS was originally designed, the investigators as well as various reviewers felt that 20 years of follow-up would be adequate to document major adverse effects of wartime exposure to herbicides (AFHS, 1982). However this time period may be insufficient to detect effects that may take several decades to develop. The average subject age at the first examination cycle in 1982 was about 44 years; in 2005 it is approximately 67. Chronic diseases are occurring more often among study participants and mortality has increased as the population has aged.

The latest AFHS mortality update (Ketchum and Michalek, 2005) reported an elevated relative risk for all-cause mortality among all Ranch Hand veterans and a statistically significant increase in the risk of death from circulatory system diseases among veterans with the highest serum dioxin levels. If confirmed by further follow-up, these trends could have implications for health monitoring of the study's participants and possibly for compensation decisions regarding Vietnam veterans in general.

Appendix D of this report presents a calculation of the expected number of deaths over the next 10 years among the participants of the morbidity study. These calculations were made under the assumption that statistical bias was not present. Whether or not such bias will be an issue in any future analyses will depend on the outcome being examined and the characteristics of the population for whom data are available.[14] The rough estimates presented in the appendix suggest that, even in analyses limited to the subjects who participated in one or more cycle exams, the AFHS cohort is large enough to detect moderate to large associations in future mortality analyses of health outcomes of potential interest to Vietnam veterans.

The vital status of the AFHS cohort can be updated periodically without too much difficulty or expense using the National Death Index (NDI). The NDI (2005) provides information on underlying and contributing causes of death, coded to various revisions of the International Classification for Diseases (ICD), so that continuing follow-up of the cohort can be carried out expeditiously. It should be noted, though, that there are inherent limitations regarding the accuracy of certain underlying causes of death reports in the NDI—particularly, noncancer outcomes.

It may also be possible to follow up on other endpoints through the use of administrative databases—for example, examining cancer incidence through record linkage with U.S. state tumor registries or hospital discharges through Medicare and private insurance health plans. However, such work would be more difficult because there is no central data source comparable to the NDI. The committee did not investigate this in detail, but the feasibility of this approach depends, among other factors, on the extent to which subjects reside in states where there are cancer registries and whether they participate in a federal or private health provider program that systematically collects relevant information.

Nevertheless, data acquisition using administrative databases in future years could increase the statistical power of analyses for some outcomes that have been identified as being possibly related to exposure to herbicides or dioxin. Other outcomes related to the health of veterans and new questions regarding aging in the population could also be explored.

Additional Follow-Up of Health Outcomes in AFHS Participants Can Be Carried Out

There are several mechanisms for acquiring additional morbidity data on AFHS participants if a decision is made to actively maintain the cohort. New

[14]Selection bias, for example, could be a factor if the participation rate of subjects with a particular health outcome depended on their herbicide exposure status.

general physical examinations of the cohort are one means. However, as noted in Chapter 2, these are highly resource-intensive exercises, costing more than $20 million for examinations, specimens' analysis, questionnaire administration, coding, and other database activities in Cycle 6. Epidemiologic studies of other cohorts, including veterans' cohorts, have used more focused data gathering. These include surveys conducted by mail, phone, or on the World Wide Web (with or without independent verification of information through contact with physicians), contracting with local health professionals to administer limited physical exams, and establishing central sites for examinations in cohort population centers or at events where groups of participants gather, such as veterans service organization annual meetings. Such data collection could involve the entire cohort or subgroups with particular characteristics of interest to the researchers (only veterans with a confirmed polyneuropathy, for example).

The range of such studies is limited only by the initiative and imagination of potential investigators and their ability to identify funds to conduct the work. For example, one association that has been found in the AFHS is a relationship between exposure to Agent Orange and type 2 diabetes. As the incidence of diabetes increases with age, it may be useful to reexamine this association or other age-related health outcomes. Assuming that the number of new cases increases as the study population ages, it will become increasingly more likely that underlying exposure–response patterns will be detected, should they exist. If detected, thorough analysis of such patterns may require the collection of additional data. One cost-effective method to gather simple, yet substantial, additional data would be to administer questionnaires to living subjects and surrogate respondents to obtain physician diagnoses and treatments administered, notably antiglycemic therapies. This kind of questionnaire follow-up also reduces the burden placed on unwell subjects to attend complex health evaluation sessions and hence is less likely to be subject to differential participation due to health status. Other postservice influences could be investigated as well, including diet (which was surveyed in the Cycle 4 questionnaire) and occupational and leisure activities (which would serve as indicators of sedentary and active lifestyles).

A major strength of the AFHS is its longitudinal component and therefore investigations of associations with outcomes such as diabetes across time can provide some picture as to whether drop outs are influencing study results. The committee believes that the data in this study are probably sufficient to evaluate selection bias through various sensitivity analyses.

Any further collection of data would entail establishing a mechanism for contacting study subjects in a manner that would be respectful of their privacy and of ethical and legal constraints.[15] Chapter 6 touches on this issue in the context of the committee's discussions of options for further study and consent issues.

---

[15]Goldberg et al. (2002) describe one such mechanism that is in place for gathering data from participants in the Vietnam Era Twins Registry.

There is very little scientific literature on the long-term effects of herbicide or dioxin exposure so any further follow-up of the cohort—if pursued—would add to the medical knowledge base on this topic, whether or not specific health impacts were identified.

PRIVACY AND SECURITY CONCERNS RELATED TO THE RETENTION AND MAINTAINANCE OF THE AFHS DATA ASSETS

As noted in the interim letter report (IOM, 2005b) and Chapters 3 and 4, the committee has concluded that the present state of the documentation and organization of the AFHS medical records, other study data, and laboratory specimens is an obstacle to retaining and maintaining these materials after the currently scheduled termination date of the study. Several recommendations intended to address these obstacles were offered. The committee was also charged with evaluating whether the retention and maintenance of these assets raise any "privacy concerns." It interpreted this component of the charge to cover what the public health and research communities generally refer to as *ethical, legal, and social issues* (ELSI) considerations.

Any disposition of the resources of the AFHS must address the related but distinct requirements of privacy, confidentiality, and security. Though often used interchangeably, these terms have distinct legal and ethical meanings as they relate to health information (Hodge, 2004). Health information *privacy* refers to an individual's right to control the acquisition, uses, or disclosures of his or her identifiable health data. *Confidentiality*, which is closely related, refers to the obligations of those who receive information to respect the privacy interests of those to which the data relate. In a legal sense, duties of confidentiality arise from specific relationships (e.g., doctor and patient, or researcher and subject). From an ethical perspective, health information privacy rights (grounded in individual autonomy) include a corresponding duty of confidentiality that others must adhere. *Security* is altogether different. It refers to technological or administrative safeguards or tools to protect identifiable health data from unwarranted access or disclosure. Maintaining information security is becoming increasingly complex in the modern era of digitized exchanges of health information within a national electronic information infrastructure (Hodge et al., 1999). To the committee's knowledge, there have been no breaches of security in the AFHS.

Once the study reaches its scheduled end date of September 30, 2006, there are three possible destinies for its data assets: destruction, retention by the AFHS as part of an extension of the study, or transfer to some other custodian(s). Proper destruction of the data or samples would eliminate further privacy, confidentiality, and security concerns; transferring these resources to one or more new custodians would pose challenges and raise questions regarding the informed consent of the participants. The committee believes such ELSI considerations must play a central role in decisions regarding the future disposition of the AFHS; it does not, however, believe that any would necessarily prevent further study. ELSI considerations thus are addressed in Chapter 6 in the context of the committee's recommendations for further study.

CONCLUSIONS AND OBSERVATIONS

On the basis of its review of AFHS reports, its site visit to the study facility, the scientific literature, and other information presented in this and previous chapters, the committee has reached the following conclusion:

> There is scientific merit in retaining and maintaining the medical records, other study data, and laboratory specimens collected in the course of the Air Force Health Study after the study's currently scheduled termination date.

Although it was not part of its evaluation of their scientific merit, the committee notes that the AFHS data assets were obtained at a considerable cost to the government and represent a substantial investment in time and dedication by the study's subjects. Of course, past investment in a project does not justify future investment in it. The committee believes, though, that it is important to acknowledge that such great expenditures of taxpayer funds and participants' effort should not be treated casually, especially when it is possible to derive additional societal benefit from them.

The committee further concludes that:

> Privacy concerns and related ethical, legal, and social issues are not an intrinsic obstacle to retaining and maintaining the AFHS medical records, other study data, and laboratory specimens after the currently scheduled termination date of the study. However, attention to such concerns and issues must play a central role in decisions regarding the future disposition of these data assets.

As there is scientific merit in retaining and maintaining these assets and the committee believes that the identified obstacles are surmountable, the committee concludes that:

> Further study of the AFHS medical records, other study data, and laboratory specimens is advisable. The potential value and relevance of extending the study of the AFHS data assets rests in the application of the results of future research on the assets. This research could encompass:
>
> • reanalysis of the herbicide or dioxin exposures and health outcomes examined by the AFHS using different assumptions and approaches than have been applied to date;
>
> • new analyses of the medical records and other study data that examine questions that were not addressed in the AFHS;
>
> • new studies of the collected biospecimens that take advantage of advances in technology and science to conduct analyses that were not contemplated in the AFHS protocol;

- expansion of the study's period of analysis through follow-up of the cohorts using publicly available information; and
- additional follow-up of health outcomes in AFHS participants.

As already noted in Chapters 2 and 3, the AFHS dataset has several weaknesses that may limit its utility as a means of evaluating the health impacts of exposure to Agent Orange. These include the inherently small size of the cohort, lack of any biomarkers of herbicide exposure other than 2,3,7,8-TCDD, little information on subjects' locations in-theater, unavailability of a detailed exposure history, and possible herbicide exposures in the comparison population. The reproductive outcomes and mortality-only components of the study have larger sample populations but far less detailed data on the subjects. It would thus be a mistake to view the committee's conclusions here as an indication that the AFHS data assets are a definitive source of information on the topic of Vietnam veterans' health—they are not. Instead, the data and specimens are pieces of evidence that can be put to use in the effort to understand the determinants of good and ill health in Vietnam veterans and to address other scientific questions.

REFERENCES

AFHS (Air Force Health Study). 1982. *An Epidemiologic Investigation of Health Effects in Air Force Personnel Following Exposure to Herbicides: Study Protocol, Initial Report.* Brooks AFB, TX: USAF School of Aerospace Medicine. SAM-TR-82-44.

AFHS. 1987. *An Epidemiologic Investigation of Health Effects in Air Force Personnel Following Exposure to Herbicides. First Follow-up Examination Results.* 2 vols. Brooks AFB, TX: USAF School of Aerospace Medicine. USAFSAM-TR-87-27.

AFHS. 2005. *An Epidemiologic Investigation of Health Effects in Air Force Personnel Following Exposure to Herbicides. 2002 Followup Examination Results.* Brooks AFB, TX: Epidemiologic Research Division. Armstrong Laboratory. AFRL-HE-BR-SR-2005-0003.

AFIP (Armed Forces Institute of Pathology). 2005. *National Pathology Repository.* [Online]. Available: http://www.afip.org/Departments/repository/npr.html [accessed Nov. 9, 2005].

Aylward LL, Brunet RC, Carrier G, Hays SM, Cushing CA, Needham LL, Patterson DG Jr, Gerthoux PM, Brambilla P, Mocarelli P. 2005. Concentration-dependent TCDD elimination kinetics in humans: toxicokinetic modeling for moderately to highly exposed adults from Seveso, Italy, and Vienna, Austria, and impact on dose estimates for the NIOSH cohort. *Journal of Exposure Analysis and Environmental Epidemiology* 15:51–65.

Bell B, Rose CL, Damon A. 1972. The Normative Aging Study: An interdisciplinary and longitudinal study of health and age. *Aging and Human Development* 3:5–17.

Bossé R, Spiro A III. 1995. The Normative Aging Study. In Maddox G, ed. *Encyclopedia of Aging.* 2nd ed. New York: Springer Press. Pp. 688–690.

Caudill SP, Pirkle JL, Michalek JE. 1992. Effects of measurement error on estimating biological half-life. *Journal of Exposure Analysis and Environmental Epidemiology* 2:463–476.

Chan CY, Kim PM, Winn LM. 2004. TCDD-induced homologous recombination: the role of the Ah receptor versus oxidative DNA damage. *Mutation Research* 563(1):71–79.

Chen R, Pan S, Brentnall TA, Aebersold R. 2005. Proteomic profiling of pancreatic cancer for biomarker discovery. *Molecular and Cellular Proteomics* 4(4):523–533.

Chou PH, Chen SH, Liao HK, Lin PC, Her GR, Lai AC, Chen JH, Lin CC, Chen YJ. 2005. Nanoprobe-based affinity mass spectrometry for selected protein profiling in human plasma. *Analytic Chemistry* 77:5990–5997.

Coriell Institute for Medical Research. 2005. *Coriell Cell Repositories Overview.* [Online]. Available: http://www.coriell.org/ccr/ccrsumm.html [accessed November 9, 2005].

Domon B, Broder S. 2004. Implications of new proteomics strategies for biology and medicine. *Journal of Proteome Research* 3(2):253–260.

Eiseman E, Haga SB. 1999. *Handbook of Human Tissue Sources: A National Resource of Human Tissue Samples.* RAND Corporation. RAND Document No: MR-954-OSTP. [Online]. Available: http://www.rand.org/publications/MR/MR954/ [accessed October 7, 2005].

Emond C, Michalek JE, Birnbaum LS, DeVito MJ. 2005. Comparison of the use of a physiologically based pharmacokinetic model and a classical pharmacokinetic model for dioxin exposure assessments. *Environmental Health Perspectives* 113(12):1666–1668.

Figeys D. 2003. Proteomics in 2002: a year of technical development and wide-ranging applications. *Analytic Chemistry* 75(12):2891–2905.

Goldberg J, Curran B, Vitek ME, Henderson WG, Boyko EJ. 2002. The Vietnam Era Twin Registry. *Twin Research* 5(5):476–481.

Henderson WG, Eisen S, Goldberg J, True WR, Barnes JE, Vitek ME. 1990. The Vietnam Era Twin Registry: a resource for medical research. *Public Health Reports* 105(4):368–373.

Henriksen GL, Ketchum NS, Michalek JE, Swaby JA. 1997. Serum dioxin and diabetes mellitus in veterans of Operation Ranch Hand. *Epidemiology* 8(3):252–258.

Hirsch LR, Jackson JB, Lee A, Halas NJ, West JL. 2003. A whole blood immunoassay using gold nanoshells. *Analytic Chemistry* 75(10):2377–2381.

Hodge JG. 2004. Health information privacy and public health. *Journal of Law, Medicine, and Ethics* 31(4):663–671.

Hodge JG, Gostin LO, Jacobson PD. 1999. Legal issues concerning electronic health information: privacy, quality, and liability. *Journal of the American Medical Association* 2829(15):1466–1471.

Horak S, Polanska J, Widlak P. 2003. Bulky DNA adducts in human sperm: relationship with fertility, semen quality, smoking, and environmental factors. *Mutation Research/Genetic Research Toxicology and Environmental Mutagenesis* 537(1):53–65.

Huang P, Ceccatelli S, Håkansson H, Grandison L, Rannug A. 2002. Constitutive and TCDD-induced expression of Ah receptor-responsive genes in the pituitary. *Neurotoxicology* 23(6):783–793.

IOM (Institute of Medicine). 1994. *Veterans and Agent Orange: Health Effects of Herbicides Used in Vietnam.* Washington, DC: National Academy Press.

IOM. 1996. *Veterans and Agent Orange: Update 1996.* Washington, DC: National Academy Press.

IOM. 1999. *Veterans and Agent Orange: Update 1998.* Washington, DC: National Academy Press.

IOM. 2000. *Veterans and Agent Orange: Herbicide/Dioxin Exposure and Type 2 Diabetes.* Washington, DC: National Academy Press.

IOM. 2001. *Veterans and Agent Orange: Update 2000.* Washington, DC: National Academy Press.

IOM. 2003. *Veterans and Agent Orange: Update 2002.* Washington, DC: The National Academies Press.

IOM. 2005a. *Veterans and Agent Orange: Update 2004.* Washington, DC: The National Academies Press.

IOM. 2005b. *Disposition of the Air Force Health Study—Interim Letter Report.* Washington, DC: The National Academies Press. [Online]. Available: http://www.nap.edu/catalog/11483.html [accessed December 1, 2005].

Kahl KG, Bens S, Ziegler K, Rudolf S, Dibbelt L, Kordon A, Schweiger U. 2006. Cortisol, the cortisol-dehydroepiandrosterone ratio, and pro-inflammatory cytokines in patients with current major depressive disorder comorbid with borderline personality disorder. *Biological Psychiatry* 59(7)667–671.

Kang HK, Dalager NA, Needham LL, Patterson DG Jr, Matanoski GM, Kanchanaraksa S, Lees PS. 2001. U.S. Army Chemical Corps Vietnam Veterans Health Study: preliminary results. *Chemosphere* 43(4–7):943–949.

Kelly RT, Woolley AT. 2005. Microfluidic systems for integrated, high-throughput DNA analysis. *Analytic Chemistry* 77(5):97A–102A.

Ketchum NS, Michalek JE. 2005. Postservice mortality of Air Force veterans occupationally exposed to herbicides during the Vietnam War: 20-year follow-up results. *Military Medicine* 170(5): 406–413.

Kingman A, Albers JW, Arezzo JC, Garabrant DH, Michalek JE. 2005. Amalgam exposure and neurological function. *Neurotoxicology* 26(2):241–255.

Landi MT, Bergen AW, Baccarelli A, Patterson DG Jr, Grassman J, Ter-Minassian M, Mocarelli P, Caporaso N, Masten SA, Pesatori AC, Pittman GS, Bell DA. 2005. CYP1A1 and CYP1B1 genotypes, haplotypes, and TCDD-induced gene expression in subjects from Seveso, Italy. *Toxicology* 14: 207(2):191–202.

Lenaz G, Bovina C, Formiggini G, Castelli GP. 1999. Mitochondria, oxidative stress, and antioxidant defences. *Acta Biochimica Polonica* 46(1):1–21.

Liu Y, Michalek JE, Lian M, Dickerson RL, Frame LT. 2005 (June 10). *Reported Sleep Disorders and Dioxin in Veterans of Operation Ranch Hand.* PowerPoint presentation before the Ranch Hand Advisory Committee, Rockville, MD. [Online]. Available: www.fda.gov/ohrms/dockets/ac/05/slides/2005-4146s1_05_Michalek%20slides.ppt [accessed February 10, 2006].

Longnecker MP, Michalek JE. 2000. Serum dioxin level in relation to diabetes mellitus among Air Force veterans with background levels of exposure. *Epidemiology* 11(1):44–48.

MAVERIC (Massachusetts Veterans Epidemiology Research and Information Center). 2001 (November 10). *MAVERIC Project Detail—Normative Aging Study.* [Online]. Available: http://www.maveric.org/route/maveric/news/readnew.asp?id=27 [accessed October 24, 2005].

Michalek J. 2005. *Air Force Health Study Update; June 10, 2005.* [Online]. Available: http://www.fda.gov/ohrms/dockets/ac/05/slides/2005-4146s1_05_Michalek%20slides.ppt [accessed November 13, 2005].

Michalek JE, Tripathi RC. 1999. Pharmacokinetics of TCDD in veterans of Operation Ranch Hand: 15-year follow-up. *Journal of Toxicology and Environmental Health* 57:369–378.

Michalek JE, Tripathi RC, Caudill SP, Pirkle JL. 1992. Investigation of TCDD half-life heterogeneity in veterans of Operation Ranch Hand. *Journal of Toxicology and Environmental Health* 35:29–38.

Michalek JE, Pirkle JL, Caudill SP, Tripathi RC, Patterson DG Jr, Needham LL. 1996. Pharmacokinetics of TCDD in veterans of Operation Ranch Hand: 10-year follow-up. *Journal of Toxicology and Environmental Health* 47(3):209–220.

Michalek JE, Tripathi RC, Kulkarni PM, Gupta PL, Selvavel K. 1998. Correction for bias introduced by truncation in pharmacokinetic studies of environmental contaminants. *Environmetrics* 9:165–174.

Michalek JE, Pirkle JL, Needham LL, Patterson DG Jr, Caudill S, Tripathi RC, Mocarelli P. 2002. Pharmacokinetics of 2,3,7,8 tetrachlorodibenzo-*p*-dioxin in Seveso adults and veterans of Operation Ranch Hand. *Journal of Exposure Analysis and Environmental Epidemiology* 12:44–53.

NDI (National Death Index). 2005. [Online]. Available: http://www.cdc.gov/nchs/ndi.htm [accessed November 22, 2005].

Paoli DP. 2005. Biobanking in microbiology: from sample collection to epidemiology, diagnosis and research. *FEMS Microbiology Reviews* 29:897–910.

Pavuk M, Michalek JE, Ketchum NS. 2005a. Prostate cancer in US Air Force veterans of the Vietnam War. *Journal of Exposure Analysis and Environmental Epidemiology.* [Online]. Available: http://www.nature.com/jea/journal/vaop/ncurrent/pdf/7500448a.pdf [accessed July 27, 2005].

Pavuk M, Michalek JE, Schecter A, Ketchum NS, Akhtar FZ, Fox KA. 2005b. Did TCDD exposure or service in Southeast Asia increase the risk of cancer in Air Force Vietnam veterans who did not spray Agent Orange? *Journal of Occupational and Environmental Medicine* 47(4):335–342.

Pfizer, Inc. 2005. *Pfizer Health Publications: Pfizer Facts—the health profile of United States Air Force Retirees: 1982–1997.* [Online]. http://www.pfizer.com/pfizer/download/health/pubs_facts_airforce.pdf [accessed January 12, 2006].

Piacitelli L, Marlow D, Fingerhut M, Steenland K, and Sweeney MH. 2000. A retrospective job exposure matrix for estimating exposure to 2,3,7,8-tetrachlorodibenzo-*p*-dioxin. *American Journal of Industrial Medicine* 38(1):28–39.

Pirkle JL, Wolfe WH, Patterson DG, Needham LL, Michalek JE, Miner JC, Peterson MR, Phillips DL. 1989. Estimates of the half-life of 2,3,7,8-tetrachlorodibenzo-*p*-dioxin in Vietnam veterans of Operation Ranch Hand. *Journal of Occupational and Environmental Medicine* 27(2):165–171.

RHAC (Ranch Hand Advisory Committee). 2004. *Certified Verbatim Transcript: Ranch Hand Advisory Committee Meeting, April 30, 2004.* [Online]. Available: http://www.fda.gov/ohrms/dockets/ac/04/transcripts/2004-4041t1.doc [accessed December 4, 2005].

RHAC. 2005. Record of the Proceedings. Ranch Hand Advisory Committee Meeting, Department of Health and Human Services, June 10, 2005, Rockville, Maryland. [Online]. Available: http://www.fda.gov/ohrms/dockets/ac/05/minutes/2005-4146m1.htm [accessed February 10, 2006].

Ryan L, Huang W, Thurston SW, Kelsey KT, Wiencke JK, Christiani DC. 2004. On the use of biomarkers for environmental health research. *Statistical Methods in Medical Research* 13(3): 207–225.

SAIC (Science Applications International Corporation). 2005. *Longitudinal Summary.* [Online]. Available: http://www.fda.gov/ohrms/dockets/ac/05/slides/2005-4146s1_03_SAIC%20Response.pdf [accessed October, 25 2005].

Seattle ERIC (Epidemiologic Research and Information Center). 2005. *Seattle ERIC Home Page.* [Online]. Available: http://www.eric.seattle.med.va.gov/ [accessed October, 24 2005].

Shertzer HG, Clay CD, Genter MB, Chames MC, Schneider SN, Oakley GG, Nebert DW, Dalton TP. 2004. Uncoupling-mediated generation of reactive oxygen by halogenated aromatic hydrocarbons in mouse liver microsomes. *Free Radical Biology and Medicine* 36(5):618–631.

Shevkoplyas SS, Yoshida T, Munn LL, Bitensky MW. 2005. Biomimetic autoseparation of leukocytes from whole blood in a microfluidic device. *Analytic Chemistry* 77(3):933–937.

Srivastava S, Srivastava RG. 2005. Proteomics in the forefront of cancer biomarker discovery. *Journal of Proteome Research* 4(4):1098–1103.

Steenland K, Deddens J, and Piacitelli L. 2001. Risk assessment for 2,3,7,8-tetrachlorodibenzo-*p*-dioxin (TCDD) based on an epidemiologic study. *American Journal of Epidemiology* 154(5): 451–458.

Stellman SD, Stellman JM. 2004. Exposure opportunity models for Agent Orange, dioxin, and other military herbicides used in Vietnam, 1961–1971. *Journal of Exposure Analysis and Environmental Epidemiology* 14(4):354–362.

Stellman JM, Stellman SD, Christian R, Weber T, Tomasallo C. 2003a. The extent and patterns of usage of Agent Orange and other herbicides in Vietnam. *Nature* 422(6933):681–687.

Stellman JM, Stellman SD, Weber T, Tomasallo C, Stellman AB, Christian R. 2003b. A geographic information system for characterizing exposure to Agent Orange and other herbicides in Vietnam. *Environmental Health Perspectives* 111(3):321–328.

Sun G, Kaushal R, Pal P, Wolujewicz M, Smelser D, Cheng H, Lu M, Chakraborty R, Jin L, Deka R. 2005. Whole-genome amplification: relative efficiencies of the current methods. *Legal Medicine* 7(5):279–286.

VA. 2001 (May 8). *Rules Published for VA's Diabetes-Agent Orange Benefits* (press release). [Online]. Available: http://www1.va.gov/pressrel/aodiab01.htm. [accessed February 10, 2006].

Warner M, Eskenazi B, Patterson DG, Clark G, Turner WE, Bonsignore L, Mocarelli P, Gerthoux PM. 2005. Dioxin-like TEQ of women from the Seveso, Italy, area by ID-HRGC/HRMS and CALUX. *Journal of Exposure Analysis and Environmental Epidemiology* 15(4):310–318.

Wolfe WH, Michalek JE, Miner JC, Rahe A, Silva J, Thomas WF, Grubbs WD, Lustik MB, Karrison TG, Roegner RH. 1990. Health status of Air Force Veterans occupationally exposed to herbicides in Vietnam. I. Physical health. *Journal of the American Medical Association* 264(14): 1824–1831.

Wolfe WH, Michalek JE, Miner JC, Pirkle JL, Caudill SP, Needham LL, Patterson DG Jr. 1992. Dioxin half-life in veterans of Operation Ranch Hand. *Organohalogen Compounds* 10: 239–242.

Wolfe WH, Michalek JE, Miner JC, Pirkle JL, Caudill SP, Patterson DG Jr, Needham LL. 1994. Determinants of TCDD half-life in veterans of Operation Ranch Hand. *Journal of Toxicology and Environmental Health* 41(4):481–488.

Wolfe WH, Michalek JE, Miner JC, Rahe AJ, Moore CA, Needham LL, Patterson DG Jr. 1995. Paternal serum dioxin and reproductive outcomes among veterans of Operation Ranch Hand. *Epidemiology* 6(1):17–22.

6

Options and Recommendations for Further Study of the AFHS Data Assets

This final chapter of the report draws on the material presented previously to draw conclusions and recommendations regarding the disposition of the medical records, other study data, and laboratory specimens collected in the course of the Air Force Health Study (AFHS) after its currently scheduled termination date. The charge to the committee set forth a set of interrelated questions to be addressed in relation to future research using the AFHS data assets: in brief, whether—and if so in what form—the study should be extended, whether the data assets should be made available for independent research, and whether—and if so, in what form—independent oversight of these activities should be provided. The committee was also asked to evaluate the potential value and relevance of further research, and its potential cost. Assessing the potential value and relevance of future research is integral to the question of whether there is scientific merit to retaining and maintaining the data assets—this was addressed in Chapter 5. The remaining issues are dealt with here.

In answering these questions, the committee took a broad view of what constituted extension of the AFHS. It thus considered a number of options for the future of the AFHS data assets, including rendering the assets to the National Archives, dissemination of the existing assets by a research entity, continuation of data collection through publicly available sources or from the study subjects, and the extension of the AFHS in its current form.

DISPOSITION OF THE AFHS NONELECTRONIC DATA ASSETS

Hard Copy Records

The AFHS's collection of hard copy originals of cycle physical exam reports and completed questionnaires; the subject' medical, military administrative, and vital status records; research reference materials; and copies of the study's reports and papers take up ~5,350 cubic feet of records storage systems space (AFHS, 2005b). All have been scanned and the images[1] stored in electronic files in Portable Document Format (PDF).

The two primary considerations in evaluating the disposition of the hard copy records are compliance with the Federal Records Act and retention for further research purposes. These are addressed below.

Compliance with Records Retention Requirements

The U.S. Air Force (USAF) has regulations (termed *instructions*) defining records management responsibilities (USAF, 2003) and the proper disposition of records (USAF, 1994). The latter document directs that no records be disposed of "without the specific authority of the Archivist of the United States" (§ 1.1.1) and indicates that "valuable research records" are generally sent to the Archive's Washington National Records Center for evaluation and either transfer to permanent storage or destruction (§ 2.12.2.6).

A threshold issue is thus whether any of the resources of the AFHS are subject to the requirements of the Federal Records Act, which requires agencies to "make and preserve records containing adequate and proper documentation of the . . . decisions, procedures, and essential transactions of the agency . . . designed to furnish the information necessary to protect the legal and financial rights of the Government and of persons directly affected by the agency's activities" (44 USC § 3101). As defined by the Act, records include the following:

> All books, papers, maps, photographs, machine-readable materials, or other documentary materials, regardless of physical form or characteristics, made or received by an agency of the United States Government under Federal law or in connection with the transaction of public business and preserved or appropriate for preservation by that agency or its legitimate successor as evidence of the organization, functions, policies, decisions, procedures, operations, or other activities of the Government or because of the informational value of data in them. (44 USC § 3301)

Using this definition, the biologic specimens collected during the AFHS are not subject to the Act and can be handled pursuant to the recommendations of-

---

[1]The committee was told by AFHS staff that the text in these files is not, in general, searchable.

fered later in this chapter. Because the findings of the AFHS have been a basis for certain disability determinations,[2] an argument can be made that the data and supporting documentary materials created during the study (the medical records) are covered by the Act.

If these resources are records within the statutory definition, the National Archivist must determine whether they "have sufficient administrative, legal, research, or other value to warrant their continued preservation by the Government" (44 USC § 3303a). If not, and the vast majority of materials are not judged worthy of retention, the Archivist may dispose of them following notice in the Federal Register and opportunity to comment. Separately, the AFHS must meet other applicable Department of Defense (DOD) and USAF records retention and disposal requirements.

In the event that the Archivist concludes that the data and supporting documentary materials are records that should be retained, either the original hard copy documents or the PDF copies could be stored (NARA, 2006). Documents stored in the National Archives[3] are subject to the requirements of the Federal Privacy Act of 1974, discussed below, as well as all the protections that were provided in the research protocol (36 CFR § 1228.274).

Committing the records to the National Archives would not preclude using them for research in the future. The Archivist can—again, subject to Privacy Act requirements—make the PDFs, other electronic files, and the hard copy documents available to researchers at one of their facilities or via the World Wide Web. Alternatively, the Archivist can place the materials with another entity within or outside the federal government (44 USC § 2107(3)). The Federal Records Act does not preclude additional copies of the dataset being placed with, used by, or managed by other entities.

Retention for Further Research Purposes

The committee believes the major obstacles to retaining the AFHS hard copy records are the costs to securely store and manage the paper and the possibility that these records may be improperly disclosed to third persons. The committee has not explicitly estimated costs for hard copy records storage, as this varies considerably by location. Further, assuming that the scanned images are of acceptable quality and that sufficient electronic backup procedures will be established to ensure the integrity of these electronic records, the committee does not

[2]AFHS research has been cited in the National Academy of Sciences' Veterans and Agent Orange series reports, which are in turn a source of information used by the Department of Veterans Affairs in making determinations of whether certain health outcomes are service connected for Vietnam veterans.

[3]Formally, the agency is known as the National Archives and Records Administration.

believe that it is necessary to retain hard copy records in order to conduct further research on the AFHS cohort. Modern privacy concerns suggest secure destruction of unnecessary medical records held by government bodies.

Recommendations Regarding the AFHS Hard Copy Records

Given the legal, regulatory, and logistic considerations discussed above, the committee recommends the following:

> **All of the hard copy originals of AFHS documents that have been saved in electronic form should be destroyed unless the National Archivist concludes that these records must be maintained or they are subject to other records retention requirements. No matter what decision is made by the National Archives regarding the retention of the records produced during the AFHS, a separate complete set of electronic copies of these records should be kept for possible placement with another custodian.**

These recommendations are predicated on the assumption that the electronic images (PDFs) accurately represent the hard copy records. The committee was informed that the PDF files were subjected to quality control checks for readability, and that special attention was given to poor quality originals[4] to try to enhance the scanned images (J. Robinson, Air Force Health Study, personal communication, January 10, 2006).

Facilitating Future Use of Other Nonelectronic Assets

The committee's interim letter report (IOM, 2005a) offered several recommendations for organizing and documenting the serum, whole blood, urine, and semen specimens collected by the AFHS that would facilitate their future use. These recommendations are reiterated in Chapter 4 of this report.

There are three other components of the AFHS data collection that are neither in traditional paper nor electronic form: the electrocardiogram (ECG) strips, X-ray films, and Super-VHS (SVHS) video tapes collected during the cycle exams. If there is to be further study of the AFHS data assets, then the committee believes that consideration should be given to taking additional steps to render these assets in a form and format that facilitates their use in the future.

ECG Strips and X-Ray Images

As Chapter 3 notes, 12-lead, scalar, resting ECGs were obtained from subjects during all six physical exam cycles. The ECGs were evaluated and informa-

[4]These include records dating from World War II and those printed on thermofax or other unstable media.

tion regarding various parameters[5] and evidence and type of prior myocardial infarction were coded and placed into the electronic database. There are also over 15,000 X rays, primarily chest films captured during Cycles 2–6.

Chest X rays are objective evidence of lung pathology (at least by one measure), and ECGs serve the analogous function for cardiovascular pathology. Both of these could be important endpoints for herbicide or dioxin exposure, and both are likely to show findings well in advance of symptoms or medical diagnoses. Because these measures are largely standardized, in the sense that chest X rays and ECGs are taken in more or less the same way for everyone and have been for decades, they provide a potentially valuable resource defining preclinical health endpoints that may relate to subjects' exposures. The serial nature of these data provides critical time-point information and allows for the analysis of changes over the 20 years in which data were taken. It also lessens concerns about confounding from intercurrent disease that might affect one cycle of measurements. The X-ray films and ECGs are thus valuable components of the database.

The major obstacles to retaining these materials are the costs to index and store them and the possibility that these records may be inappropriately disclosed to third persons. Means exist for converting paper ECGs to digital format (Badilini et al., 2005; Moody, 2005) but the technologies are not widespread, and the committee cannot offer any observations on their utility or costs. The X-ray films could be housed in a repository, but the committee believes it makes more sense to convert them to digital format: this will allow them to be more compactly stored and more easily made available for research purposes. Conversion is a mature and widely available technology, and the committee estimates that the labor and materials cost to digitize the X-ray films is on the order of $35,000.[6] The cost of proper disposal of the original films may be mitigated through silver recovery.

The committee thus recommends that:

> **All electrocardiogram strips collected in the course of the AFHS should be retained; their documentation should be reviewed and, if needed, supplemented to ensure easy retrieval.**
>
> **All X-ray films collected in the course of the AFHS should be digitized with acceptable quality control, this resource properly documented, and thereafter the original films be disposed of according to standard practices. The digitized records should be retained and handled in accor-**

---

[5]Depending on the exam cycle, these parameters included ST-T, P, U, and Q wave morphology; QRS and QT interval; axis deviation; and evidence of bradycardia, tachycardia, arrhythmia, and abnormal sinus rhythm.

[6]This estimate is based on information provided to the committee by the Vanderbilt University Medical Center Department of Radiology on September 8, 2005, and was calculated as follows: ((5 minutes labor/film × $10.15/hour) + ($1.31 materials/film)) × 15,400 films.

dance with the recommendations for the disposition of the AFHS data assets.

SVHS Video Tapes

There are 3,074 Super-VHS (SVHS) format video tapes in the AFHS data collection, comprising high-resolution images of subjects' teeth taken during the Cycle 4 and 5 exams. The tapes were made as part of a National Institute of Dental and Craniofacial Research (NIDCR) adjunct to the study examining the association between exposure to elemental mercury via dental amalgams and measures of neurologic function (Kingman et al., 2005).

The major obstacles to retaining these records are, again, the costs to index and store them and the possibility that any personal information on the tapes might be disclosed to third persons. The committee does not have any suggestions for future research employing the videos but understands that such material, in combination with other data on the subjects, can be useful in oral epidemiology studies.

As this data asset was gathered under a contract with NIDCR and would be of primary interest to the oral epidemiology community, the committee suggests that the NIDCR be consulted on whether the tapes can be usefully exploited by the research community. If the decision is made to retain them, then their usefulness will depend on their linkage to the rest of the AFHS data assets, and it thus makes sense for them to be a part of the collection. In this circumstance, the SVHS tapes—which are in a little-used and largely-obsolete format—should be digitized and written to a medium such as DVD for ease of long-term storage. The cost of this would be ~$50,000, based on $15/tape for the conversion. Additional costs would be incurred in documenting and indexing the materials.

The committee therefore recommends that:

The AFHS should consult with the National Institute of Dental and Craniofacial Research on whether the video tapes of subjects' teeth collected in the course of the study have future research value. If the tapes have value for future research, they should be digitized with appropriate quality control, written to an acceptable long-term storage medium, properly documented, and thereafter the original tapes be disposed of according to standard practices. The digitized records, if created, should be retained and handled in accordance with the recommendations for the disposition of the AFHS data assets.

Concluding Remarks Concerning the AFHS Nonelectronic Data Assets

In summary, the committee believes that the (nonbiologic) data assets of the AFHS that are not already in electronic form should be converted to this form where a mature technology exists to do so and where the assets have future research value. Federal regulations addressing the preparation of electronic records for transmittal to the National Archives (36 C.F.R. § 1228.270) contain specific information about file formats and media that are appropriate for long-term storage. These assets must be stored in a manner that ensures their integrity and security, and protects the privacy of study subjects.

ALTERNATIVES FOR THE FUTURE OF THE AFHS DATA ASSETS

This section addresses two closely interrelated issues: the alternatives for administering the AFHS data assets and the parameters of future research using those assets. Five alternatives were identified for administering the assets after the currently scheduled termination date of the study in September 2006. The committee's conclusions on the preferred means for carrying out future research on the assets and the scope of that work—including potential future data gathering—are in turn driven by their consideration of these alternatives.

Alternatives for Administering the AFHS Data Assets

Render the Data Assets to the National Archives for Evaluation and Possible Retention

As noted above, federal law and USAF regulations require that the National Archives make a determination of whether it will retain the data collected in the course of the AFHS. Rendering the assets to the Archives is thus the default option.

In this alternative, any further research on the assets would be dependent on the Archives deciding to preserve the data and make them available to the public—the latter decision subject to applicable privacy and other laws. It could choose to make the data accessible as it has for other epidemiologic datasets in its collection such as the *Hill Air Force Base Study Files* (NARA, 2000) which includes electronically encoded information on the health status of persons whose job at the base exposed them to hazardous substances and potential diseases (Blair et al., 1998). The Archives also holds data from the Vietnam Experience Study (VES), another study that included a medical examination, laboratory tests, and a psychologic evaluation of a cohort of Vietnam veterans. However, the Archives website indicates, without further explanation, that the VES records cannot be released (NARA, 2005).

Privacy considerations might lead to a decision to restrict access to the AFHS data for an extended time period—possibly 75 years or more—intended to ensure that all study subjects are deceased before information on them is made public. Work on any publicly available materials would need to be done without any research support to investigators as the Archives does not provide this service.

The Archives does not maintain biospecimens. A 2001 GAO congressional briefing (GAO, 2001) mentioned that the AFHS was considering transmitting biospecimens to the Armed Forces Institute of Pathology (AFIP), but it is not known whether this option was actively pursued or whether the AFIP would have an interest in the samples.[7] The National Archives sometimes chooses to manage materials through *disposal by donation*, in which case they would be passed on to one or more entities that would assume responsibility for them. The data assets would then presumably be handled in accordance with one of the alternatives below.

This option is separate from the others discussed in this section because it would involve no action on the part of the Congress and no additional funding. The National Archives already has the mission to evaluate—and where appropriate to preserve and make publicly available—documents and materials created in the course of business conducted by the United States federal government. It does not, however, have exclusive rights to the data. No matter what the Archives decides, copies of the data can be made available through other channels.

Identify or Establish a Research Entity for Dissemination of Existing Data Assets

This alternative would require a research entity with the funding and mission to carry out responsible management of the assets. Management responsibilities would include the ability to securely store materials, to conduct or manage the appropriate review of requests for data access, and ensure that subjects' privacy was maintained. It could also include aiding investigators in understanding and exploiting the assets, collaborating with outside investigators, and preparing custom data sets for analysis by those researchers.

Specimens could be disposed of, maintained by the research entity, or stored by a separate entity. It should be noted, however, that the specimens have little value without the detailed medical and questionnaire data collected. Access and linkage to subjects' data are thus necessary components to the retention of the specimens.

Identify or Establish a Research Entity to Continue Passive Data Collection on AFHS Subjects

Under this alternative, the activities described above would be expanded to include the collection of data on the AFHS morbidity or mortality cohort through publicly available sources such as the National Death Index. Such work could

[7]It should also be noted that the AFIP was slated for closure as part of the DOD Base Realignment and Closure 2005 initiative (Kaiser, 2005). It is unclear how the specimens in its collection would be affected by this.

take place under one or both of two circumstances. It could be part of an explicit research project conducted by the entity holding the existing data assets. Alternatively or additionally, one-time studies could be pursued by outside investigators.

If the entity holding the data assets were to carry out this work, there would be the need for a specific research plan with a data manager or principal investigator and some assurance of research funding for the period covered by the plan. An outside investigator could carry out the same work, although there would be no assurance that data would be collected systematically or consistently over time.

Identify or Establish a Research Entity to Maintain Contact with the AFHS Subjects and Conduct or Facilitate Further Active Data Collection

This alternative would extend the passive data collection option above to also encompass active following of and contact with AFHS cohort participants. Active administration of an epidemiologic cohort entails far more effort and cost than the previously identified options. It would require regular communication with study subjects to ensure that contact information remained current and to ensure that they were vested members of the research team.

Active data collection could take many forms, including questionnaires seeking self-reported health or sociodemographic data, or ascertaining vital status from all or parts of the cohort; as well as conducting limited physical examinations of subjects. New tests results could be obtained and medical imagery or specimens could be collected. Data gathering could be accomplished through outside investigator initiatives or through an explicit research plan carried out by the entity responsible for holding the assets.

Extend the AFHS

Extension of the AFHS would entail a decision by Congress to provide funds to continue the administration of periodic, extensive data and biospecimen gathering through cohort-wide physical examinations and questionnaires. Support for a dedicated staff to maintain contact with the cohort and manage and analyze these data assets would also be required. This alternative could be accomplished with the existing AFHS infrastructure or by assigning responsibility and funding to some other entity.

Parameters of Future Research on the AFHS Data Assets

Means of Carrying out Future Research on the Data Assets

There are two means of carrying out any of the research options listed above: through the work of a dedicated research staff, as the AFHS is currently conducted; or via a custodian that makes the assets available to independent researchers. The committee believes that the second of these options is more desirable because it taps the creativity, expertise, and motivation of the entire research community to pursue promising applications. This custodian should not act as a passive repository of the data but should play an active role in fostering its use. Such activities should at minimum include collaboration with outside researchers to ensure the assets are used effectively and with proper respect for the participants. Depending on the scope of future research, the custodian's responsibilities could also include the preparation of restricted datasets or managing interactions between researchers and the study subjects for the collection of new data. Work done on behalf of outside investigators should be compensated, of course—a cost that these parties can factor into their requests for research support. In addition to facilitating the work of others, the persons responsible for managing the assets may also seek funding for their own research on them.

Scope of Future Research on the Data Assets

Developing a future research agenda or setting research priorities for the AFHS data assets is beyond the charge of the committee. However, it is possible to talk about the scope of such work in general terms.

In Chapter 5, the committee indicated that while AFHS analyses focused on the effects of herbicide or dioxin exposure, data were collected on a wide range of potential influences on disease and health status, and that a number of outcomes not addressed in the AFHS reports could potentially be studied with them. Given the nature of the cohort, all studies of the data assets are arguably studies of veterans' health. It may, thus, be more appropriate to view the range of studies possible with the data as a function of how closely they conform to the original intent of the AFHS. Potential studies could be classified, for example, by whether they address the health consequences of wartime exposure to herbicides or dioxin, service in Vietnam, service in the military during the Vietnam era, aging in males, or general health and well-being. A less specific construction might define the Cycle 6 consent form term *military health* and add a category for all other studies.

Depending on the objective of the specific investigation, the AFHS's division of the cohort into Ranch Hand and comparison subjects might or might not be relevant—research might combine the two or only use one of the subcohorts. Other studies might need to identify a different comparison cohort because all of the subjects were in-theater veterans. Researchers conducting work under one of these rubrics would, of course, need to factor the relevant limitations of the cohort.

The committee believes that the issues of military and veterans' health should be paramount in future research but that other applications are also appropriate. Taking a broader view of applications for AFHS data assets will allow the study to generate results that could potentially inform a greater range of VA compensation and health delivery issues—not just those related to wartime exposure to herbicides. It may also allow a better understanding of health issues that can best be explored in a population for whom detailed longitudinal data are available. Other studies using cohorts of veterans have taken this broader view and done so in a manner that respects the study participants. The Normative Aging Study, for example, has recently addressed the relationship between lead exposure and changes in cognition (Weisskopf et al., 2004) and the effects of air pollution on heart rate variability (Park et al., 2005) while the Vietnam Era Twins (VET) Registry database has been used to examine the genetic and dietary influences on nephrolithiasis (Goldfarb et al., 2005) and the links between depression symptoms, hypertension, and heart disease (Scherrer et al., 2003).

The decision on the scope of future research is ultimately in the hands of the participants who contributed the data—their informed consents will define the span of the work. It is important, then, that the consent request clearly communicate the options and what research might flow from them—a topic that is addressed below.

Future Data Gathering

The AFHS's current collection of data and specimens is rich and could be a source for studies for several years. However, there are also options for supplementing the collection. One of these is for the custodian to collect or facilitate the collection of data from publicly available sources. Chapter 5 and Appendix D discuss the possibility of expanding the study's period of analysis through a mortality follow-up of the cohorts using the National Death Index and other data sources. Rough estimates presented in the appendix suggest that, even in analyses limited to the subjects who participated in one or more cycle exams, the AFHS cohort is large enough to detect associations of realistic magnitude in future mortality analyses of health outcomes of potential interest to Vietnam veterans. The information needed to do such work could be obtained for no more than a few thousand dollars.

A second, more detailed level of involvement is to engage in further data gathering from the participants. Questionnaires administered through the mail, over the phone, or even via the web could be used to obtain information from all or from subsets of the cohort. Third parties could be contracted to administer limited physical exams to selected participants via in-home visits, or centralized locations could be used in areas where there were concentrations of subjects.

The committee believes that there is merit is keeping open the possibility of further data gathering, allowing future investigators to consider and pursue the additional avenues of research. As indicated above, compiling publicly available data is relatively straightforward and inexpensive, and serious consideration should be given to pursuing this. It is unclear whether further active data gathering efforts will be practicable—this will depend on whether enough study participants consent to be contacted to make this work worthwhile. The committee already recommends that the future custodian develop and implement strategies for apprising the research subjects about the ways in which their information is used and the scientific discoveries that result. Continuing communication with study subjects will help ensure that up-to-date contact information is available for the cohort for use in any data collection activities.

Conclusions Regarding the Future of the AFHS Data Assets

Given the discussions and findings presented above, the committee has reached the following conclusion:

> It is advisable to extend the study of the AFHS assets by making the database and associated biospecimen collection available for study via a custodian. This custodian should take an active role in fostering research on the assets.

The committee is thus not recommending that the AFHS be extended in its current form as a research study characterized by periodic, cohort-wide data and biospecimen collection, and analysis by a dedicated team of researchers. Instead, the committee believes that the present data assets should be made available to the whole of the research community so that its collective creativity, expertise, and motivation can be tapped. This should be done in a manner that respects the privacy of the study subjects and the confidentiality of their data—a topic that is addressed later in this chapter.

The committee also concludes:

> It is advisable to allow for the possibility of collecting additional data and specimens, work that could be conducted by the custodian or by independent researchers.

The committee does not explicitly endorse the collection of further morbidity or mortality data but believes that it is appropriate to leave the option open should both the need and support for such work be identified. Developing a future research agenda or setting research priorities is beyond the charge of the committee.

CHARACTERISTICS OF A GOOD CUSTODIAN OF THE AFHS DATA ASSETS

Any future custodian of the AFHS database and biospecimens needs to demonstrate the ability to properly house and manage these assets. It should have the capacity for data management, security, and backup data storage of very large and complex databases. For biospecimens, it should be able to show that these would be stored in appropriate conditions in a secure location. Persons staffing these functions must be trained to understand the importance of privacy, and protocols must be in place to assure compliance with all relevant legal and ethical requirements.

The following sections address the technical; ethical, legal and social issues (ELSI); and other characteristics of a good custodian.

Technical Characteristics of a Good Custodian

A good future custodian of the AFHS research materials must be able to satisfy several operational requirements related to the supervision of and access to the data and biologic materials.

Data Considerations

Data are only useful if used, and investigators are far less likely to pursue research on materials that present high barriers to access. The interim letter report (IOM, 2005a) offered several recommendations for organizing and documenting the AFHS medical records and other study data in ways that facilitates their management. If these are implemented, they will significantly ease the job of any custodian to supervise the data and share it with others.

The database currently resides on two servers—an IBM 580 (Kiowa) and a Compaq ProLiant ML370. Data take up ~525 GB of space on the machines, including operating system and backup files. A new custodian will need to have comparable hardware to store, access, and back up the files. These physical requirements are not unusual or remarkable, and the committee does not believe there is a need to offer specific recommendations regarding them. There are also, however, related considerations that pertain to maintaining the security and privacy of the data. These are addressed below in the discussion of ethical, legal, and related considerations.

Biospecimen Considerations

The utility of the AFHS biospecimens in future research is influenced in part by the availability of evidence that they are being maintained in a manner consistent with current laboratory best practices. At present, they are contained in 21 Revco ultralow temperature freezers (model ULT-2186-5A), each with 20.2 ft^3 (572 liter) capacity; two additional freezers are kept as backup should one of the primary units fail.

The committee recommends that their future custodian either possess or demonstrate the ability to provide the following:

- **A secure facility for –70°C or colder freezers, with controlled access and redundant power supplies (e.g., backup generators). Approximately**

425 ft^3 of freezer capacity is required to contain the AFHS biospecimen collection

- **Established protocols for continuous monitoring of freezer function as well as other quality control/assurance practices for long-term specimen preservation, including appropriate internal audits**
- **Appropriate local and remote alarm systems to ensure the preservation and integrity of specimens**
- **Staff trained to respond to freezer breakdowns, power outages, or other emergencies at any hour**
- **A plan detailing specimen access and residual return policies. This plan should clearly document the entire specimen access application process, including the application review process, decision-making criteria, specimen processing and shipping costs, dissemination of results, and final disposition of specimens.**

The committee also believes that the future custodian will need a mechanism for assessing requests to access these finite resources. This is taken up in a section on the oversight of the future uses of the AFHS data assets below.

Ethical, Legal, and Other Characteristics of a Good Custodian

Although using medical information and biologic samples independently for research each raise ethical, legal, and social issues, the combination of both types of collections into what are now sometimes called *biobanks* is widely acknowledged to be particularly complex (Rothstein and Knoppers, 2005). Proper future management of the AFHS resources will thus pose challenges and it is important to understand not only the safeguards required by the law but also the additional protections warranted by ethical and policy considerations.

In its analysis of such issues, the committee drew upon a variety of perspectives, ranging from legal to ethical and prudential. Legal requirements, such as those of the federal Policy for the Protection of Human Subjects (Common Rule[8]) and the federal Privacy Act, are essential to the disposition of the AFHS assets. Additional privacy standards like the Freedom of Information Act and the Public Health Service Act provide additional guidance for the disclosure of specific information collected or maintained by the federal government. Ethical precepts both underlie legal rules and provide additional guidance regarding the conduct of research.

---

[8]The *Common Rule* is the colloquial name used for the Department of Health and Human Services core regulations concerning IRBs and human-subject protections that form the basis of U.S. federal policy on human-subject protections.

Issues Presented by Collections of Data and Biologic Samples

In 2005, the Committee on the Review of the National Immunization Program's Research Procedures and Data Sharing Program of the Institute of Medicine reviewed mechanisms for sharing data with other investigators. These range from the creation of public use datasets, through the developments of restricted use agreements, to the establishment of limited access data enclaves (IOM, 2005d). As a general rule, in order to protect privacy and confidentiality, the greater the access to the public, the less information can be contained with the dataset. In other words, access is inversely related to utility for research. The immunization program review committee identified several common characteristics governing resource access and use in major data enclaves:

- Researchers must be specific about the variables needed.
- Researchers must justify the need for and relevance of confidential data and state why public data will not suffice.
- Researchers must provide a plan to protect the privacy of the individually identifiable information in the dataset.
- Final proposals must be reviewed for feasibility, relevance to the purpose or mission of the organization, and risk of disclosure of confidential information.
- A responsible person or board oversees a defined proposal review process.
- Institutional Review Board (IRB) approval is required.
- Researchers access data at designated data enclaves.
- Only minimal data analysis assistance, if any, is offered; limited technical assistance is available in the data center.
- Disclosure review for all information taken out of the data enclave is required. (p. 57)

Although not entirely applicable to the current case, these characteristics point to a number of areas that warrant attention if the AFHS resources are to be continued to be used. These include protection of the data and oversight of use.

As Chapter 5 notes, any disposition of the resources of the AFHS must address the related, but distinct requirements of privacy, confidentiality, and security. There are a number of possible future custodians for the resources of the AFHS, including federal agencies, universities, and other nongovernmental research institutions. These entities are subject to different legal rules, the varying requirements of which may be relevant to the ultimate disposition of the AFHS.

A maze of laws affects the protection of privacy and confidentiality of health data held by the federal government for research purposes. These laws include the Freedom of Information Act (FOIA) of 1966, the federal Privacy Act of 1974, and specific provisions of the Public Health Service Act. FOIA (5 U.S.C. § 552 (1988)) requires federal agencies to disclose certain federal government records kept by the executive branch on written request, unless an exemption applies.

FOIA stipulates nine exemptions in which information can be withheld, including, in particular, requests for information from personnel, medical, and other files involving personal privacy. The government may completely withhold such information, or may release the information with any potential identifiers removed or redacted.

The Privacy Act (5 U.S.C. § 552(a) (1988)) applies to any information that is maintained by a federal agency in a system of records.[9] The Privacy Act protects individual privacy by specifying conditions under which an individual's health information can be disclosed without that individual's consent. In all other situations, consent must be obtained before information can be disclosed. The Privacy Act also prohibits the maintenance of identifiable health information by a governmental agency that is not relevant to the agency's purposes, and requires agencies to publish notice about each record system, describing its purposes and identifying disclosures outside the agency. The National Academies' Institute of Medicine is also subject to these provisions when it manages large datasets that have been obtained from other federal agencies (Berkowitz and Santangelo, 1999; IOM, 2005c).

The Public Health Service Act (42 U.S.C.A. § 242) contains specific provisions that protect the privacy of research and other health data. Section 308(d) protects individuals' privacy in research and nonresearch projects and protects institutions in research and nonresearch projects by authorizing the execution of assurances of confidentiality. Section 301(d) protects individuals' privacy in research projects by authorizing the execution of certificates of confidentiality.[10] In combination, these sections provide mechanisms through which public health service agencies can assure research participants and other individuals that the confidentiality of their health data will be protected by restricting others from accessing the data.

Some of the above laws act to protect information, while others permit or even mandate disclosure and use. Which ones apply to any particular collection of information depend to a significant degree on the identity of the custodian. For example, in discussions leading to the creation of the AFHS, USAF leadership vowed to make every effort to protect the participants' information, relying on the Privacy Act (AFHS, 1982). At the same time, the USAF concluded that it was unable to promise absolute protection, recognizing the possibility of requests under FOIA, judicial and other subpoenas, and the risk that medical examinations might uncover conditions that posed a serious risk to the health of the public and would thus have to be reported to appropriate authorities. These sorts of disclo-

---

[9]That is, records under the control of a federal agency from which information is retrieved by an individual's name, an identifying number or symbol, or any other identifying factor.

[10]Such certificates grant a right to researchers to prevent the disclosure of records pursuant to legal processes; subjects do not have the right to invoke the certificate if the researcher fails to do so.

sures may be curtailed through protections like those available through the Public Health Service Act, although the custodian must take specific steps to seek these protections.

If the data were transferred in an identifiable format to a *covered entity* under the Health Insurance Portability and Accountability Act (HIPAA) (Pub. L. No. 104-191, 110 Stat. 1936 (1996)), such as an academic medical center performing covered functions, the privacy and security regulations of the HIPAA Privacy Rule may be implicated. The HIPAA Privacy Rule, which had a compliance date of April 14, 2003, for most covered entities, protects most individually identifiable health information that is created or received by a covered entity (a health plan, health care clearinghouse, or health care provider that conducts transactions electronically, or others performing *covered functions*) (Hodge, 2004). Covered entities are required to establish and adhere to privacy protections including notification of individuals regarding their privacy rights and the use and disclosure of their health information, the implementation of internal privacy policies, and the establishment of administrative, technical, and physical safeguards to protect identifiable health information.

In general, a covered entity may not disclose identifiable health information[11] without individual written authorization outside of standard health care transactions. However, the Privacy Rule provides a few exceptions under which a covered entity may disclose such information. These include broad disclosures for public health purposes (CDC, 2003). The Privacy Rule also expressly excludes three types of research from its coverage: studies done in preparation for research so long as the protected health information is not removed from the institution and is necessary to develop the protocol; studies involving decedents so long as living individuals will not be studied (45 CFR § 164.512(i)); and research involving *limited data sets*, defined as those from which 16 of the 18 identifiers (listed in the Rule) have been removed, so long as the investigator executes a data use agreement (45 CFR § 164.514(e)(1)). The Privacy Rule also allows for waivers of written authorization for research purposes under standards that mimic Common Rule provisions (45 CFR § 164.512(i)). Thus, even under national privacy standards, identifiable health data may be shared for research purposes without individual informed consent under specific circumstances.

Geographic location of the new repository may be important because a number of states have enacted specific privacy laws. Most states have statutory provisions similar to FOIA and the federal Privacy Act that regulate the disclosure of specific health data. However, some states feature comprehensive privacy protections like those set forth in the HIPAA Privacy Rule (Hodge, 2004). States may also feature genetic-specific or other topical privacy laws that apply to tissue samples or genetic information contained in the electronic records (Gostin and

[11]Referred to as *protected health information* or *PHI*.

Hodge, 1999). Thus, the legal implications of any proposed repository would need to be analyzed individually according to federal, state, and even local regulations of the jurisdiction in which it would exist.

The future custodian must also adhere to current standards for data security practices. Modern security requirements developed by the Department of Health and Human Services (DHHS) pursuant to HIPAA (45 CFR Parts 160, 162, and 164) require that covered entities ensure the confidentiality, integrity, and availability of all electronic, identifiable health information; protect against any threats to the security or integrity of such information; and protect against any uses or disclosures of such information not permitted by the Privacy Rule. Specific security standards require development of appropriate electronic or physical safeguards to limit the potential for data theft, inadvertent disclosures, or unlawful acquisitions.

Other Considerations

Different types of AFHS resources present different challenges to efforts to protect privacy and confidentiality and ensure security, although these challenges are not intrinsically different from other large-scale studies. The collection's medical records on paper are interwoven with identifying information that would require considerable effort to remove. Even if such an effort were undertaken, the information would have to be removed piece-by-piece, inherently intruding to some extent on the subjects' privacy. Paper, however, is difficult to search and it is relatively easy to protect such documents from outside intruders. As the committee noted above, modern privacy and security practices indicate that unneeded hard copy records should be disposed of in a manner that prevents the opportunity for unwarranted acquisitions, uses, or disclosures. It therefore recommends that the AFHS paper records be destroyed unless the National Archivist concludes they must be retained.

Electronic records have different liabilities and strengths. Greater effort is required to protect such resources from outside hacking, but much progress has been made in developing strategies to provide the necessary security.[12] The committee noted in its discussion of procedural limitations to retaining the AFHS database (Chapter 3) that the exceptionally large amount of information available on each subject may make it possible for their identities to be determined through triangulation of the data with public sources. It is possible, though, to reduce the opportunity for this by only allowing limited datasets with one-time-use case numbers to be analyzed, or enforcing signed confidentiality agreements. In other circumstances, it may be appropriate not to disclose certain results on the ground that the cell size is so small that it increases the risk to privacy. The National

[12]These include keeping machines with data off of networks or placing them behind firewalls.

Academies reports *Protecting Data Privacy in Health Services Research* (IOM, 2000), *Protecting Participants and Facilitating Social and Behavioral Sciences Research* (NRC, 2003), and *Expanding Access to Research Data: Reconciling Risks and Opportunities* (NRC, 2005) address the topic of privacy protections in greater detail; *Vaccine Safety Research, Data Access, and Public Trust* (IOM, 2005d) contains an extended discussion of the use of enclaves to securely manage data access.

One of the strengths of the AFHS is the availability of biospecimens, which can have identifying information removed. Concerns that DNA is inherently identifiable are misplaced. Although each individual's DNA sequence is unique, no one can be identified simply by examining their genetic makeup. To be identifiable, another known sequence must be available. Nonetheless, it is critical that the biospecimens and medical records be coded in a way that permits information from them to be combined after identifiers are removed.

Recommendations Regarding the Characteristics of a Future Custodian of the AFHS Assets

Given the ethical, legal, and social issue considerations discussed above, the committee recommends:

> **The future custodian of the resources of the AFHS should be able to demonstrate in advance its capacity to protect the privacy and security of the research participants and their data to the greatest extent possible. It should thereafter manage access to the electronic data resources of the AFHS in a manner that accomplishes these goals.**
>
> **The custodian should comply with the information and publication restrictions in Section 308(d) of the Public Health Act and should seek a certificate of confidentiality under Section 301(d) of the Public Health Act.**

CONSENT ISSUES REGARDING FUTURE USES OF THE AFHS DATA ASSETS

Respect for persons is the main ethical principle underlying the requirement of specific informed consent. This concept is particularly salient in the setting of the AFHS where thousands of research participants devoted a great deal of time and underwent significant inconvenience and discomfort to contribute to this study. Their wishes must be considered in deciding whether and how to use these data in future research. Thus, it is important to examine whether the existing consent obtained from the subjects provides an adequate foundation for the relocation and future uses of the AFHS data assets. In the last round of examinations for the AFHS (Cycle 6), the study participants were asked to sign a document containing the following language regarding future use of information and biologic samples that they had provided (AFHS, 2005c):

> **PURPOSE OF THIS CONSENT DOCUMENT**
>
> During the period 1982 to 2002, you have participated in the Air Force Health Study. Since the study is projected to end in October 2006, we would like to know if your data and biologic samples may be used for future research. If you agree, your data and samples may be used for medical research. Research that may be done with your data and samples may not help you personally.
>
> **RISKS/INCONVENIENCES**
>
> The greatest risk to you is the release of information from your study records. However, Privacy Act and laws and regulations governing health studies will protect your privacy.
>
> **ALTERNATIVES/IMPLICATIONS OF YOUR CHOICE**
>
> In the choices below, please indicate your decision regarding the use of your data. No matter what you decide, your decision will not affect your participation in the Air Force Health Study. If you decide now that your samples can [be] used for future research, you can change your mind at any time by contacting the Air Force at (210) 536-2600.
>
> After 30 Sept. 2006, your data and biological samples may
>
> [ ] Be used for Agent Orange research or other military health issues
> [ ] Be used for research relating to only Agent Orange research (*sic*)
> [ ] Not be used for any purpose

Almost all of the participants (94.1 percent of Ranch Hand subjects and 96.9 percent of comparison subjects; 95.8 percent overall) elected the first option, while 2.8 percent (4.1 percent of Ranch Hand subjects and 2 percent of comparison subjects) opted for Agent Orange research only (Michalek, 2005).

This language demonstrates laudable anticipation by the AFHS investigators and the IRB responsible for the study, but it also presents a number of challenges for the potential future uses discussed in this report.[13] The most notable is that even the most permissive option addresses only use for research regarding Agent Orange and other military health issues. The term *military health* is nowhere defined, but even a generous reading probably would not include the full range of future investigations that might be conducted with the resources of the AFHS. Personnel associated with the study offered the opinion that many of the research participants would have chosen to give broader permission had that option been

[13]According to current ethical and regulatory standards, this consent form has a number of other shortcomings as well. It fails to define what is meant by "data and biological samples," which is important since some of these were collected decades ago. The form also does not state that the data and biological samples are personally identifiable and that non-AFHS researchers may have access to the samples and information (as in fact has occurred).

available (Michalek, 2005), which suggests that the subjects, too, understood the consent document to be limited in its scope.

More generally, the last decade has seen an enormous amount of debate regarding the ethical and legal requirements of informed consent for the use of medical information and human biologic materials for research (Clayton et al., 1995; Knoppers et al., 1997; NBAC, 1999; Clayton, 2005; NCI, 2005a). Among the issues that are often addressed in current consent forms are what types of research may be conducted; who is going to hold and have access to these resources; what privacy and security protections are going to be used; under what conditions, if any, individuals may be recontacted either to obtain further consent or to be provided specific health-related results; and the possibility that intellectual property may be developed.[14] None of these matters were addressed in any depth in the consent document that the AFHS research participants received regarding future use.

A topic that has generated a particularly large amount of controversy in recent years is whether research participants should be permitted to provide so-called *blanket consent* for future research uses. The committee feels that the application of the oversight and ELSI provisions recommended in this chapter provide sufficient protection to the interests of research participants to make such broad-based consent ethically permissible. Some members of the National Bioethics Advisory Commission, however, have opined that it was not possible to give meaningful consent for future unspecified uses (NBAC, 1999). Were the new custodian to be subject to the HIPAA Privacy Rule, an argument could be made that authorization for unspecified future research use would be forbidden as a matter of law (45 CFR § 164.508(f)). A number of commentators have urged that the Privacy Rule and the Common Rule be harmonized in this regard (Clayton, 2005; Rothstein and Knoppers, 2005). There is ongoing debate, however, about the reach of the HIPAA Privacy Rule in academic medical centers. These centers often include medical and public health components that perform what the Privacy Rule refers to as *covered functions*. A covered function is "any function the performance of which makes the performer a health plan, a health care provider, or a health care clearinghouse" (NIH, 2004)—providing and seeking electronic reimbursement for medical care, for example. To distinguish between their covered and non-covered (e.g., research) functions, most centers elect to become so-called *hybrid entities* under the Privacy Rule. The practical effect of this status is that only those designated parts of the center performing covered functions are subject to the Privacy Rule (45 C.F.R. § 164.504). Some confusion remains within medical centers as to what may constitute a covered function, and specifically who is responsible (or not) for adhering to the Privacy Rule. Although these issues

[14]The National Cancer Institute (NCI) has posted a model informed consent form for researchers' reference (NCI, 2005b).

are in stages of resolution, such factors may be relevant in identifying a new custodian for the AFHS data assets.

In the course of the AFHS, information was collected about the health status of the research participants' wives, partners, and children. Separate consent needs to be sought from these women and the children who have reached maturity for retaining this information. For children who are not yet capable of providing informed consent, their assent and parental permission should be obtained in accordance with subpart D of the Common Rule.

The committee believes that the optimal course is to obtain new consent for future research that reflects the changes that will occur in the control and possibly the use of the resources of the AFHS. Such an effort would provide a more solid basis for new investigations and honor the significant commitment these research participants have made to this project over the years.

The committee recognizes that timing is a serious problem. The AFHS is likely to end before a new custodian is identified, and participants may understandably be wary of renewing their consent before a new custodian is named. At the same time, it seems at best imprudent to let the current study expire and then have the new custodian approach the participants seemingly out of the blue. Recognizing that complexity can be confusing, the committee recommends the following two part process to ensure a smooth transfer:

Prior to the end of the study, the Air Force Health Study should notify the participants of the following:

- **The study, as currently constituted, is ending.**
- **The assets will be transferred to a successor custodian, the characteristics of which will be described to the extent feasible.**
- **The successor custodian will seek additional informed consent for future research involving identifiable data from the research participants, which will cover the topics enumerated below, prior to conducting any research.**

This notification should offer the participants the opportunity to decide that information and specimens relating to them should not be transferred.

The successor custodian should obtain new informed consent that includes at least the following topics:

- **Their identity.**
- **Notice of the types of participant data and samples that will be maintained by the custodian.**
- **The procedural protections that will be provided for the data and specimens, including access policies, and oversight.**

• The specific privacy and security protections that will protect the data and specimens.

• The types of studies that the participant is willing to have his data and specimens used for.

• Whether the participant is willing to be approached in the future by investigators to seek participation in additional studies, including information regarding notice and recontact criteria.

• Which individual study results the participant will and will not receive.

If health information regarding the wives and children of the AFHS research participants is made available for future research, consent, and where appropriate, parental permission and assent, must be sought from these individuals.

OVERSIGHT OF THE FUTURE USES OF THE AFHS DATA ASSETS

To comply with the Common Rule and ethical precepts, research projects must be scientifically sound: that is, designed so that they can achieve valid results. At the same time, projects should be designed so as to minimize intrusion on the interests of the research participants. Independent oversight of the conduct of a research study and the specific applications to which its data assets are put is a means of assuring that these principles are adhered to.

This section focuses on the committee's charge to evaluate "[t]he advisability of providing independent oversight of the medical records, other study data, and laboratory specimens [and] the mechanism for providing such oversight." The committee concludes that

> Independent oversight of the medical records, other study data, and laboratory specimens collected in the course of the Air Force Health Study is advisable.

Indeed, such oversight is common in the conduct of major epidemiologic studies. The discussion that follows addresses three mechanisms for providing it, via an IRB, an advisory and oversight board, and communications with study's subjects.

The Role of an Institutional Review Board

An IRB is "a specially constituted review body established or designated by an entity to protect the welfare of human subjects recruited to participate in biomedical or behavioral research" (OHRP, 1993). By the authority granted through the DHHS and Food and Drug Administration (FDA) Protection of Human Subjects regulations—45 CFR part 46 [HHS] and 21 CFR parts 50 and 56 [FDA]—IRBs can approve or reject any research activities involving human subjects that are conducted or funded by participating federal agencies. The AFHS has been subject to DOD and USAF regulations regarding research on human subjects. These requirements,[15] which parallel the civilian strictures, are under the aegis of the USAF Office of the Surgeon General's Division of Biomedical Research and Regulatory Compliance (USAF, 2004). The IRB responsible for reviewing and approving AFHS activities is located in the Human Effectiveness Directorate of the Air Force Research Laboratory at Brooks City-Base in Texas.

The committee notes that future IRB review of research on the AFHS data assets is not guaranteed. According to recent guidance from the DHHS Office of Human Research Protections (OHRP), it would be possible to exclude research using the resources of the AFHS for studies beyond those initially contemplated in that project from IRB review so long as the resources were coded to limit the possibility of identification of subjects. Specifically, the guidance states that:

> OHRP does not consider research involving **only** [emphasis original] coded private information or specimens to involve human subjects as defined under 45 CFR 46.102(f) if the following conditions are both met:
>
> (1) the private information or specimens were not collected specifically for the currently proposed research project through an interaction or intervention with living individuals;
>
> and
>
> (2) the investigator(s) cannot readily ascertain the identity of the individual(s) to whom the coded private information or specimens pertain because, for example:
>
> (a) the key to decipher the code is destroyed before the research begins;
>
> (b) the investigators and the holder of the key enter into an agreement prohibiting the release of the key to the investigators under any circumstances, until the individuals are deceased (note that the HHS regulations do not require the IRB to review and approve this agreement);
>
> (c) there are IRB-approved written policies and operating procedures for a repository or data management center that prohibit the release of the key to the investigators under any circumstances, until the individuals are deceased; or
>
> (d) there are other legal requirements prohibiting the release of the key to the investigators, until the individuals are deceased (OHRP, 2004).

Notwithstanding this guidance, which in some ways is more permissive than the requirements of HIPAA, the committee believes that review by an IRB must be required in order to honor the commitments made by these research partici-

---

[15]The requirements include 32 CFR Part 219—*Federal Policy for the Protection of Human Subjects* (the DOD version of the Common Rule) and DODD 3216.2—*Protection of Human Subjects in DoD-Supported Research* (USAF, 2004).

pants and to ensure optimal use of these resources. The committee thus recommends that:

> **The successor custodian of the AFHS data and biospecimens should commit to review of future research involving the assets by an Institutional Review Board constituted in accordance with the Common Rule. This commitment should be a prerequisite to the transfer of the assets.**

The Role of an Advisory and Oversight Board

Currently, the work of the AFHS is overseen by the Ranch Hand Advisory Committee[16] (RHAC), a body constituted in January 1981 to provide independent monitoring and oversight to the epidemiologic studies by the USAF on the Ranch Hand personnel and related research (Coene, 2000). The committee is made up of nine members, one-third of who are nominated by veterans' organizations as specified in the committee's charter (NCTR-FDA, 2001). The mandate of the RHAC expires with the scheduled end of the AFHS in September 2006.

The resources of the AFHS study consist of vast quantities of clinical, lifestyle, and environmental data, as well as biospecimens collected over a 20-year period. The specimens, including repeated serum and urine collections, are both a unique and finite resource. It is increasingly common that advisory and oversight boards are constituted for complex studies where multiple scientists may wish to use the data, particularly those with finite biologic resources. Examples include the advisory bodies for the Nurses' Health Study (NHS, 2002), Health Professionals Follow-up Study (HPFS, 2005), and the Multiethnic/Minority Cohort Study (MMCS, 2005).

An advisory and oversight board would provide several important benefits to the future custodian of the AFHS data assets. It would serve as a gatekeeper to help assure appropriate and scientifically valid use of the materials. Responsibilities in this arena would be to review and approve (or disapprove) study proposals submitted by investigators to utilize the preexisting resources or possibly to collect additional data or biologic samples from study participants. The board would make decisions not only regarding the feasibility, conformity to subjects' consent, and scientific merit of particular proposals, but also, where use of the biologic samples is proposed, whether the quantity of sample to be used is appropriate given the nature of the questions being asked and the finite nature of the resource. For example, any single proposal that would lead to the depletion of a specific type of biologic sample would in all likelihood not be approved even if

[16]The formal name of the body is *The Advisory Committee on Special Studies Relating to the Possible Long-term Health Effects of Phenoxy Herbicides and Contaminants.*

the question posed was generally meritorious.[17] Board members might also suggest additional areas of research that are important and to which the AFHS resources could potentially contribute, hence, helping to maximize the overall scientific contribution of the study.

There is no set formula for determining the proper size, membership, and operation of an advisory and oversight board.[18] The committee suggests that the board's membership should consist of 8–12 established scientists representing a range of appropriate disciplines. Such disciplines would include, for example, experts on herbicide exposure health effects, military health, epidemiology (including molecular epidemiology), biostatistics, and aging. Two lay members, study subjects if possible, should be included to provide insights from the participant and veteran perspectives. The committee does not believe that a federally administered advisory committee like the RHAC is necessary to obtain independent advice on the future conduct of studies of the AFHS data assets and cohort. Other ongoing studies of veterans' health appear to operate in a scientifically sound and objective manner, and with respect for their subjects, without this form of oversight. The salient issue is that such a board operates in a manner that is transparent to the subjects and public, and that outside parties have the opportunity to present information for its consideration.

The committee recommends that:

> **The new custodian of the AFHS data and biospecimens should commit to constituting and maintaining an independent advisory and oversight board to provide guidance on the conduct of future research and to review and evaluate proposals for use of the data and biologic samples. This commitment should be a prerequisite to the transfer of the assets.**

The Role of Communication with Study Subjects

The increasing emphasis on transparency in research reflects the interest of research participants and of the public at large in knowing what is being done and accomplished. The committee has already recommended several steps that promote this transparency. A central one is obtaining new consent from the participants. This will ensure that they know about and agree to the change in the custodian and to any expansion in the use of the AFHS data assets. The committee has also recommended that all future research protocols be reviewed at least by an

---

[17]There would not be the same concerns over depletion for DNA-based studies since, once isolated from the samples, this is a renewable resource.

[18]Experience teaches that large numbers of members dilute a board's effectiveness while increasing the cost and logistic complexity of its operation; this is to be avoided.

IRB and an independent advisory and oversight board, both of which will have public representation.

Additional steps are warranted as well. If a participant chooses to have further communications with the custodian, efforts should be made to inform him about new findings. Among the strategies that can be employed are sending each participant periodic newsletters, making presentations at meetings of or attended by these people, and creating a website with the newsletters as well as links to other information and research publications for those who are interested.

Ongoing communication with the research participants is important for another reason as well. Great controversy exists about whether to reveal individual research results to participants. Both participants and investigators often express interest in this, but research laboratory practices differ from those of clinical laboratories, and people often choose not to get results when the opportunity arises. Informing participants of general research results reconciles much of this tension by enabling the participants to decide with their clinicians about whether to undergo testing in the clinical setting.

Increasingly, custodians of medical information and biologic materials are establishing relationships with lay groups to increase the transparency of the research process and to recognize the interests of research participants in the outcomes of the research (Rothstein, 2005). Such groups can contribute to informing the research participants of new findings and, to that end, some of these custodians provide modest support for the lay bodies. The Coriell Institute for Medical Research, for example, provides up to $1,000 per year to the community advisory groups for the International HapMap Project, which have played a large role in educating their populations (International HapMap Consortium, 2004).

The committee recommends that:

> **The new custodian of the AFHS data and biospecimens should commit to developing and implementing strategies for apprising the research subjects about the ways in which their information is used and the scientific discoveries that result. This commitment should be a prerequisite to the transfer of the assets.**

One of the primary sources of information on the AFHS is the website it maintains, which describes the study and provides links to or summaries of its reports, papers, presentations, testimony, and the like. This site is an important conduit for communication between the AFHS and its study subjects and the general public. The committee thus recommends that:

> **The AFHS website (http://www.brooks.af.mil/AFRL/HED/hedb/default.html) and associated pages, files, and linkages should be maintained by the USAF until such a time that its contents and the responsibility for managing such a site can be turned over to a custodian. After the turnover takes place, the committee recommends that the**

USAF maintain a link to the successor site from the URL(s) of the AFHS website.

The Mechanism for Providing Independent Oversight of Future Research

The sections above thus recommend a three-pronged approach to providing independent oversight for future research using the AFHS data assets: the review of proposals for scientific merit and adherence to ethical, legal, and related considerations by an IRB and, separately, an advisory and oversight board. In addition, the committee recommends that steps be taken to ensure that the research is carried out in a manner transparent to study subjects, through systematic communication of research plans and results.

It is difficult to assess the cost of such oversight. Some entities that conduct research involving human subjects have essentially no-cost access to an IRB through their home institution. Universities do not typically charge nonprofit enterprises or academic researchers for this service. However, in other circumstances fees are assessed. These vary widely depending on several factors such as the location of the institution, if the submission is new or a renewal, or whether a full or expedited review is needed—and the committee cannot offer an estimate of the cost of implementing this recommendation. Investigators budget the cost of IRB review into their proposals where required.

Advisory and oversight boards also differ in their costs, depending on their size, the frequency of their meetings, and the logistics involved in convening them. The estimated annual operating cost of the RHAC, a body organized under the Federal Advisory Committees Act (Pub. L. 92-463) and subject to its requirements, was ~$106,000 in 2001 (NCTR-FDA, 2001). As already noted, the committee does not believe that such an expenditure is needed—or is desirable for budget reasons—in order to obtain independent advice and oversight. Some custodians may already maintain advisory and oversight boards that could take on this responsibility with the appropriate augmentation of their membership for a fraction of the cost of establishing a new body. Communications with study subjects can be done quite inexpensively and at the same time still result in the provision of large amounts of information.

The committee notes that some institutions impose oversight requirements additional to those discussed here: for example, approval of studies using biospecimens by a biologic safety committee.

OPTIONS FOR THE FUTURE MANAGEMENT OF THE AFHS DATA ASSETS

The committee considered seven possible alternatives for future access to and management of AFHS data assets. The alternatives, addressed below, are based on the committee's research into the range of entities administering large epidemiologic databases, workshop presentations, and their own experience as researchers.

Generally speaking, the committee believes that it would be desirable for the future custodian of the AFHS assets to have a demonstrated track record of publishing epidemiologic research on databases that contain large amounts of complex data and associated biospecimens. The organization should also be, or have the capability to be, highly visible to the research community, with a record of attracting interest in and funding for new research initiatives. The committee also believes that the AFHS assets will be best served by an entity that has the management and support of scientific research activities as a core function. An experienced entity will be better able to manage the complex logistic requirements for managing data flow and biospecimen inventories.

Utilize the National Archives Data Management and Distribution Mechanisms

The role of the National Archives in evaluating and possibly storing and disseminating the AFHS data was addressed earlier in this chapter in discussions of records retention requirements and alternatives for future research. The Archives will make its own determination of whether it will retain the data and make it available to researchers upon acquisition or at some point in the future. This determination does not affect the ability of another custodian to hold and disseminate the resources.

The primary advantages of having the National Archives as the custodian of the AFHS data are that they have the mission and—unlike any other potential custodian—the funding to act as a repository. The Archives manages access to other epidemiologic databases, and have legal mandates to protect privacy and provide security for the data. However, it is uncertain whether the Archives will decide to make AFHS data a part of their collection and, even if they do, make it available to the public. The Archives does not provide research support, so investigators would not have the benefit of a consulting or collaborative relationship with the custodian. There is no means for the National Archives to store biospecimens, and this asset would be lost.

Utilize the Existing AFHS Infrastructure

The AFHS has evaluated the parameters of a 5-year extension to the study and developed cost estimates for a number of alternatives, including conducting another full physical exam and analysis cycle; collecting and analyzing participant provided morbidity and mortality data only; performing a morbidity follow-up only; and acting as a data clearinghouse for the existing assets (AFHS, 2005a). The budget projections for these options varied widely. A 5-year continuation of the study as it is presently constituted was anticipated to cost ~$47 million, over $24 million of which were exam-related expenses associated with an outside prime contractor (AFHS, 2005b). Acting as a clearinghouse for the dissemination of data and specimens was estimated to run ~$1.4 million per year in FY 2007 dollars. These expenses appear to reflect the use of dedicated staff and space—that is, 100% of time and overhead. No assumption of a home institution is listed, but this presumably would be at Brooks City-Base in San Antonio, Texas.

Current AFHS staff, if retained for such an extension, would clearly have an advantage over other potential custodians in terms of their familiarity with the data assets and perhaps their rapport with the study subjects. Extending the AFHS would also eliminate or at least simplify consent issues. However, the committee notes that the study has already lost its long-standing principal investigator and that further attrition is likely. The high estimated cost of extending the AFHS and the reported lack of interest by the USAF in conducting epidemiologic studies of veterans (RHAC, 2000) are other significant factors in considering this option.

Utilize DOD Epidemiologic Data Management and Distribution Mechanisms

The DOD and the individual military services conduct a number of epidemiologic studies of personnel and—in some circumstances—civilians involved in support functions. Although most of these address persons on active duty, there is at least one current DOD study other than AFHS that addresses postservice health: the Millennium Cohort Study (MCS), which is following both active duty and postservice health of Army, Navy, and USAF personnel for up to 21 years (MCS, 2005). The study is using questionnaires and linkages to supplemental medical and administrative information as their data-gathering instruments (Gray et al., 2002), one model for further data AFHS cohort data collection. The MCS is being conducted in collaboration with the VA.

AFHS is consistent with the mission of the DOD Center for Deployment Health Research, whose portfolio includes studies of the effects of exposure to pesticides, oil well smoke, and nerve agents (Naval Health Research Center, 2005). The DOD also has experience with large-scale, long-term biologic specimen storage and management. The Department of Defense Serum Repository maintains ~35,000,000 specimens, along with relevant demographic, occupational, and medical information (Army Medical Surveillance Activity, 2005). The AFIP National Pathology Repository "comprises written records and over 50 million microscopic slides, 30 million paraffin tissue blocks, and 12 million preserved wet tissue specimens" (AFIP, 2005).

DOD thus appears to have the capacity to serve as a manager and analyst of the AFHS data assets, and—separately or in addition—function as a repository for the specimens. Debatably, maintenance of these resources falls under the Department's obligation to understand the health consequences of military service. As noted above, though, the USAF has not expressed an interest in continuing to serve as custodian, and the DOD's focus is on those currently in its ranks rather than veterans populations.

Utilize VA or VA-Affiliated Epidemiologic Data Management and Distribution Mechanisms

The U.S. Department of Veterans Affairs (VA) mission—first articulated by Abraham Lincoln during his second inaugural address—is "[t]o care for him who shall have borne the battle and for his widow and his orphan" (VA, 2005b). In partial fulfillment of that mission, the VA carries out or funds a number of epidemiologic studies of veterans' health and well-being. These include[19] an ongoing examination of the health of members of the Army Chemical Corps who were responsible for ground-based herbicide handling and spraying during the Vietnam War (Kang et al., 2001).

Studies are conducted both in-house and by collaborators based in other institutions. In-house research is carried out by the Environmental Epidemiology Service. The service, among other activities, does the following:

> conducts health surveillance of . . . Vietnam veterans and or other veterans exposed to environmental hazards, i.e., phenoxy herbicides . . . [and] creates and maintains unique databases which may lend themselves to research of veterans and promote their use in collaboration with other interested researchers. (VA, 2003)

The VA also maintains three Epidemiologic Research and Information Centers (ERICs) under their Cooperative Studies Program (CSP) whose primary mission is "to enhance VA health care delivery by promoting VA-based population research and to convert those results into a format that [Veterans Health Administration] providers and administrators can apply to improve patient care" (VA, 2005a). Two of the centers[20]—the Massachusetts Veterans Epidemiology Research and Information Center (MAVERIC) and the Seattle Epidemiologic Research and Information Center (Seattle ERIC)—manage data assets that are in some respects similar to AFHS's and make these assets available to independent, outside researchers under controlled circumstances. They are described below.

---

[19]Appendix C cites and summarizes VA epidemiologic studies of Vietnam veterans that were reviewed in the Institute of Medicine's Veterans and Agent Orange series of reports through *Update 2004* (IOM, 2005e).

[20]The other center is the Durham ERIC, which is affiliated with the Duke University School of Medicine and the University of North Carolina School of Public Health. A clinical epidemiology research center, clinical research pharmacy, and health economics resource center are also a part of the CSP (VA, 2005a).

MAVERIC

MAVERIC is a collaboration between the CSP, the VA Boston health care system, and the Boston University and Harvard University schools of medicine and public health. It is the home of the *VA Normative Aging Study*, a continuing longitudinal investigation of the biomedical and psychosocial parameters of normal aging. The study cohort comprises 2,280 initially healthy men from the Boston, Massachusetts area, almost all of whom are veterans of World War II or the Korean War. The investigation began in 1963 and, over most of this time period, participants have been subject to exams every three years. Among the data collected over the course of the study are basic physical examination parameters, serum samples, anthropometric data, information on health behaviors (smoking, alcohol intake, and the like), sociodemographic data, and the results of a number of standardized psychosocial tests (Niaura, 2000). Approximately half of the cohort also participate in a companion investigation of oral health.

MAVERIC identifies itself as "a national resource to foster epidemiologic research in the VA" and "a clearinghouse for VA and non-VA databases [with] the expertise to harvest them for epidemiologic research projects" (MAVERIC, 2005a). Studies must be approved by an IRB and pass scientific review prior to initiation. A MAVERIC collaborator is required to be among the investigators in order to both assure the appropriate use of the data assets and to facilitate access to them. The facility's core laboratory stores ~200,000 specimens from multiple collections—including transferred archived collections—comprising serum, plasma, urine, buffy coats, DNA, and immortalized cell lines (MAVERIC, 2005b). The laboratory also carries out DNA and RNA extraction, genotyping, and other analyses.

Over the more than 40 years of the Normative Aging Study, some 400 papers, book chapters, and books have been generated. A small amount of the study's published research directly addresses military health issues—a study of combat exposure, post-traumatic stress disorder (PTSD) symptoms, and health behaviors as predictors of self-reported physical health, for example (Schnurr and Spiro, 1999). Most, though, deal with general health and aging issues that are relevant to veterans as aging males, including diabetes (Cassano et al., 1992; Lazarus et al., 1998) and coronary heart disease (Todaro et al., 2003; Scott et al., 2004).

Seattle ERIC

Seattle ERIC—a collaboration between VA and the University of Washington—is the home of the *Vietnam-Era Twins (VET) Registry* (Seattle ERIC, 2005). The registry was conceived in the early 1980s as a means of evaluating the long-term effects of wartime service on Vietnam veterans' health. Its cohort consists of 7,369 male–male twin pairs, both of whom served in the military during the Vietnam era (1965–1975) (Goldberg et al., 2002). There have been five data collection initiatives that involved the entire cohort: the initial compilation of information from military records; a survey of combat exposure, physical and mental health, health-related behaviors, and demographic information in 1987; a cardiovascular survey conducted for NIH's National Heart, Lung, and Blood Institute in 1990; a substance abuse and psychiatric disorders survey funded by the National Institute on Drug Abuse in 1993; and a two-page questionnaire focused on male health problems in 1999. There have also been several rounds of data collection using subsets of the cohort, some including clinical or laboratory testing. Since 2003, the registry has required all newly funded projects that involve in-person examinations to seek participants' consent to draw blood and submit it to a DNA repository. They estimate that this effort will accumulate DNA specimens on approximately 1,000 twin pairs by 2008.

The registry database and cohort are in demand by researchers because of the value of twins in epidemiologic studies.[21] Strict protocols are applied to protect participants' privacy and confidentiality. Investigators seeking access must have their own source(s) of funding and their proposals reviewed by registry staff, a scientific advisory committee, and an IRB. No direct access to participants is allowed: if contact is required for data-gathering purposes, it must be managed through either the registry or an approved third-party contractor, and identifying information must be destroyed after use. Registry policy also requires a respite period between contacts with the participants. Collected data are integrated into the database for possible future use in other studies.

Several studies of Vietnam War combat exposure and PTSD have been conducted using the cohort (Koenen et al., 2003, 2005; Roy-Byrne et al., 2004). Other research has examined Vietnam veteran status and insomnia (McCarren et al., 1994), self-reported health status (Eisen et al., 1991), and alcohol consumption (Richards et al., 1990). A study of the health effects of wartime exposure to herbicides was contemplated in the 1980s but was not carried out (Goldberg et al., 2002). There have also been several studies related to more general male health and aging issues.

Issues Regarding VA and VA-Affiliated Epidemiologic Data Management and Distribution Mechanisms

The VA Epidemiologic Research and Information Centers—both the existing ERICs and the general ERIC concept—have several attributes that are desirable in a future custodian of the AFHS data assets. The centers have mechanisms in place for the collection, management, analysis, and dissemination of veterans' health data. Funding mechanisms to support their work are established. As VA

[21]Studies of twins—in particular, monozygotic ("identical") twins—facilitate the separation of genetic factors from environmental and other influences.

collaborators, they have the mission to address veterans' health issues; however, they do so outside of the functional control of that agency. MAVERIC and Seattle ERIC have track records for successfully maintaining subject's privacy and confidentiality; managing contacts with their veterans cohorts; providing data to and collaborating with outside investigators; and yielding peer-reviewed scientific publications. Both maintain biospecimens as part of their collections.

However, it is uncertain whether the VA would want to establish a new ERIC or whether the existing centers would be interested in taking on responsibility for the AFHS data assets. Unless appropriate support—including start-up costs if a new center were to be established—was provided by Congress, transferring responsibility would divert funds from other, vital research efforts that are being carried out by the VA.

Utilize NIH/CDC Epidemiologic Data Management and Distribution Mechanisms

The National Center for Health Statistics (NCHS) of the Centers for Disease Control and Prevention (CDC) and several institutes of the National Institutes of Health (NIH) manage access to epidemiologic data and specimen collections as part of their missions. NCHS's National Health and Nutrition Examination Survey (NHANES), for example, is a large database of linked data and biospecimens (serum and urine) made available to researchers (NCHS, 2005a,b).

One means used to manage this dissemination is the Research Data Center[22] (RDC) (NCHS, 2005c). The RDC was established "to provide a mechanism whereby researchers can access detailed data files in a secure environment, without jeopardizing the confidentiality of respondents" (CDC, 2004). It is a form of a *data enclave*. A 2005 IOM report summarized access procedures at such enclaves as follows:

> To access data at a data enclave, researchers submit a proposal outlining their proposed study and describing why confidential or sensitive data not available in other ways are needed. Researchers conduct their analyses at the data enclave, and all output must be reviewed for the risk of disclosure before it can leave the data enclave. (IOM, 2005d)

Appendix E contains a table outlining the operation of five large enclaves in the NIH and elsewhere that is reproduced from that 2005 report. Included is information on how the application for data access is made, confidentiality protection measures, proposal review, costs and fees, and availability of assistance from program staff. This table illustrates the major considerations that go into a data dissemination program.

---

[22]The Census Bureau also maintains RDCs to manage access to their voluminous data resources (NRC, 2005).

The AFHS cohort is entering an age range where adverse pulmonary, hepatic, immunologic, cognitive, neurologic, and other outcomes are becoming more common. The detailed information available on subjects' health and personal histories over the past 20 years could thus potentially be of interest to several Institutes. Arguably, the National Institute of Aging (NIA) might be the most compatible of these, as its research programs include the broad range of issues related to "the mechanisms of aging, the processes of aging, aging and the nervous system, and aging in relation to health and disease" (NIA, 2005b). NIA maintains a list of databases of longitudinal studies (NIA, 2005a) and provides funding to researchers to study them.

The cohort's past exposure to herbicides and experience as veterans does not present a barrier to studies of them via NIH or CDC research channels,[23] and these bodies have considerable experience in managing, analyzing, and disseminating epidemiologic data and biologic specimens. They are subject to stringent statutory requirements for protecting participants' privacy and confidentiality. The interest of the NIH or CDC in managing the AFHS is uncertain, though, because of the perception of it as a veterans database and the small and unrepresentative (of the general population) nature of the cohort. It is also unclear whether the AFHS subjects would be agreeable to having—as would be inevitable in such a transfer of custodianship—the focus of study of their data change from veterans' health issues to aging, cancer outcomes, or other research areas. As was the case for the VA, transferring responsibility for the assets to the NIH or CDC would divert funding from other, vital research efforts unless appropriate support was provided by Congress.

Utilize the IOM Medical Follow-Up Agency

The IOM's Medical Follow-up Agency (MFUA) conducts epidemiologic studies of military and veterans health under DOD, VA, and other federal sponsorship. MFUA focuses on records-based research—primarily retrospective cohort studies of morbidity outcomes and mortality. Studies are subject to a multilayered review and oversight process. Proposals are subject to internal approval and IRB review; an advisory panel (drawn from a standing board of senior medical, epidemiology, and public health researchers) oversees the conduct of the major studies; and the final product(s) are subject to scientific review before publication. IOM maintains a web-based information outlet that provides summary information to the public on study conduct and allows comments to be submitted. During some studies, public meetings are conducted that collect information from

[23]The NIDCR, for example, collaborated with the AFHS in the 1990s in an investigation of the association between exposure to elemental mercury via dental amalgams and measures of neurologic function (Kingman et al., 2005).

outside researchers and stakeholders. Veterans service organizations (VSOs) are advised of studies and results on an informal basis.

MFUA also maintains *The Cohort Catalog*, a collection of data on study populations of former military personnel (MFUA, 2005). The catalog comprised 48 cohorts as of December 2005 that range from the specific (Vietnam War battle-injured Marines who received blood transfusions, plus controls) to the general (all persons admitted to military hospitals from 1941 to 1944).[24] Outside investigators wishing to analyze the data may only do so in collaboration with MFUA researchers, and studies are subject to the approvals, reviews, and oversight delineated above. MFUA does not maintain any biospecimens collections but collaborates with federal agencies and universities that do. One cohort in their catalog[25] has an associated serum collection that is housed at an academic institution, and these assets have been jointly analyzed (Seeff et al., 2000).

Although it is not an agency of the federal government, MFUA has been granted some privileges that are typically available only to such entities. It is designated as a "routine user" of military medical and personnel records, allowing it more ready access to these materials. Additionally, MFUA operates an office at the National Personnel Records Center in St. Louis, Missouri, to facilitate research involving materials in the National Archives' primary repository for service, health, and medical information on discharged and deceased veterans.

Established in 1946, MFUA has produced a number of National Academy of Sciences reports, and written or collaborated in over 460 papers published in the peer-reviewed scientific literature. Its early work consisted primarily of clinical follow-up studies of the aftereffects of injuries and diseases of World War II veterans. Later studies have a broader scope, and include recent reports and papers regarding veterans of other conflicts (Rollison et al., 2004; Wallin et al., 2004; Mathes et al., 2005), biowarfare agents countermeasures (IOM, 2004), and a long-running set of studies of health, behavior, and socioeconomic status of pairs of twins who served in the military (Gurland et al., 2004; Page et al., 2003) derived from data in their twin registry (IOM, 2005b).

Among the alternatives listed here, MFUA is the nongovernmental body with the longest history of veterans' health research. It has proven track records of protecting participants' privacy and confidentiality; managing, analyzing, and disseminating epidemiologic data; and maintaining channels of communication with stakeholders. However, MFUA does not store biologic specimens, so a home and

---

[24]Among the cohorts is the National Academy of Sciences/National Research Council (NAS/NRC) Twin Registry, which consists of 15,924 pairs of white male twins who were born during the period 1917–1927 and who served in the U.S. armed forces. A separate advisory and oversight subcommittee is used to review studies regarding this large and well-documented cohort.

[25]The cohort, designated *R87: Biomarkers*, comprises 9,427 Korean War-era veterans; morbidity and mortality data on the subjects are available.

funding would need to be found for the AFHS collection if it were to be maintained. Because it does not have a federally appropriated or independent funding stream,[26] MFUA could not take responsibility for the assets unless external support was provided.

Identify a New Custodian Through a Competitive Process

The above described options for future access to and management of AFHS data assets all involve designating an existing institution as either the custodian itself or as the parent body for a new custodian established under its aegis. However, one could alternatively open up the management of the data assets to a competitive process wherein universities, nonprofit or private research entities, research consortia, and the like could submit proposals. These would be evaluated according to announced criteria and the strongest candidate chosen to carry the work forward.

Such an approach would permit a high degree of control over the characteristics of the custodian. The request for proposals (RFP) could impose whatever requirements and constraints thought appropriate: for example, the qualifications of the data administrators, what types of research would be allowed, and how the subjects' privacy and confidentiality would be protected.[27] This approach would ensure that a motivated party with an explicit data management plan would assume responsibility. It would, though, require significant planning, time, and costs. A body would need to be designated and funded to write the RFP, circulate it, choose who would review responses, conduct the review, choose the custodian, and perhaps oversee the custodian's operation. A multiyear commitment to supporting the custodian would likely be required in advance to attract candidates to apply. The cost of establishing a new body would likely exceed that of utilizing an already existing entity or means of management. And, the extended period between the end of the AFHS and the beginning of the new custodian's responsibility might weaken the cohesiveness of the cohort and thus result in lowered participation rates.

OBSERVATIONS AND RECOMMENDATIONS REGARDING THE CHOICE OF A FUTURE CUSTODIAN

Decisions by the National Archives regarding the retention of the AFHS materials and their availability to the public under the Archives' auspices are outside the scope of this study. Uncertainties concerning their actions, and their

---

[26]MFUA receives some core funding from DOD and VA, but this is not a guaranteed source of support.

[27]The recommendations contained in this report could serve as a foundation for these requirements.

inability to deal with biologic specimens and provide an infrastructure to facilitate research make the Archives an inappropriate choice as sole future custodian of the AFHS data. It should also be reiterated that the National Archives does not have exclusive rights to the data assets of the AFHS.

Thus, the committee recommended (above) that, no matter what decision is made by the National Archives regarding the retention of the records, a separate complete set of electronic copies of these records should be kept for possible placement with another custodian. Even if the data were to be made publicly available, the committee believes it is unlikely that their research potential would be realized if they were only available from a custodian that neither promoted their use nor supported analysis of them.

The committee found that the AFHS staff has properly maintained the data assets over the course of the study. However, it does not believe that continuation of the study under their custodianship is the best option. There is no assurance that the AFHS staff who are most knowledgeable about the data assets would be a part of a continuing effort and—even if they were—they do not have the experience in administrating a data dissemination effort[28] that other potential custodians do. USAF has not indicated an interest in continuing the work, which addresses a population that is no longer on active duty and exposures that are unlikely to be an issue for future operations. Continuation of work on the cohort via other DOD epidemiologic research channels does not appear to be a strong candidate for these same reasons.

The committee believes that one viable option is to develop a competitive process to identify a new custodian and that institutions that have data enclaves or biobanks—and this includes many universities across the country—may be interested in such an opportunity. The committee is, however, concerned about the logistic difficulties involved in going forward with this process. Such an effort would require Congress—as a first step—to make a commitment to funding the search, designating who would be responsible for carrying it out, and presumably specifying what the parameters of the request for proposals would be. The committee believes that, even with the swiftest action and best intentions, that the effort could not be completed in less than a year and would likely take longer. Any extended gap between the end of the AFHS and the beginning of a new custodianship has the potential to weaken the bond between the subjects and the study, possibly making future work more problematic.

The National Center for Health Statistics of the CDC and the NIH have extensive infrastructures in place to manage the dissemination of epidemiologic data and biospecimens. Statutory constraints and agency practices would ensure that ethical, legal, and social issues in handling the AFHS data assets were taken into account. The major issue in the eyes of the committee is whether there is

[28]As compared to the data analysis operation that they currently conduct.

interest in either side of an agency/subject relationship in going forward. For all of its positive attributes, the AFHS data assets remain a small and highly circumscribed sample, unrepresentative of the population at large. To be sure, there are other datasets that have similar limitations, but AFHS suffers from the two additional disadvantages. It was collected outside of the CDC or NIH, leaving it without a known internal advocate or natural home. And, the database describes a military population.

The committee notes anecdotally that there appears to be reluctance on the part of funding agencies outside of the DOD and VA to support research on military populations, even if that research addresses topics that do not relate directly to the military experience. This reluctance may well result in less interest in and support for future studies of the AFHS database than would otherwise be the case for a cohort for which such detailed information is available. Consent for any change in the primary focus of the study away from Vietnam service or military health engendered by a CDC/NIH custodianship[29] would have to be sought beforehand, as the database would be of little use if a large number of subjects chose not to participate further. If the study subjects were comfortable with any focus change and if a champion for the data assets stepped forward, one of these agencies could be an appropriate home for the data assets.

The VA's ERICs and IOM's MFUA share several positive attributes. MAVERIC, Seattle ERIC, and MFUA all have prior experience in veterans' health studies: collecting and storing epidemiologic data; disseminating it to independent researchers; fostering collaborations with those researchers; maintaining quality control over the studies that use their datasets; and publishing results in the peer-reviewed literature. All have military or veterans health issues as the central focus of their operations, but also conduct other types of studies with their data assets. To the committee's knowledge, none has experienced a breach in their system of protecting subjects' privacy and the security of their data. There are some differences among them. MAVERIC and Seattle ERIC manage biospecimen collections; MFUA cooperates with another institution that maintains a biospecimen collection related to one of their datasets. MFUA is a part of the independent, nongovernmental Institute of Medicine of the U.S. National Academy of Sciences; the ERICs are affiliated with universities and operate under the umbrella of the VA's Cooperative Studies Program.

The committee believes the ERICs—either one of the existing centers or a new one created on the ERIC model—are good candidates for custodianship, and that the IOM's MFUA is also a good candidate. These entities are not, however, without weaknesses.

Although the ERICs are not under the formal control of the VA, there could be stakeholder concerns with VA involvement with a study management mecha-

---

[29]Changing the focus to some other issue would not prevent future studies of Vietnam service or military-related questions by researchers but might serve to discourage them.

nism where the results involve compensation issues related to herbicide exposure, given the very sensitive nature of this topic among veterans. It is also unknown whether or how the AFHS data assets could be integrated into the existing ERICs or whether those entities would welcome the prospect. Establishing a new ERIC to administer the assets would entail start-up costs and uncertainties about the qualifications and experience of the administrators. A new entity would additionally have to establish an identity with funding sources and within the community of scholars.

Because MFUA is not a government entity, it cannot be instructed by the Congress or an agency to take responsibility for the AFHS data assets. Instead, a request would have to be made to and approved by the National Academy of Sciences. There would also be logistic challenges involved in assuming responsibility for the biospecimens as MFUA does not have direct access to a repository. Although management of the specimens could be contracted out to a commercial firm, this would be a relatively expensive option. The alternatives would be finding a collaborating institution willing and able to offer their services at a reduced fee, having a governmental body take responsibility for the specimens, or choosing not to retain them.

A common issue for these entities is a secure source of funding. The committee notes above that assigning responsibility for the assets to a component of the VA without a budget allocation would sap funds in a time of constrained resources, and that MFUA has no independent support that it could use to cover expenses. Cost issues in administrating the data and storing the biospecimens are addressed below.

The committee thus does not believe there is any clearly superior candidate(s) that it can recommend to be the future custodian of the AFHS data assets. The considerations listed above should inform the decision of what entity should take on this responsibility. The charge to the committee did not specify where the authority to make decisions regarding a new custodian will rest, and the committee has not made any assumptions regarding this. It believes that, no matter whom the decision maker is, that party needs to take action expeditiously. If a custodian is not identified prior to the scheduled end of the AFHS, the committee believes that it is incumbent on the USAF—as the custodian of the AFHS research materials—to properly preserve them until a decision is made on their disposition. This will entail expenses as the maintenance of the biospecimens requires a secure and continuously monitored facility and support personal that can respond to equipment failures. The medical records and other study data must also be securely stored.

As the discussion of options shows, there is no one ideal candidate to assume custodianship of the AFHS data assets. All of the alternatives have advantages and disadvantages, and all of the options could be made to work with the appropriate provision of funds, commitment on the part of the new custodian, and application of requirements on the management of the resources.

Therefore, the committee cannot offer a specific recommendation on the federal or nonfederal entity best suited to continue the AFHS, if extended, but has identified a number of options that could be pursued successfully.

COST ISSUES IN EXTENDING STUDY OF THE AFHS DATA ASSETS

The committee was charged with evaluating the potential costs of extending the AFHS and of conducting research on its data assets. Such costs fall into four broad categories:

1. Costs associated with preparing the data assets for use by researchers outside of the AFHS and transferring them to the successor custodian
2. Costs associated with managing the database
3. Costs associated with managing the biospecimen collection
4. Costs associated with conducting research on the data assets

These categories are addressed in turn below. As the committee recommended that the AFHS be extended by making the database and associated biospecimen collection available for study via a custodian, potential costs are considered from this perspective.

If the decision is made to identify a new custodian through a competitive process, additional costs would be incurred in managing this process. The Congress would need to allocate funding to cover these costs, which would depend on which agency or institutional body was assigned the task and how much time was allotted to complete it.

Costs Associated with Preparing the Data Assets for Use by Researchers Outside of the AFHS and Transferring Them to the Successor Custodian

Preparation of the data assets for analysis by researchers outside of the AFHS entails documenting and reorganizing them in a form and format that allows them to be easily understood, evaluated, managed, or analyzed by persons who are not already familiar with them. This topic was addressed in the committee's interim letter report (IOM, 2005a) and in Chapters 3 and 4.

The interim letter report stated that it was difficult to estimate the potential cost of implementing the documentation and reorganization recommendations. These costs would depend on several factors, including the ease with which existing documentation could be adapted to satisfy the recommendations,[30] whether

[30]The committee reviewed a great deal of AFHS electronic and paper material but could not perform a detailed examination of all of it. The difficulty of determining the extent to which appropriate records currently exist underscores the need for the documentation actions it proposes.

the AFHS personnel performed the work themselves or contracted it out, and the amount of time available to accomplish the tasks once the decision was made to undertake them. However, at least some of the actions recommended by the committee were already planned by the AFHS investigators and may be underway. Other work may well fall under existing budget items and should thus not represent an incremental cost to the study. As noted in Chapter 2, the AFHS Fiscal Year 2006 (FY06) budget (DTIC, 2005) includes allocations to perform documentation and organization of the data assets in anticipation of their future disposition. It also includes funds to prepare for and complete turnover of the assets. These activities are contained in the descriptions of two overlapping tasks:

> Continue to process and document examination data and to verify the physical examination database. Continue new medical records coding and verify existing medical records coding. . . . Process and document Cycle 6 examination data to include updating of the participant database. . . . Prepare for project termination and turnover of archives/biological samples to designated agencies. Terminate project in FY06.

> Continue to process and document examination data. Continue archiving previous cycles' examination data and digitize and archive the Cycle 6 data as received. Conduct medical records coding and verification of examination database and Cycles 1 through 6 coding. . . . Prepare for and complete transition or turnover of archives and specimens to designated agencies. Terminate project in FY06.

A total of $3,289,000 was assigned to these and other data analysis and support tasks.[31]

The committee believes that it is incumbent on the USAF, as the current custodian of the AFHS research materials, to ensure their proper documentation and organization. As stated in Chapters 3 and 4, the committee recommended that—if available AFHS program funds are not sufficient to accomplish the documentation and reorganizations actions they elucidated—supplemental funding should be provided to carry out such work in a complete and timely manner. Funding for activities related to the turnover of the database and biospecimen collection to the successor custodian appear to be explicitly covered in the existing AFHS budget. Should that party not be identified by the end of FY06, the USAF's custodial obligations include properly maintaining the assets until they can be turned over.

---

[31]The other tasks specified in the items were support of the annual mortality analysis, conduct of data analyses for journals and reports to Congress, completion of collaborative studies with other institutions, and continued maintenance of the study's local area network.

Costs Associated with Managing the Database

The primary costs of maintaining AFHS's medical records and other study data are associated with storage and handling of the electronic materials. The custodian will need to have or obtain sufficient space on servers to contain at least ~525 GB of files. Software for database management and possibly analysis will be required and a modest amount of file cabinet space needed. If collaborating researchers are allowed direct access to the electronic files, a secure room will be needed for this purpose. There will also be some one-time costs associated with the start of the custodianship, including those connected with transferring files, setting up storage, creating protocols for managing the data, and obtaining new consent from the subjects for the continued use of the materials. Earlier in the chapter, the committee recommended that all of the hard copy records of the AFHS that have been saved in PDF form be destroyed unless the National Archivist concludes that these records must be maintained or they are subject to other records retention requirements. There is no need for the custodian to hold the hard copy versions of these materials.

The primary means for providing data to researchers for studies are to create public use databases, prepare custom data sets for specific research projects, and supply access via a limited access data enclave mechanism. Chapter 3 notes that, for a time in the early 2000's, deidentified data from physical examination Cycles 2–5 were available to the public. However, AFHS later withdrew access, owing to questions over whether the study subjects had given consent for the posting. Explicitly obtaining such consent would allow relatively limited amounts of data to be freely available for research without the need for staff time after the datasets and associated documentation were created. The limitations imposed by the need to protect the interests of subjects would, however, greatly limit the kind and scope of research that would be permitted with these data. Preparation of custom datasets allows for far greater flexibility in type and scope of available data at the expense of the time to assemble them.[32] This approach used by Seattle ERIC, MAVERIC, and MFUA as a mechanism for data dissemination. Limited access data enclaves, which are discussed earlier in this chapter and in Appendix E, require staff time for supervision of researchers and secure space and equipment for their use.

Generally speaking, the ease with which data can be retrieved and correspondingly the cost of pulling data for research purposes depends on the quality of the assets' documentation. If the committee's documentation recommendations are followed, there will be abundant information for prospective researchers

[32]Only qualified researchers who execute privacy and confidentiality agreements and who conform to data security requirements would be able to request a dataset like this because it could contain information that could be used to discern subjects' identities.

to use in planning studies and for the custodian's staff to use in facilitating that work. Less time and effort will be expended by both parties in the mechanics of getting research done, leading to lower labor costs per study. However, better documentation may well lead to more demand for the data assets and thus greater time commitments from the staff.

The custodian will also incur costs associated with implementing the committee's recommendations for providing independent oversight of future research. A three-pronged approach was put forward: the review of proposals for scientific merit and adherence to ethical, legal, and related considerations by an IRB and, separately, an advisory and oversight board, and systematic communication of research plans and results to study subjects. In brief, the boards will require time from the custodian's staff for managing applications for data access and interactions with board members, while communications with subjects will involve the development and dissemination of newsletters, websites, or other media. Details of the committee's observations on this topic are presented earlier in this chapter in a section entitled "Oversight of the Future Uses of the AFHS Data Assets."

Expenses related to database management are best expressed in terms of workforce needs, as the allocations required to cover direct and indirect costs vary by location and type of institution (government, nonprofit, commercial) as well as over time. The committee spoke with investigators responsible for other epidemiologic datasets that permit public access. They indicated that typical needs would be for time from a principal investigator or project director, database manager, programmer(s), clerical personnel, and perhaps a webmaster or participant liaison. With the possible exception of a database manager, there would be no need to allocate an entire full-time equivalent (FTE)[33] to any of these tasks.

Roughly speaking, the committee estimates that $150,000–300,000 per year would be required to support a data management and access operation of the type proposed here. The actual amount would depend critically on the custodian chosen and the number and type of studies proposed for and conducted with the data assets (which would in turn influence the amount of staff time required to support those studies). At least some of these funds would presumably be derived from fees assessed to researchers seeking access to the resources. It is important, especially in the early years of this new phase in the life of the AFHS resources, that such fees be set a level that will facilitate use of the resource.

Costs Associated with Managing the Biospecimen Collection

The costs associated with the maintenance of the biospecimen collection are related to its physical maintenance and retrieval of materials for research purposes.

---

[33]FTE is a standard means of characterizing personnel needs. One FTE is one job at 100% time.

Physical Maintenance of the Collection

The cost for physical maintenance of the AFHS biospecimens vary considerably depending upon the setting in which the collection is housed. A research university with a large capacity biospecimens repository may impose relatively modest costs to store materials for a project that has some affiliation with it. A government repository would incur costs in accepting and storing specimens, but there is no set means for factoring how this would be handled for budgeting purposes. Informal discussions with commercial repositories suggest that such institutions would charge $200,000 or more per year to house a collection the size of the AFHS's. Biospecimens may need to undergo inventorying and labeling (barcoding, for example) upon receipt so that they can be integrated into a repository's management system. This would result in additional costs in the range of dollars per vial in the first year of the custodian's operation.[34] It is not clear whether secure transfer of the biospecimen collection under cryogenic conditions is covered under AFHS funds allocated for the "turnover of archives/biological samples to designated agencies" (DTIC, 2005).

If the specimens are instead maintained by a freestanding entity that does not have oversight for other biologic materials, costs for establishing and maintaining the repository will be higher than if the materials are received and maintained by an entity with an existing repository. Expenses such as rental space for freezers will vary, depending upon where in the country[35] and possibly the type of institution at which the specimens are maintained. Other expenditures related to the set-up of a new facility—the purchase or rental of laboratory-quality ultralow temperature freezers and creation of a specimen inventory management system, for example—will also be required.

Regardless of where the specimens are housed, maintenance of the collection requires space for the 23 freezers currently used for specimen storage and backup freezers or the equivalent volume in comparable storage conditions, space for additional freezers for future aliquots, personnel to monitor freezer function, costs for preventive maintenance and repair when compressors fail, and electricity costs. An alarm system must also be used to monitor freezer function and alert personnel of problems whether or not they are on site. If the specimens were housed in a preexisting facility, then monitoring would be subsumed into the staff's existing responsibilities and could be accomplished with only a nominal increase in existing overhead costs that would be covered in the storage fee. In a freestanding facility, sufficient staff to respond to failures at all times would be required.

[34]Over 86,000 specimens have been collected over the course of the study.

[35]State, local, and institutional regulations that affect biospecimens can be additional sources of regional variation in cost.

Retrieval of Materials for Research Purposes

Costs associated with the retrieval of biospecimens from storage may include those related to locating, pulling, realiquoting, packing, and proper shipping. In addition, time from a database manager may be needed to select the study subjects and exam cycles to be included in a specific project, identify locations of the specimens requested and to update the repository database when specimens are removed. If the custodian maintains its own repository, laboratory space will be required for the technical staff to work on dry ice to maintain the specimens during handling and do any realiquoting. Associated laboratory supplies (e.g., pipettes and tips, gloves) will also be needed. For specimens labeled with the subject's name, it will be necessary to relabel or carefully delete the identifying information before shipment, if complete vials are being sent. A source of specimens for use in quality control for laboratory testing will also need to be identified. If new specimens are collected, additional freezers or space will be required. Realiquoting the specimens into smaller volume vials might result in some space saving, at the expense of a freeze-thaw cycle.

Repositories do not, in general, publicly post the amount they charge for their services, making cost estimates difficult. Informal discussions with such organizations suggest it will cost between dollars and tens of dollars per specimen for samples to be extracted and shipped from a repository. Economies of scale may be realized with larger numbers of samples. Many, but not all, repositories can carry out in-house laboratory testing, obviating the need for shipment and lowering the access cost.

Laboratory testing costs, which are in addition to retrieval fees, vary quite widely depending on the procedure. Simple clinical parameters—many of which, it should be noted, were already measured and coded in the AFHS database[36]—cost tens of dollars per sample; newer and more complex tests, hundreds of dollars per sample. University and government laboratories may have different cost structures for resident researchers; this also affects estimates.

The committee assumes that the custodian would follow the practice of other repositories and impose fees for biospecimens access that would recover at least some their costs. As the committee noted in its discussion of database access management, it is important—especially in the early years of this new phase in the life of the AFHS resources—that such fees be set a level that will facilitate use of the resource.

Costs Associated with Conducting Research on the AFHS Data Assets

The committee recommends that further study of the AFHS medical records, other study data, and laboratory specimens be accomplished by making these

[36]Table B-14 in Appendix B provides a partial list of the laboratory analyses coded in the database and which cycle(s) the specimens were collected in.

materials available for research via a custodian that takes an active role in fostering use of the assets. It does not propose that particular studies or type of studies be conducted nor does it put forward a research agenda. A number of possible topics for future work are listed in Chapter 5.

The cost of conducting new studies will greatly depend on their scope and whether they need to use other databases, analyze biospecimens, or contact subjects. Pilot studies and empirical analyses of the existing AFHS dataset could have relatively modest needs for support—tens of thousands of dollars—while investigations that include gathering additional data and specimens from all of the subjects in the cohort could easily cost millions of dollars. The studies that will be conducted on the data assets will depend on the initiative and imagination of prospective researchers, as tempered in the crucible of funding, institutional, and scientific review.

The committee believes that funds are needed to establish the AFHS data assets as a resource for independent researchers. Its judgment is that a limited-life, small grant program is the best way to accomplish this goal. The committee anticipates that this program will stimulate prospective researchers to also seek external funding from other existing sources for further or more in-depth projects. Such an approach has been successfully used by the federal government in other circumstances. The committee therefore recommends that:

> **The Congress should allocate a minimum of $250,000 per year of direct costs for three years for small grants for secondary data analysis or pilot projects using the data assets of the AFHS. These funds should be *in addition to* already-planned or contemplated support of Vietnam veterans' health research—funding should not be diverted from other research efforts for this initiative.**

An allocation of at least $250,000 per year will provide at least partial support to one to three research projects. This seed money is intended to raise the visibility of the AFHS data assets in the research community and stimulate prospective researchers to seek additional sources of support. Such sources could include the National Institutes of Health, Centers for Disease Control and Prevention, Department of Veterans Affairs, and private foundations. MAVERIC provides a listing of these for prospective users of their assets (MAVERIC, 2006). The Seattle ERIC program has administered a pilot study grant program, details of which are available at their website (Seattle ERIC, 2006). It is the committee's judgment that a 3-year trial will be sufficient to establish the AFHS assets as a research resource and that, thereafter, it is appropriate that research projects that propose to use them obtain support through customary funding channels.

The committee has no recommendation regarding the mechanism by which the support proposed here should be administered. This could take place through a federal entity such as the NIH or VA, or the responsibility could be assigned to the custodian. Outreach activities by the custodian—conference presentations, articles in professional journals, or informational workshops, and the like—would help ensure that the scientific community is made aware of the small grant program and, more generally, the research possibilities presented by the data assets.

Although the committee is enthusiastic about the potential for future studies of the AFHS data assets, it understands that the viability of such work is not assured. It therefore believes that it is appropriate to revisit the question of support for further work after the committee's recommendations have been implemented and have had time to play out in the research realm. A 5-year commitment—that is, two years after the last small grants proposed above are made—should be sufficient to establish whether the AFHS resources have value and relevance as a resource. The committee therefore recommends that:

> **Five years after the chosen custodian assumes responsibility, a committee should be convened to evaluate the potential value and relevance of extending further support to the maintenance of access to the data or the biospecimens collected in the course of the AFHS.**

Summary Remarks Regarding the Costs Associated with Extending the AFHS

As the discussion above makes clear, there are a number of uncertainties and variables in the costs associated with extending the AFHS as a data resource managed by a custodian. It is therefore difficult for the committee to present a bottom-line estimate for the total cost of implementing its recommendations. The major fixed costs for the custodian are those related to the management of the database and biospecimens. *Roughly speaking*, the committee estimates that $150,000–300,000 per year would be required to support database management responsibilities and an additional $200,000 or more per year for proper maintenance of the biospecimens. First year costs would be higher because a number of one-time only tasks would have to be performed to set up the operation. Re-inventorying of the biospecimens, if required, would be a major component of such start-up costs. Estimates of the fixed costs could be refined once a decision is made on the custodian.

The committee also recommends that a minimum of $250,000 per year of direct costs be allocated to a limited-life small-grants program to stimulate interest in and awareness of the AFHS data assets within the research community. The program should span the first three years after the successor custodian establishes operations. Other than the limited-life grant program figures, no estimate can be offered of the costs associated with conducting research on the AFHS data assets as these depend so heavily on the form of research contemplated. However, these costs are the responsibility of prospective researchers, who will need to obtain their own support from funding sources.

The committee believes that the costs of properly documenting the data assets, making them available to the research community, and implementing the proposed 5-year program to encourage their use are small in comparison with the government's investment of ~$143 million to date. The potential benefits of these actions, while subject to considerable uncertainty, appear to greatly outweigh the costs.

REFERENCES

AFHS (Air Force Health Study). 1982. *An Epidemiologic Investigation of Health Effects in Air Force Personnel Following Exposure to Herbicides: Study Protocol, Initial Report.* Brooks AFB, TX: USAF School of Aerospace Medicine. SAM-TR-82-44.

AFHS. 2005a (January 20). *Air Force Health Study Post-End-of-Protocol Options.* Memorandum to the Committee on the Disposition of the Air Force Health Study by the AFHS.

AFHS. 2005b (January 28). *Ranch Hand II Follow-On Effort.* Spreadsheet provided to the Committee on the Disposition of the Air Force Health Study by the AFHS.

AFHS. 2005c (January 26). Consent form provided to the Committee on the Disposition of the Air Force Health Study by the AFHS.

AFIP (Armed Forces Institute of Pathology). 2005. *National Pathology Repository.* [Online]. Available: http://www.afip.org/Departments/repository/npr.html [accessed August 30, 2005].

Army Medical Surveillance Activity. 2005. *The Department of Defense Serum Repository.* [Online]. Available: http://amsa.army.mil/DoDSR_Items/DoDSR_Overview.htm [accessed August 29, 2005].

Badilini F, Erdem T, Zareba W, Moss AJ. 2005. ECGScan: a method for conversion of paper electrocardiographic printouts to digital electrocardiographic files. *Journal of Electrocardiology* 38(4):310–318.

Berkowitz ED, Santangelo MJ, eds. 1999. *The Medical Follow-Up Agency: The First Fifty Years 1946–1996.* Washington, DC: National Academy Press.

Blair A, Hartge P, Stewart PA, McAdams M, Lubin J. 1998. Mortality and cancer incidence of aircraft maintenance workers exposed to trichloroethylene and other organic solvents and chemicals: extended follow up. *Occupational and Environmental Medicine* 55(3):161–171.

Cassano PA, Rosner B, Vokonas PS, Weiss ST. 1992. Obesity and body fat distribution in relation to the incidence of non-insulin-dependent diabetes mellitus. A prospective cohort study of men in the Normative Aging Study. *American Journal of Epidemiology* 136(12):1474–1486.

CDC (Centers for Disease Control and Prevention). 2003. HIPAA Privacy Rule: guidance for public health. *Morbidity and Mortality Weekly Report* 52(1):1–24.

CDC. 2004. Procedures and costs for use of the research data center: notice and request for action. *Federal Register* 69(222):67584–67592.

Clayton EW. 2005. Informed consent and biobanks. *Journal of Law, Medicine, and Ethics* 33(1): 15–21.

Clayton EW, Steinberg KK, Khoury MJ, Thomson E, Andrews L, Kahn MJ, Kopelman LM, Weiss JO. 1995. Informed consent for genetic research on stored tissue samples. *Journal of the American Medical Association* 274(22):1786–1792.

Coene R, Deputy Director for Washington Operations, National Center for Toxicological Research, FDA. 2000. Statement at the March 15, 2000, hearing of the Subcommittee on National Security, Veterans Affairs, and International Relations Committee on Government Reform, U.S. House of Representatives. [Online]. Available: http://www.fda.gov/ola/2000/ranchhand.html [accessed November 28, 2005].

DTIC. February 2005. *RDT&E Budget Item Justification Sheet, Ranch Hand II Epidemiology Study, PE number: 0605306F.* [Online]. Available: //www.dtic.mil/descriptivesum/Y2006/AirForce/0605306f.pdf [accessed August 31, 2005].

Eisen SA, Goldberg J, True WR, Henderson WG. 1991. A co-twin control study of the effects of the Vietnam War on the self-reported physical health of veterans. *American Journal of Epidemiology* 134(1):49–58.

GAO (General Accounting Office). 2001. *Agent Orange Awareness, Education, and Outreach.* Briefing at the September 6, 2001, hearing of the Subcommittee on National Security, Veterans Affairs, and International Relations, Committee on Government Reform, U.S. House of Representatives.

Goldberg J, Curran B, Vitek ME, Henderson WG, Boyko EJ. 2002. The Vietnam Era Twin Registry. *Twin Research* 5(5):476–481.

Goldfarb DS, Fischer ME, Keich Y, Goldberg J. 2005. A twin study of genetic and dietary influences on nephrolithiasis: a report from the Vietnam Era Twin (VET) Registry. *Kidney International* 67(3):1053–1061.

Gostin LO, Hodge JG. 1999. Reforming state public health law. *Transformations in Public Health* 2:1–4.

Gray GC, Chesbrough KB, Ryan MA, Amoroso P, Boyko EJ, Gackstetter GD, Hooper TI, Riddle JR, Millennium Cohort Study Group. 2002. The millennium cohort study: a 21-year prospective cohort study of 140,000 military personnel. *Military Medicine* 167(6):483–488.

Gurland BJ, Page WF, Plassman BL. 2004. A twin study of the genetic contribution to age-related functional impairment. *Journals of Gerontology Series A: Biological Sciences and Medical Sciences* 59(8):859–863.

Hodge JG. 2004. Health information privacy and public health. *Journal of Law, Medicine, and Ethics* 31(4):663–671.

HPFS (Health Professionals Follow-Up Study). 2005. *About the Study.* [Online]. Available: http://www.hsph.harvard.edu/hpfs/ [accessed November 29, 2005].

International HapMap Consortium. 2004. Integrating ethics and science in the International HapMap Project. *Nature Reviews. Genetics* 5(6):467–475

IOM (Institute of Medicine). 2000. *Protecting Data Privacy in Health Services Research.* Washington, DC: National Academy Press.

IOM. 2004. *Giving Full Measure to Countermeasures: Addressing Problems in the DOD Program to Develop Medical Countermeasures Against Biological Warfare Agents.* Washington, DC: The National Academies Press.

IOM. 2005a. *Disposition of the Air Force Health Study—Interim Letter Report.* Washington, DC: The National Academies Press. [Online]. Available: http://www.nap.edu/catalog/11483.html [accessed December 1, 2005].

IOM. 2005b. *IOM Studies of U.S. Veteran Twins.* [Online]. Available: http://www.iom.edu/project.asp?id=4907 [accessed December 4, 2005].

IOM. 2005c. *The Medical Follow-up Agency Cohort Catalog.* [Online]. Available: http://www.iom.edu/project.asp?id=4903 [accessed September 5, 2005].

IOM. 2005d. *Vaccine Safety Research, Data Access, and Public Trust.* Washington, DC: The National Academies Press.

IOM. 2005e. *Veterans and Agent Orange: Update 2004.* Washington, DC: The National Academies Press.

Kaiser J. 2005. Pathology institute hit in base-closing plan. *Science* 308:101.

Kang HK, Dalager NA, Needham LL, Patterson DG, Matanoski GM, Kanchanaraksa S, Lees PSJ. 2001. US Army Chemical Corps Vietnam veterans health study: preliminary results. *Chemosphere* 43:943–949.

Kingman A, Albers JW, Arezzo JC, Garabrant DH, Michalek JE. 2005. Amalgam exposure and neurological function. *Neurotoxicology* 26(2):241–255.

Knoppers BM, Laberge C, Robertson G, eds. 1997. *DNA Sampling and Genetic Research: Ethical, Legal and Policy Aspects.* The Hague, Netherlands: Kluwer Law International.

Koenen KC, Lyons MJ, Goldberg J, Simpson J, Williams WM, Toomey R, Eisen SA, True W, Tsuang MT. 2003. Co-twin control study of relationships among combat exposure, combat-related PTSD, and other mental disorders. *Journal of Traumatic Stress* 16(5):433–438.

Koenen KC, Hitsman B, Lyons MJ, Niaura R, McCaffery J, Goldberg J, Eisen SA, True W, Tsuang M. 2005. A twin registry study of the relationship between posttraumatic stress disorder and nicotine dependence in men. *Archives of General Psychiatry* 62(11):1258–1265.

Lazarus R, Sparrow D, Weiss S. 1998. Temporal relations between obesity and insulin: longitudinal data from the Normative Aging Study. *American Journal of Epidemiology* 147(2):173–179.

Mathes RW, Page WF, Crawford HM, McBean AM, Miller RN. 2005. Long-term sequelae of hemorrhagic fever with renal syndrome attributable to hantaan virus in Korean War veterans. *Military Medicine* 170(4):315–319.

MAVERIC (Massachusetts Veterans Epidemiology Research and Information Center). 2005a. *About MAVERIC.* [Online]. Available: http://www.maveric.org/route/maveric/Home.asp [accessed October 8, 2005].

MAVERIC. 2005b. *Laboratory Facilities for Blood Storage.* [Online]. Available: http://www.maveric.org/route/maveric/info/Blood%20Storage%20-%20MAVERIC%20Resources.htm [accessed October 8, 2005].

MAVERIC. 2006. *Relevant Funding Opportunities.* [Online]. Available: http://maveric.org/route/maveric/Resources/Funding.asp [accessed January 31, 2006].

McCarren M, Goldberg J, Ramakrishnan V, Fabsitz R. 1994. Insomnia in Vietnam era veteran twins: influence of genes and combat experience. *Sleep* 17(5):456–461.

MCS (Millennium Cohort Study). 2005. *What is the Millennium Cohort Study?* [Online]. Available: http://www.millenniumcohort.org/about.html [accessed November 29, 2005].

MFUA (Medical Follow-up Agency, Institute of Medicine). 2005. *The Medical Follow-up Agency Cohort Catalog.* [Online]. Available: http://www.iom.edu/project.asp?id=4903 [accessed December 1, 2005].

Michalek, JE. 2005 (January 5). *The Air Force Health Study: An Overview and Update.* PowerPoint presentation before the Committee on the Disposition of the Air Force Health Study, Washington, DC.

MMCS (The Multiethnic/Minority Cohort Study). 2005. *Current Research: Multiethnic/Minority Cohort Study of Diet and Cancer.* [Online]. Available: http://epi.grants.cancer.gov/ResPort/Multiethnic.html [accessed November 29, 2005].

Moody GB. 2005. *Digitizing Paper ECGs and Other Plots.* [Online]. Available: http://www.physionet.org/physiotools/digitizing/ [accessed November 22, 2005].

NARA (National Archives and Records Administration). 2000. *Hill Air Force Base Study Files, 1982–1990.* Archival Research Catalog identifier 605131, Accession Number NN3-443-98-005.

NARA. 2005. *Electronic Records from the Defense Department* [Online]. Available: http://www.archives.gov/research/electronic-records/defense-dept.html [accessed December 5, 2005].

NARA. 2006. *Expanding Acceptable Transfer Requirements: Transfer Instructions for Permanent Electronic Records—Records in Portable Document Format (PDF).* [Online]. Available: http://www.archives.gov/records-mgmt/initiatives/pdf-records.html [accessed January 31, 2006].

Naval Health Research Center. 2005. *Deployment Health Research Studies.* [Online]. Available: http://www.nhrc.navy.mil/rsch/code25/projects/deploymenthealth.htm [accessed August 30, 2005].

NBAC (National Bioethics Advisory Commission). 1999. *Research Involving Human Biological Materials: Ethical Issues and Policy Guidance.* Vol. 1. Rockville, MD: National Bioethics Advisory Commission.

NCHS (National Center for Health Statistics). 2005a. *NHANES Stored Biologic Specimens.* NCHS, Centers for Disease Control, National Institutes of Health. [Online]. Available: http://www.cdc.gov/nchs/about/major/nhanes/serum1b.htm [accessed December 2, 2005].

NCHS. 2005b. *Procedures and Costs for Use of the Research Data Center.* NCHS, Centers for Disease Control, National Institutes of Health. [Online]. Available: http://www.cdc.gov/nchs/r&d/rdcfr.htm [accessed December 2, 2005].

NCHS. 2005c. *Research Data Center.* NCHS, Centers for Disease Control, National Institutes of Health. [Online]. Available: http://www.cdc.gov/nchs/r&d/rdc.htm [accessed December 2, 2005].

NCI (National Cancer Institute). 2005a. *Human Specimens for Research; Legal and Ethical Issues.* [Online]. Available: http://www.cancerdiagnosis.nci.nih.gov/specimens/legal.html [accessed November 27, 2005].

NCI. 2005b. *Model Informed Consent.* [Online]. Available: http://www.cancerdiagnosis.nci.nih.gov/specimens/model.pdf [accessed November 27, 2005].

NCTR-FDA (National Center for Toxicological Research—Food and Drug Administration). 2001. *Charter—Advisory Committee on Special Studies Relating to the Possible Long-Term Health Effects of Phenoxy Herbicides and Contaminants.* [Online]. Available: http://www.fda.gov/nctr/science/committees/rhcharter.doc [accessed November 28, 2005].

NHS (Nurses' Health Study). 2002. *Guidelines for Use of the Nurses' Health Study: External Collaborators.* [Online]. Available: http://www.channing.harvard.edu/nhs/questionnaires/nhs-data-use.doc [accessed November 28, 2005].

NIA (National Institute of Aging). 2005a. *Database of Longitudinal Studies.* [Online]. Available: http://www.nia.nih.gov/ResearchInformation/ScientificResources/LongitudinalStudies.htm [accessed December 2, 2005].

NIA. 2005b. *Research Information.* [Online]. Available: http://www.nia.nih.gov/Research Information/ [accessed December 2, 2005].

Niaura R, Banks SM, Ward KD, Stoney CM, Spiro A III, Aldwin CM, Landsberg L, Weiss ST. 2000. Hostility and the metabolic syndrome in older males: the Normative Aging Study. *Psychosomatic Medicine* 62(1):7–16.

NIH (National Institutes of Health). 2004. *HIPAA Privacy Rule and Its Impacts on Research.* [Online] Available: http://privacyruleandresearch.nih.gov/pr_06.asp [accessed January 9, 2006].

NRC (National Research Council). 2003. *Protecting Participants and Facilitating Social and Behavioral Sciences Research.* Washington, DC: The National Academies Press.

NRC. 2005. *Expanding Access to Research Data: Reconciling Risks and Opportunities.* Washington, DC: The National Academies Press.

OHRP (Office of Human Research Protections, Department of Health and Human Services). 1993. *Protecting Human Research Subjects: Institutional Review Board Guidebook.* [Online]. Available: http://www.hhs.gov/ohrp/irb/irb_guidebook.htm [accessed November 28, 2005].

OHRP. 2004. *Guidance on Research Involving Coded Private Information or Biological Specimens.* [Online]. Available: http://www.hhs.gov/ohrp/humansubjects/guidance/cdebiol.pdf [accessed November 28, 2005].

Page WF, Hoaglund FT, Steinbach LS, Heath AC. 2003. Primary osteoarthritis of the hip in monozygotic and dizygotic male twins. *Twin Research* 6(2):147–151.

Park SK, O'Neill MS, Vokonas PS, Sparrow D, Schwartz J. 2005. Effects of air pollution on heart rate variability: the VA Normative Aging Study. *Environmental Health Perspectives* 113(3): 304–309.

RHAC (Ranch Hand Advisory Committee). 2000. Ranch Hand Advisory Committee Meeting, Department of Health and Human Services, October 19–20, 2000, Day Two, Conference Center, Hilton Palacio del Rio, San Antonio, Texas. [Online]. Available: http://www.fda.gov/ohrms/dockets/ac/00/transcripts/3654t2.pdf [accessed November 29, 2005].

Richards MS, Goldberg J, Anderson RJ, Rodin MB. 1990. Alcohol consumption and problem drinking in Vietnam era veterans and non-veterans. *Journal of Studies on Alcohol* 51(5):396–402.

Rollison DE, Page WF, Crawford H, Gridley G, Wacholder S, Martin J, Miller R, Engels EA. 2004. Case-control study of cancer among US Army veterans exposed to simian virus 40-contaminated adenovirus vaccine. *American Journal of Epidemiology* 160(4):317–324.

Rothstein MA. 2005. Expanding the ethical analysis of biobanks. *Journal of Law, Medicine, and Ethics* 33(1):89–101.

Rothstein MA, Knoppers BM. 2005. Introduction (Regulation of Biobanks). *Journal of Law, Medicine, and Ethics* 33(1):6.

Roy-Byrne P, Arguelles L, Vitek ME, Goldberg J, Keane TM, True WR, Pitman RK. 2004. Persistence and change of PTSD symptomatology—a longitudinal co-twin control analysis of the Vietnam Era Twin Registry. *Social Psychiatry and Psychiatric Epidemiology* 39(9):681–685.

Scherrer JF, Xian H, Bucholz KK, Eisen SA, Lyons MJ, Goldberg J, Tsuang M, True WR. 2003. A twin study of depression symptoms, hypertension, and heart disease in middle-aged men. *Psychosomatic Medicine* 65(4):548–557.

Schnurr PP, Spiro A III. 1999. Combat exposure, posttraumatic stress disorder symptoms, and health behaviors as predictors of self-reported physical health in older veterans. *The Journal of Nervous and Mental Disease* 187(6):353–359.

Scott TE, Mendez MV, LaMorte WW, Cupples LA, Vokonas PS, Garcia RI, Menzoian JO. 2004. Are varicose veins a marker for susceptibility to coronary heart disease in men? Results from the Normative Aging Study. *Annals of Vascular Surgery* 18(4):459–464.

Seattle ERIC. 2005. *Seattle ERIC Home Page.* [Online]. Available: http://www.eric.seattle.med.va.gov/index.html [accessed November 30, 2005].

Seattle ERIC. 2006. *Pilot Study Grant Applications.* [Online]. Available: http://www.eric.seattle.med.va.gov/index.html [accessed January 31, 2006].

Seeff LB, Miller RN, Rabkin CS, Buskell-Bales Z, Straley-Eason K, Smoak BL, Johnson LD, Lee SR, Kaplan EL. 2000. Forty-five year follow-up of hepatitis C virus infection among healthy young adults. *Annals of Internal Medicine* 132(2):105–111.

Todaro JF, Shen BJ, Niaura R, Spiro A III, Ward KD. 2003. Effect of negative emotions on frequency of coronary heart disease (the Normative Aging Study). *The American Journal of Cardiology* 92(8):901–906.

USAF (US Air Force). 1994. *Records Disposition—Procedures and Responsibilities.* Air Force Instruction 37-138. [Online]. Available: http://www.e-publishing.af.mil/pubfiles/af/37/afi37-138/afi37-138.pdf [accessed November 23, 2005].

USAF. 2003. *Records Management Program.* Air Force Instruction 33-322. [Online]. Available: http://www.e-publishing.af.mil/pubfiles/af/33/afi33-322/afi33-322.pdf [accessed November 23, 2005].

USAF. 2004. *An Overview of the USAF Human Subjects Protection Program.* USAF Office of the Surgeon General's Division of Biomedical Research and Regulatory Compliance (SGRC). [Online]. Available: https://mrmc.detrick.army.mil/docs/rcq/HSRRBOffSite04/An%20Overview%20of%20the%20USAF%20Human%20Subjects%20Protection%20Program%20-%20MAJ%20Donnamarie%20Robinson.ppt [accessed November 28, 2005].

VA (Department of Veterans Affairs). 2003. *Environmental Epidemiology.* [Online]. Available: http://www.vethealth.cio.med.va.gov/epidemiology.htm [accessed November 28, 2005].

VA. 2005a. *Cooperative Studies Program. VA Research and Development, Veterans Health Administration.* [Online]. Available: http://www1.va.gov/resdev/programs/blrd-csrd/csp.cfm [accessed August 25 2005].

VA. 2005b. *Mission, Vision, Core Values & Goals.* [Online]. Available: http://www.va.gov/about_va/mission.asp [accessed November 28, 2005].

Wallin MT, Page WF, Kurtzke JF. 2004. Multiple sclerosis in US veterans of the Vietnam era and later military service: race, sex, and geography. *Annals of Neurology* 55(1):65–71.

Weisskopf MG, Wright RO, Schwartz J, Spiro A III, Sparrow D, Aro A, Hu H. 2004. Cumulative lead exposure and prospective change in cognition among elderly men: the VA Normative Aging Study. *American Journal of Epidemiology* 160(12):1184–1193.

Appendixes

A

Agendas of Public Meetings Held by the Committee on the Disposition of the Air Force Health Study

First Public Meeting

Friday, February 4, 2005
Keck Building, Room 101
500 Fifth Street NW
Washington, DC

- **Welcome, opening remarks and introduction**
  David Tollerud, M.D., M.P.H.
  Committee Chair

- **Charge to the committee**
  Mark A. Brown, Ph.D.
  Director, Environmental Agents Service
  U.S. Department of Veterans Affairs

- **Overview of the Air Force Health Study**
  Joel Michalek, Ph.D.
  Principal Investigator, Air Force Research Laboratory

SECOND PUBLIC MEETING

Thursday, April 14, 2005
Board Room, National Academy of Sciences Building
2101 Constitution Ave., NW
Washington, DC

- **Welcome, opening remarks, and introduction**
  David Tollerud, M.D., M.P.H.
  Committee Chair

- *Mark A. Brown, Ph.D.*
  Director of Environmental Agents Service
  U.S. Department of Veterans Affairs

- **Disposition of the Air Force Health Study**
  Michael Stoto, Ph.D.
  Chair, Ranch Hand Advisory Committee

- **Amalgam study design**
  Albert Kingman, Ph.D.
  Chief Biostatistician and Head of the Biostatistics Core
  National Institute of Dental and Craniofacial Research, NIH

- **Uses and usefulness of data and specimen resources from the Air Force Health Study**
  Teri Manolio, M.D., Ph.D.
  Director, Epidemiology and Biometry Program
  Division of Epidemiology and Clinical Applications
  National Heart, Lung and Blood Institute, NIH

- *Richard M. Suzman, Ph.D.*
  Associate Director, Behavioral and Social Research Program
  National Institute on Aging, NIH

- *Marie Haring Sweeney, Ph.D.*
  Health Attaché, United States Embassy
  Hanoi, Vietnam

- *Mary Ellen McCarthy*
  Minority Staff Director, House Veterans Affairs Committee
  Subcommittee on Benefits

- **Testimony on the behalf of The American Legion**
  Shannon Middleton
  The American Legion

- **Testimony on the behalf of the Vietnam Veterans of America**
  Rick Weidman
  Vietnam Veterans of America

Third Public Meeting

Monday, June 20, 2005
Keck Building, Room 204
500 Fifth Street, NW
Washington, DC

- **Welcome, opening remarks and introduction**
  David Tollerud, M.D., M.P.H.
  Committee Chair

- **The MAVERIC database of veterans' health information**
  Pantel S. Vokonas, M.D.
  Principal Investigator, The VA Normative Aging Study

- **Management and analysis of the MFUA veterans' health databases**
  William Page, Ph.D.
  Medical Follow-Up Agency, Institute of Medicine
  The National Academies

- **NCHS's experiences with the administration and dissemination of epidemiologic data and biologic samples**
  Geraldine McQuillan, Ph.D. and *Kathryn Porter, M.D., M.S.*
  National Center for Health Statistics, Centers for Disease Control

- **Lessons learned from the "Vaccine Safety Research, Data Access, and Public Trust" study**
  Andrea Pernack Anason, M.P.H. and *John Bailar, M.D., Ph.D.*
  Committee on the Review of the National Immunization Program's Research Procedures and Data Sharing Program

B

Air Force Health Study Data

Section 602(c) of Pub. L. 108-183 called for this committee to evaluate "[t]he scientific merit of retaining and maintaining the medical records, other study data, and laboratory specimens collected in the course of the Air Force Health Study after its currently scheduled termination date in 2006" and to determine "[w]hether or not any obstacles exist to retaining and maintaining the medical records, other study data, and laboratory specimens."

Pursuant to this charge, the committee reviewed data and specimen collection as reported in the original study protocol (AFHS, 1982), official AFHS morbidity cycle reports (AFHS, 1984, 1987, 1990, 1995, 2000, 2005), the *Serum Dioxin Analysis of 1987 Examination Results* (AFHS, 1991), AFHS mortality (AFHS, 1983, 1984, 1985, 1986, 1989, 1991, 1993, 1994, 1996) and reproductive outcomes reports (AFHS, 1992, 1998), as well as various AFHS analyses reported in scientific journals as cited in preceding chapters. AFHS data dictionaries and clinical collection and laboratory processing protocols were also reviewed where available.

The purpose of this appendix is to provide a sense of the scope and magnitude of the data collected and analyzed throughout the course of the AFHS. The following tables are not intended to serve as an exhaustive accounting of data collected or archived. Data collected in the mortality arm of the study are not represented in this appendix. The information contained in Tables B-1 through B-13 was derived primarily from analyses reported in AFHS morbidity cycle reports (cited above). Hence, they generally represent those outcomes included in morbidity analyses for a particular cycle and not necessarily all outcomes recorded or measured in AFHS clinical and laboratory evaluations or those obtained from private medical and dental records or military records.

The myriad laboratory tests performed (by the Kelsey-Seybold Clinic for Cycle 1 and Scripps Clinic for Cycles 2–6) on subject blood, urine, and semen were provided by AFHS investigators by committee request and are listed in Table B-14. Dioxin assays are not included in this list as they were performed separately at the Centers for Disease Control and Prevention.

A summary of covariates used in various analyses throughout the AFHS is provided in Table B-15 to further characterize available subject data.

Table B-16 provides a brief overview of the types of data gathered through questionnaire administration as well as the major changes made to questionnaire (baseline and interval) content over time.

Additional details relating AFHS data resources and analyses are can be found in Chapters 2–4.

TABLE B-1 General Health Assessment

Cycle	1	2	3	4	5	6
Examination Year	1982	1985	1987	1992	1997	2002
Analyzed Endpoints						
Self-perception of health (Q)	X	X	X	X	X	X
Appearance of illness or distress as assessed by physician (PE)	X	X	X	X	X	X
Relative age appearance as assessed by physician (PE)	X	X	X	X	X	X
Calculated body fat (percentage) (PE)	X	X	X	X	X	
BMI (PE)						X
Erythrocyte sedimentation (mm/hour) (LAB)	X	X	X	X	X	X
Covariates						
Age (years) (MIL)	X	X	X	X	X	X
Race (MIL)	X	X	X	X		
Military occupation (MIL)	X	X	X	X	X	X
Current cigarette smoking (cigarettes/day) (Q)					X	X
Lifetime cigarette smoking history (pack-years) (Q)					X	X
Current alcohol use (2 weeks prior to physical exam) (drinks/day) (Q)						X
Current alcohol use (drinks/day) (Q)					X	
Lifetime alcohol history (drink-years) (Q)					X	X
Personality type (PE)		X	X	X	X	
Caloric intake (Q)				X		

NOTES: Data sources: (Q) questionnaires; (PE) physical examination; (LAB) laboratory tests; (MRV) medical records verified; (MIL) military records.

Areas in gray indicate that either an endpoint was not analyzed for a particular cycle or that it was unclear from the cycle report if an endpoint was analyzed. Gray areas do not indicate that an endpoint was not measured or recorded for a particular cycle. Shaded boxes with an X indicate that the endpoint was measured but not included in section analyses.

TABLE B-2 Neurological Assessment

Cycle Examination Year	1 1982	2 1985	3 1987	4 1992	5 1997	6 2002
Analyzed Endpoints						
Inflammatory diseases (MVR)	X	X	X	X	X	X
Hereditary and degenerative diseases (MRV)	X	X	X	X	X	X
Peripheral disorders (MRV)	X	X	X	X	X	X
Disorders of eye (MRV)	X	X	X			
Disorders of ear (MRV)	X	X	X			
Other neurological disorders (MRV)		X	X	X	X	X
Smell (PE)	X	X	X	X	X	X
Visual fields (PE)	X	X	X	X	X	X
Light reaction (PE)	X	X	X	X	X	X
Ocular movement (PE)	X	X	X	X	X	X
Facial sensation (PE)	X	X	X	X	X	X
Corneal reflex (PE)	X	X	X	X	X	X
Jaw clench (PE)	X	X	X	X	X	X
Smile (PE)	X	X	X	X	X	X
Palpebral fissure (PE)	X	X	X	X	X	X
Balance/Romberg sign (PE)	X	X	X	X	X	X
Gag reflex (PE)	X	X	X	X	X	X
Speech (PE)	X	X	X	X	X	X
Tongue position relative to midline (PE)	X	X	X	X	X	X
Palate and uvula movement (PE)	X	X	X	X	X	X
Shoulder shrug (PE)						X
Cranial nerve index without range of motion (PE)		X	X	X		
Cranial nerve index (PE)		X	X	X	X	X

continues

TABLE B-2 *Continued*

Cycle Examination Year	1 1982	2 1985	3 1987	4 1992	5 1997	6 2002
Neck range of motion (PE)	X	X	X	X	X	
Pinprick (PE)	X	X	X	X	X	X
Light touch (PE)	X	X	X	X	X	X
Muscle status (PE)	X	X	X	X	X	X
Vibratory sensation (PE)	X	X	X			
Patellar reflex (PE)	X	X	X	X	X	X
Achilles reflex (PE)	X	X	X	X	X	X
Biceps reflex (PE)	X	X	X	X	X	X
Babinski reflex (PE)	X	X	X	X	X	X
Any symmetrical peripheral abnormality (PE)						X
Possible peripheral neuropathy (PE)						X
Probable peripheral neuropathy (PE)						X
Polyneuropathy severity index (PE)					X	
Polyneuropathy prevalence index (PE)					X	
Multiple polyneuropathy index (PE)					X	
Confirmed polyneuropathy index (PE)					X	
Vibrotactile threshold great toes (PE)				X		
Tremor (PE)	X	X	X	X	X	X
Coordination (PE)	X	X	X	X	X	X
Romberg sign (PE)	X	X	X	X	X	X
Gait (PE)	X	X	X	X	X	X
CNS index (PE)		X	X	X	X	X
Nerve conduction velocity (PE)	X					

NOTES: Data sources: (Q) questionnaires; (PE) physical examination; (LAB) laboratory tests; (MRV) medical records verified; (MIL) military records.

Areas in gray indicate that either an endpoint was not analyzed for a particular cycle or that it was unclear from the cycle report if an endpoint was analyzed. Gray areas do not indicate that an endpoint was not measured or recorded for a particular cycle.

TABLE B-3 Psychology Assessment

Cycle Examination Year	1 1982	2 1985	3 1987	4 1992	5 1997	6 2002
Analyzed Endpoints						
Psychoses (MRV)	X	X	X	X	X	X
Alcohol dependence (MRV)	X	X	X	X	X	X
Drug dependence (MRV)			X	X	X	X
Anxiety (MRV)	X	X	X	X	X	X
Other neuroses (MRV)	X	X	X	X	X	X
Fatigue (Q)	X					
Depression (Q)	X					
Anxiety (Q)	X					
Erosion of skills (Q)	X					
Social isolation (Q)	X					
Aggressive or impulsive behavior (Q)	X					
Trouble falling asleep (Q)			X			
Waking up during the night (Q)			X			
Waking up too early and can't go back to sleep (Q)			X			
Waking up unrefreshed (Q)			X			
Involuntarily falling asleep during the day (Q)			X			
Great disabling fatigue during the day (Q)			X			
Frightening dreams (Q)			X			
Talking in sleep (Q)			X			
Sleepwalking (Q)			X			
Abnormal movement/activity during the night (Q)			X			
Sleep problems requiring medication (Q)			X			
Snore loudly in all sleeping positions (Q)			X			

continues

TABLE B-3 *Continued*

Cycle	1	2	3	4	5	6
Examination Year	1982	1985	1987	1992	1997	2002
Insomnia (Q)			X			
Overall sleep disorder index (Q)			X			
Average sleep each night (hours) (Q)			X			
SCL-90-R: Symptom Checklist-90—Revised (PE)			X	X	X	X
WMS-R: Wechsler Memory Scale—Revised (PE)						X
MCMI: Millon Clinical Multiaxial Inventory (PE)			X			
MMPI: Minnesota Multiphasic Personality Inventory (PE)	X	X				
CMI: Cornell Medical Index (PE)		X				
HRB: Halstead-Reitan Neuropsychological Test Battery (PE)	X	X				
CI: Cornell Index (PE)	X					
WAIS: Wechsler Adult Intelligence Scale (PE)	X					

NOTES: Data sources: (Q) questionnaires; (PE) physical examination; (LAB) laboratory tests; (MRV) medical records verified; (MIL) military records.

Areas in gray indicate that either an endpoint was not analyzed for a particular cycle or that it was unclear from the cycle report if an endpoint was analyzed. Gray areas do not indicate that an endpoint was not measured or recorded for a particular cycle. Shaded boxes with an X indicate that the endpoint was measured but not included in section analyses.

TABLE B-4 Gastrointestinal Assessment

Cycle Examination Year	1 1982	2 1985	3 1987	4 1992	5 1997	6 2002
Analyzed Endpoints						
Uncharacterized hepatitis (Q/MRV)	X	X	X[a]	X	X	X
Jaundice (unspecified) (Q/MRV)	X	X	X	X	X	X
Acute and subacute necrosis of the liver (Q/MRV)			X	X	X	X
Chronic liver disease and cirrhosis (alcohol related) (Q/MRV)	X	X	X	X	X	X
Chronic liver disease and cirrhosis (nonalcohol related) (Q/MRV)	X	X	X	X	X	X
Liver abscess and sequelae of chronic liver disease (Q/MRV)			X	X	X	X
Enlarged liver (hepatomegaly) (Q/MRV)		X	X	X	X	X
Skin bruises, patches, or sensitivity (Q/MRV)	X	X	X			
Reported/verified ulcer (Q/MRV)		X	X			
Other disorders of the liver (Q/MRV)	X[b]	X	X	X	X	X
Liver disease (lifetime history) (Q/MRV)		X				
Current hepatomegaly (PE)	X	X	X	X	X	X
AST (U/L) (LAB)	X	X	X	X	X	X
ALT (U/L) (LAB)	X	X	X	X	X	X
GGT (U/L) (LAB)	X	X	X	X	X	X
Alkaline phosphatase (U/L) (LAB)	X	X	X	X	X	X
Total bilirubin (mg/dl) (LAB)	X	X	X	X	X	X
Direct bilirubin (mg/dl) (LAB)	X	X	X	X	X	X
LDH (U/L) (LAB)	X	X	X	X	X	X
Cholesterol (mg/dl) (LAB)	X	X	X	X	X	X
HDL cholesterol (mg/dl) (LAB)			X	X	X	X
Cholesterol-HDL ratio (LAB)			X	X	X	X
Triglycerides (mg/dl) (LAB)	X	X	X	X	X	X

continues

TABLE B-4 *Continued*

Cycle Examination Year	1 1982	2 1985	3 1987	4 1992	5 1997	6 2002
Creatine phosphokinase (U/L) (LAB)			X	X	X	X
Serum amylase (U/L) (LAB)				X	X	X
Evidence of prior hepatitis A (LAB)				X	X	X
Evidence of prior hepatitis B (LAB)				X	X	X
Current hepatitis B (LAB)				X	X	
Evidence of prior hepatitis C (LAB)				X	X	X
Evidence of prior hepatitis D (LAB)					X	
Stool occult blood test (LAB)				X	X	X
Protein profile: prealbumin (mg/dl) (LAB)				X	X	X
Protein profile: albumin (mg/dl) (LAB)				X	X	X
Protein profile: α-1-acid glycoprotein (mg/dl) (LAB)				X	X	X
Protein profile: α-1-antitrypsin (mg/dl) (LAB)				X	X	X
Protein profile: α-2-macroglobulin (mg/dl) (LAB)				X	X	X
Protein profile: apolipoprotein B (mg/dl) (LAB)				X	X	X
Protein profile: C3 complement (mg/dl) (LAB)				X	X	X
Protein profile: C4 complement (mg/dl) (LAB)				X	X	X
Protein profile: haptoglobin (mg/dl) (LAB)				X	X	X
Protein profile: transferrin (mg/dl) (LAB)				X	X	X
Prothrombin time (seconds) (LAB)						X
Fasting glucose (LAB)			X			
Uroporphyrin (LAB)	X	X				

Coproporphyrin (LAB)	X	X
Aminolevulinic acid (LAB)	X	

NOTES: Data sources: (Q) questionnaires; (PE) physical examination; (LAB) laboratory tests; (MRV) medical records verified; (MIL) military records.

Areas in gray indicate that either an endpoint was not analyzed for a particular cycle or that it was unclear from the cycle report if an endpoint was analyzed. Gray areas do not indicate that an endpoint was not measured or recorded for a particular cycle. Shaded boxes with an X indicate that the endpoint was measured but not included in section analyses.

[a]In Cycle 3 *viral hepatitis* is reported versus *uncharacterized hepatitis* in other cycles.
[b]Liver necrosis and enzyme elevation included in the *other liver conditions* category.

TABLE B-5 Dermatological Assessment

Cycle Examination Year	1 1982	2 1985	3 1987	4 1992	5[a] 1997	6 2002
Analyzed Endpoints						
Acne (lifetime) (Q/MRV)	X	X	X	X		X
Post-SEA acne (Q/MRV/MIL)	X	X	X	X		X
Post-SEA acne (no pre-SEA acne) (Q/MRV/MIL)	X	X	X	X		X
Post-SEA acne (with pre-SEA acne) (Q/MRV/MIL)	X	X	X	X		X
Location of post-SEA acne (pre-SEA acne cases excluded) (Q/MRV)		X	X	X		X
Location of post-SEA acne (all post-SEA occurrences) (Q/MRV)	X	X	X	X		X
Duration of post-SEA acne (pre-SEA acne cases excluded) (months) (Q)	X	X	X			X
Duration of post-SEA acne (all post-SEA occurrences) (months) (Q)	X	X	X			X
Acneiform lesions (PE)	X	X	X			X
Acneiform scars (PE)	X	X	X			X
Comedones (PE)	X	X	X			X
Depigmentation (PE)		X	X			X
Hyperpigmentation (PE)	X	X	X			X
Inclusion cysts (PE)	X	X	X			X
Dermatology index (PE)[b]	X	X	X	X		X
Other abnormalities (PE)[c]	X	X	X	X		

NOTES: Data sources: (Q) questionnaires; (PE) physical examination; (LAB) laboratory tests; (MRV) medical records verified; (MIL) military records.

Areas in gray indicate that either an endpoint was not analyzed for a particular cycle or that it was unclear from the cycle report if an endpoint was analyzed. Gray areas do not indicate that an endpoint was not measured or recorded for a particular cycle. Shaded boxes with an X indicate that the endpoint was measured but not included in section analyses.

[a]Dermatologic assessment not reported in the Cycle 5 follow-up examination results.

[b]The dermatology index comprised counts for comedones, acneiform lesions, acneiform scars, and inclusion cysts (AFHS, 1990).

[c]Conditions comprising the other abnormalities category were jaundice, spider angiomata, palmar erythema, suspected melanoma, palmar keratoses, petechiae, ecchymoses, conjunctival abnormality, oral mucosal abnormality, fingernail abnormality, toenail abnormality, dermatographia, cutis rhomboidalis, suspected basal cell carcinoma, suspected squamous cell carcinoma, nevus, or other abnormalities (AFHS, 1990). Vitiligo was added to the list in Cycle 5 (AFHS, 1997).

TABLE B-6 Cardiovascular Assessment

Cycle Examination Year	1 1982	2 1985	3 1987	4 1992	5 1997	6 2002
Analyzed Endpoints						
Essential hypertension (Q/MRV/PE)		X	X	X	X	X
Heart disease (excluding essential hypertension) (Q/MRV/PE)	X	X	X	X	X	X
Myocardial infarction (Q/MRV/PE)	X	X	X	X	X	X
Stroke or transient ischemic attack (MRV)					X	X
Systolic blood pressure (mm Hg) (PE)	X	X	X	X	X	X
Diastolic blood pressure (mm Hg) (PE)	X	X	X	X	X	X
Heart sounds (PE)	X	X	X	X	X	X
Overall ECG (PE)	X	X	X	X	X	X
ECG: RBBB (PE)		X	X	X	X	X
ECG: LBBB (PE)		X	X	X	X	X
ECG: nonspecific ST- and T-wave changes (PE)		X	X	X	X	X
ECG: bradycardia (PE)		X	X	X	X	X
ECG: tachycardia (PE)		X	X	X	X	X
ECG: arrhythmia (PE)		X	X	X	X	X
ECG: evidence of prior myocardial infarction (PE)				X	X	X
ECG: other diagnoses (PE)		X	X	X	X	X
Funduscopic examination (PE)	X	X	X	X	X	X
Carotid bruits (PE)	X	X	X	X	X	X
Radial pulses (PE)	X	X	X	X	X	X
Femoral pulses (PE)	X	X	X	X	X	X
Popliteal pulses (PE)	X	X	X	X	X	X
Dorsalis pedis pulses (PE)	X	X	X	X	X	X
Posterior tibial pulses (PE)	X	X	X	X	X	X

continues

TABLE B-6 *Continued*

Cycle Examination Year	1 1982	2 1985	3 1987	4 1992	5 1997	6 2002
Leg pulses (PE)	X	X	X	X	X	X
Peripheral pulses (PE)	X	X	X	X	X	X
All pulses (PE)	X	X	X			
Resting pressure index (PE)						X
Hyperemic pressure index (1 minute postexercise) (PE)						X
Hyperemic pressure index (2 minutes postexercise) (PE)						X
Intermittent claudication and vascular insufficiency index (Q)				X	X	X
Kidney, urethra, and bladder (KUB) X ray excluding kidney stones (PE)				X		
Questionnaire-physical exam associations* (PE)			X			

NOTES: Data sources: (Q) questionnaires; (PE) physical examination; (LAB) laboratory tests; (MRV) medical records verified; (MIL) military records.

Areas in gray indicate that either an endpoint was not analyzed for a particular cycle or that it was unclear from the cycle report if an endpoint was analyzed. Gray areas do not indicate that an endpoint was not measured or recorded for a particular cycle.

*Measure was determined by analysis of central and peripheral PE findings and verified CVD endpoints to determine strength of correlation between PE findings and medical history (AFHS, 1990).

TABLE B-7 Hematological Assessment

Cycle	1	2	3	4	5	6
Examination Year	1982	1985	1987	1992	1997	2002
Analyzed Endpoints						
RBC count (million/mm^3) (LAB)	X	X	X	X	X	X
WBC count (thousand/mm^3) (LAB)	X	X	X	X	X	X
Hemoglobin (g/dl) (LAB)	X	X	X	X	X	X
Hematocrit (percent) (LAB)	X	X	X	X	X	X
Mean corpuscular volume (MVC) (cubic micra) (LAB)	X	X	X			
Mean corpuscular hemoglobin (MCH) (microgram) (LAB)	X	X	X			
Mean corpuscular hemoglobin concentration (MCHC) (mg/dl) (LAB)	X	X	X			
Platelet count (thousand/mm^3) (LAB)	X	X	X	X	X	X
Prothrombin time (seconds) (LAB)				X	X	
RBC morphology (LAB)				X	X	X
Absolute neutrophils (segs) (thousand/mm^3) (LAB)				X	X	X
Absolute neutrophils (bands) (thousand/mm^3) (LAB)				X	X	X
Absolute lymphocytes (thousand/mm^3) (LAB)				X	X	X
Absolute monocytes (thousand/mm^3) (LAB)				X	X	X
Absolute eosinophils (thousand/mm^3) (LAB)				X	X	X
Absolute basophils (thousand/mm^3) (LAB)				X	X	X
Fibrinogen (mg/dl) (LAB)						X
Erythrocyte sedimentation rate (ESR) (mm/hour) (LAB)	X	X	X	X	X	X

NOTES: Data sources: (Q) questionnaires; (PE) physical examination; (LAB) laboratory tests; (MRV) medical records verified; (MIL) military records.
When units are provided, they reflect the most recent cycle for which the measurement was taken.
Areas in gray indicate that either an endpoint was not analyzed for a particular cycle or that it was unclear from the cycle report if an endpoint was analyzed. Gray areas do not indicate that an endpoint was not measured or recorded for a particular cycle. Shaded boxes with an X indicate that the endpoint was measured but not included in section analyses.

TABLE B-8 Renal Assessment

Cycle / Examination Year	1 / 1982	2 / 1985	3 / 1987	4 / 1992	5 / 1997	6 / 2002
Analyzed Endpoints						
History of kidney stones (MRV/PE)						X
Occurrence of past kidney disease (MRV)	X	X	X	X		X
Blood urea nitrogen (mg/dl) (LAB)	X	X	X			X
Serum creatinine (mg/dl) (LAB)				X		X
Creatinine clearance (calculated) (LAB/PE/MIL)	X					X
Urinary microalbumin to urinary creatinine ratio (μg/mg) (LAB)						X
Urine specific gravity (LAB)	X	X	X	X		X
Urinary occult blood (cells/HPF) (LAB)	X	X	X	X		X
Urinary WBC count (cells/HPF) (LAB)	X	X	X	X		X
Urinary protein (LAB)	X	X	X	X		X
Urinary RBC count (cells/HPF) (LAB)	X	X	X	X		
Urine creatinine (LAB)	X					
Urine volume (24 Hour) (LAB)	X					
Kidney stones from KUB X ray (PE)				X		
Composite renal abnormalities (LAB)	X					

NOTES: Data sources: (Q) questionnaires; (PE) physical examination; (LAB) laboratory tests; (MRV) medical records verified; (MIL) military records.
When units are provided, they reflect the most recent cycle for which the measurement was taken.

Areas in gray indicate that either an endpoint was not analyzed for a particular cycle or that it was unclear from the cycle report if an endpoint was analyzed. Gray areas do not indicate that an endpoint was not measured or recorded for a particular cycle. Shaded boxes with an X indicate that the endpoint was measured but not included in section analyses.

TABLE B-9 Endocrine Assessment

Cycle Examination Year	1 1982	2 1985	3 1987	4 1992	5 1997	6 2002
Analyzed Endpoints						
Past thyroid disease (MRV)		X	X	X	X	X
Current thyroid function (Q)		X	X			
Composite diabetes indicator (MRV/LAB)		X	X	X		
Composite diabetes indicator (2002 AFHS diabetes definition) (MRV/LAB)						X
Composite diabetes indicator (pre-2002 AFHS diabetes definition)(MRV/LAB)					X	X
Diabetic severity (MRV)				X		
Diabetic control (MRV/LAB)				X	X	X
Time to diabetes onset (years) (MRV/LAB/MIL)				X	X	X
Thyroid gland (PE)		X	X	X	X	X
Testicular examination (PE)		X	X		X	X
Testicular volume (PE)				X		
TSH (µIU/ml) (LAB)		X	X	X	X	X
Free thyroxine index (µg/dl) (LAB)	X					
Free T4 (ng/dl) (LAB)						X
T4 (µg/dl (LAB)	X			X	X	
T3 % uptake (LAB)	X	X	X			
Antithyroid antibodies (LAB)				X	X	X
Fasting glucose (mg/dl) (LAB)				X	X	X
2-hour postprandial glucose (mg/dl) (LAB)	X	X	X	X	X	X
Fasting urinary glucose (LAB)				X	X	
2-hour postprandial urinary glucose (LAB)			X	X	X	X
Insulin (µIU/ml) (LAB)				X	X	X
2-hour postprandial insulin (µIU/ml) (LAB)						X

continues

TABLE B-9 *Continued*

Cycle Examination Year	1 1982	2 1985	3 1987	4 1992	5 1997	6 2002
Serum glucagon (pg/ml) (LAB)				X		
Hemoglobin A1c (percent) (LAB)				X	X	X
C-peptide (ng/ml) (LAB)				X		X
Proinsulin (pmol/l) (LAB)				X		X
GADA (LAB)						X
Total testosterone (ng/dl) (LAB)	X	X	X	X	X	X
Free testosterone (pg/ml) (LAB)				X	X	X
Estradiol (pg/ml) (LAB)				X	X	X
LH (mIU/ml) (LAB)				X	X	X
FSH (mIU/ml) (LAB)			X	X	X	X
Retinopathy results (diabetics only) (PE)				X		
Neuropathy results (diabetics only) (PE)				X		
Radial pulses (diabetics only) (PE)				X		
Femoral pulses (diabetics only) (PE)				X		
Popliteal pulses (diabetics only) (PE)				X		
Dorsalis pedis pulses (diabetics only) (PE)				X		
Posterior tibial pulses (diabetics only) (PE)				X		
Leg pulses (diabetics only) (PE)				X		
Peripheral pulses (diabetics only) (PE)				X		
Urine protein (diabetics only) (PE)				X		
Sex hormone-binding globulin (SHBG) (nmol/l) (LAB)				X		

Total testosterone to SHBG ratio (LAB)				X		
Cortisol (μg/dl) (initial, 2 hour, and differential) (LAB)		X				

NOTES: Data sources: (Q) questionnaires; (PE) physical examination; (LAB) laboratory tests; (MRV) medical records verified; (MIL) military records.

When units are provided, they reflect the most recent cycle for which the measurement was taken.

Areas in gray indicate that either an endpoint was not analyzed for a particular cycle or that it was unclear from the cycle report if an endpoint was analyzed. Gray areas do not indicate that an endpoint was not measured or recorded for a particular cycle. Shaded boxes with an X indicate that the endpoint was measured but not included in section analyses.

TABLE B-10 Immunology Assessment

Cycle Examination Year	1 1982	2 1985	3 1987	4 1992	5 1997	6 2002
Analyzed Endpoints						
Composite skin test (PE)		X	X	X		
CD2+ cells (total T cells) (cells/mm^3) (LAB)	X	X	X			
CD3 cells (total T cells) (cells/mm^3) (LAB)	X			X	X	X
CD4 cells (helper T cells) (cells/mm^3) (LAB)	X	X	X	X	X	X
CD5 cells (cells/mm^3) (LAB)				X		
CD8 cells (suppressor cells) (cells/mm^3) (LAB)	X	X	X	X	X	X
CD14 cells (monocytes) (cells/mm^3) (LAB)		X	X	X		
CD16+56 cells (natural killer cells) (cells/mm^3) (LAB)				X	X	X
CD20 cells (B cells) (cells/mm^3) (LAB)	X	X	X	X	X	X
CD25 cells (cells/mm^3) (LAB)			X	X		
CD4-CD8 ratio (LAB)	X	X	X	X		
HLA-DR cells (cells/mm^3) (LAB)		X	X			
CD3 with CD25 (cells/mm^3) (LAB)				X		
CD5 with CD20 (cells/mm^3) (LAB)				X		
CD4 with CD8 (cells/mm^3) (LAB)				X		
CD3 with CD16+56 (cells/mm^3) (LAB)				X		
CD3+CD4 cells (helper T cells) (cells/mm^3) (LAB)					X	X
Absolute lymphocytes (cells/mm^3) (LAB)	X		X	X	X	X
IgA (mg/dl) (LAB)			X	X	X	X
IgG (mg/dl) (LAB)			X	X	X	X
IgM (mg/dl) (LAB)			X	X	X	X
Lupus panel: ANA test (LAB)				X	X	X
Lupus panel: thyroid microsomal antibody (LAB)				X	X	X

Lupus panel: MSK antismooth muscle antibody (LAB)				X	X	X
Lupus panel: MSK antimitochondrial antibody (LAB)				X	X	X
Lupus panel: MSK antiparietal cell antibody (LAB)				X	X	X
Lupus panel: rheumatoid factor (LAB)				X	X	X
Lupus panel: B cell clones (LAB)				X		
Lupus panel: other antibodies (LAB)				X		
Lupus panel: summary index (LAB)				X		
PHA (unstimulated and net) response (LAB)		X	X			
MLC (unstimulated and net) response (LAB)		X	X			
NKCA 50:1 net response (LAB)			X			
NKCA 50:1 percent release (LAB)			X			
NKCI 50:1 net response (LAB)			X			
NKCI 50:1 percent release (LAB)			X			
PWN (pokeweed net response) (LAB)		X				

NOTES: Data sources: (Q) questionnaires; (PE) physical examination; (LAB) laboratory tests; (MRV) medical records verified; (MIL) military records. When units are provided, they reflect the most recent cycle for which the measurement was taken.

Areas in gray indicate that either an endpoint was not analyzed for a particular cycle or that it was unclear from the cycle report if an endpoint was analyzed. Gray areas do not indicate that an endpoint was not measured or recorded for a particular cycle. Shaded boxes with an X indicate that the endpoint was measured but not included in section analyses.

TABLE B-11 Pulmonary Assessment

Cycle / Examination Year	1 1982	2 1985	3 1987	4 1992	5 1997	6 2002
Analyzed Endpoints						
Asthma (MRV*/Q)		X	X	X	X	X
Bronchitis (MRV*/Q)		X	X	X	X	X
Pneumonia (MRV*/Q)		X	X	X	X	X
Pleurisy (Q)		X	X			
Tuberculosis (Q)	X	X	X			
Neoplasia (Q)	X					
Chronic sinusitis and other upper respiratory disease (Q)	X					
Thorax and lung abnormality (PE)		X	X	X	X	X
X ray interpretation (LAB)		X	X	X	X	X
Asymmetric expansion (PE)		X	X			
Hyperresonance (PE)		X	X			
Wheezes (PE)		X	X			
Rales (PE)		X	X			
Dullness (PE)		X	X			
FVC (percent of predicted) (LAB)	X		X	X	X	X
FEV_1 (percent of predicted) (LAB)	X		X	X	X	X
FEV_2 (LAB)			X			
FEV_3 (LAB)			X			
FEV MAX (LAB)			X			
Ratio of observed FEV_1 to observed FVC (LAB)	X		X	X	X	X

Loss of vital capacity (LAB)		X	X	X	X
Obstructive abnormality (LAB)		X	X	X	X

NOTES: Data sources: (Q) questionnaires; (PE) physical examination; (LAB) laboratory tests; (MRV) medical records verified; (MIL) military records.

When units are provided, they reflect the most recent cycle for which the measurement was taken.

Areas in gray indicate that either an endpoint was not analyzed for a particular cycle or that it was unclear from the cycle report if an endpoint was analyzed. Gray areas do not indicate that an endpoint was not measured or recorded for a particular cycle.

*Medical records were not verified in Cycles 2–3.

TABLE B-12 Neoplasia Assessment

Cycle Examination Year	1 1982	2 1985	3 1987	4 1992	5 1997	6 2002
Analyzed Endpoints						
Skin neoplasms (MRV/PE)						
Behavior (All Sites Combined)						
All		X	X	X	X	X
Malignant		X	X	X	X	X
Benign		X	X	X	X	X
Uncertain behavior or unspecified nature		X	X	X	X	X
Cell Type-Specific Analyses[a]						
Basal cell carcinoma	X	X	X	X	X	X
Squamous cell carcinoma	X	X	X	X	X	X
Fibrosarcoma	X					
Nonmelanoma				X	X	X
Melanoma	X	X	X[b]	X	X	X
Sun exposure-related malignancies		X	X			
Systemic neoplasms (MRV/PE)						
Behavior (All Sites Combined)						
All		X	X	X	X	X
Malignant		X	X	X	X	X
Benign		X	X	X	X	X
Uncertain behavior or unspecified nature		X	X	X	X	X
Site-Specific Analyses						
Malignant						
Eye, ear, face, head, and neck		X	X	X	X	X
Oral cavity, pharynx, and larynx	X	X	X	X	X	X
Brain			X	X	X	X
Digestive organs, peritoneum, and esophagus	X[c]	X		X	X	X[d]

Thymus, heart, and mediastinum			X	X	X	X
Thyroid gland	X	X	X	X	X	X
Bronchus and lung (includes trachea and pleura)	X	X	X	X	X	X
Liver		X			X	X
Colon and rectum (includes anus)	X	X	X	X	X	X
Urinary system	X[e]	X[f]	X[f]	X[f]	X	X
Kidney and ureter	X[e]	X[f]	X[f]	X[f]		X
Prostate	X[e]	X	X	X	X	X
Penis and other male genital organs	X[e]	X	X	X	X	X
Testicles	X[e]	X	X	X	X	X
Bone and articular cartilage	X					X
Extrahepatic bile duct					X	X
Ill-defined sites			X	X	X	
Connective and other soft tissues	X	X		X	X	X
Hodgkin's disease	X	X	X	X	X	X
Non-Hodgkin's lymphoma	X	X		X	X	
Leukemia	X	X	X	X		X
Other malignant systemic neoplasms of lymphoid and histiocytic tissue	X		X	X	X	X
Lymphoreticular sarcoma						X
Multiple myeloma				X		X
Soft-tissue sarcoma		X				
Premalignant						
Carcinoma *in situ* (breast, digestive organs, respiratory, prostate, penis and other male genitals, bladder and other, and nonspecified urinary)	X		X[g]	X	X[h]	X
Premalignant and Malignant						
Stomach (All)						X
Other and unspecified sites	X					

continues

TABLE B-12 *Continued*

	Cycle Examination Year	1 1982	2 1985	3 1987	4 1992	5 1997	6 2002
Skin and systemic neoplasms (MRV/PE)							
All							
	All sites combined		X	X	X	X	X
Malignant							
	All sites combined						X
PSA (LAB)					X	X	X

NOTES: Data sources: (Q) questionnaires; (PE) physical examination; (LAB) laboratory tests; (MRV) medical records verified; (MIL) military records.

Areas in gray indicate that either an endpoint was not analyzed for a particular cycle or that it was unclear from the cycle report if an endpoint was analyzed. Gray areas do not indicate that an endpoint was not measured or recorded for a particular cycle. Overlap in site-specific analyses occurs as in some cycles broad ICD-9 classes are used versus the specific site or organ codes used in other cycles.

[a] Site-specific analyses were conducted in Cycles 1–3 for the majority of cell types (AFHS, 1982, 1987, 1990).
[b] Sun exposure-related cases included (AFHS, 1990).
[c] Digestive organ/peritoneum is one category (AFHS, 1994).
[d] Esophagus only (AFHS, 2005).
[e] *Genitourinary* is one category (ICD 9 codes 179-189—excludes carcinoma in situ) (AFHS, 1984).
[f] *Kidney and Bladder* is the category reference (AFHS, 1987, 1990, 1995).
[g] Carcinoma *in situ* of penis and other sites listed separately (AFHS, 1990).
[h] The only site-specific reference for carcinoma in situ is penis (AFHS, 2000).

TABLE B-13 Reproductive Assessment

Year of Report	1984[a]	1992[b]	1998
Analyzed Endpoints			
Number of marriages (Q)	X		X
Duration of marital and nonmarital relationships (Q)	X		X
Number of couples with the desired number of children (Q)	X		X
Sperm count (LAB)	X		X
Sperm morphology (LAB)	X		X
Number of conceptions (Q)	X	X	X
Conception outcomes: miscarriage (Q/MRV)	X	X	X
Conception outcomes: induced abortion (Q/MRV)	X	X	X
Conception outcomes: tubal pregnancy (QMRV)		X	
Conception outcomes: stillbirth (Q/MRV)	X	X	X
Conception outcomes: live birth (Q/MRV)	X	X	X
Live birth outcomes: learning disabilities (Q/MRV)	X		X
Live birth outcomes: physical handicaps (Q/MRV)	X		X
Live birth outcomes: neonatal mortality (Q/MRV)	X		X
Live birth outcomes: infant mortality (Q/MRV)	X		X
Live birth outcomes: birth defects[c] (ICD 9 coded) (Q/MRV)	X	X	X
CDC birth defect category: total congenital anomalies (Q/MRV)		X	
CDC birth defect category: nervous system anomalies (Q/MRV)		X	
CDC birth defect category: eye anomalies (Q/MRV)		X	
CDC birth defect category: ear, face, and neck anomalies (Q/MRV)		X	
CDC birth defect category: circulatory system and heart anomalies (Q/MRV)		X	
CDC birth defect category: respiratory anomalies (Q/MRV)		X	
CDC birth defect category: digestive system anomalies (Q/MRV)		X	
CDC birth defect category: genital anomalies (Q/MRV)		X	
Birth defects: urinary system anomalies (Q/MRV)		X	
CDC birth defect category: musculoskeletal deformities (Q/MRV)		X	
CDC birth defect category: anomalies of the skin (Q/MRV)		X	
CDC birth defect category: chromosomal anomalies (Q/MRV)		X	
CDC birth defect category: other and unspecified anomalies (Q/MRV)		X	
Birth defect severity (Q/MRV)	X	X	X
Birth weight (MRV)		X	

NOTES: Data sources: (Q) questionnaires; (PE) physical examination; (LAB) laboratory tests; (MRV) medical records verified.

Analyzed endpoints in 1992 study were chosen for ease of comparison with the results from the 1989 CDC Vietnam Experience Study reproductive outcome results. Many of the outcomes in the 1992 report were included under broader variables analyzed for the 1984 and 1998 reports.

Areas in gray indicate that either an endpoint was not analyzed for a particular cycle or that it was unclear from the cycle report if an endpoint was analyzed. Gray areas do not indicate that an endpoint was not measured or recorded for a particular cycle.

[a]Data collected at Cycle 1 (1982). No outcomes verified.

[b]Data collected in 1982, 1985, and 1987.

[c]Birth defect had to match description on predetermined list to be included in analyses at the baseline.

TABLE B-14 Laboratory Analyses

	Cycle Examination Year	1 1982	2 1985	3 1987	4 1992	5 1997	6 2002
Hematology							
Cell Count/Indices		X	X	X	X	X	X
	WBC	X	X	X	X	X	X
	RBC	X	X	X	X	X	X
	RDW	X	X	X	X		
	HGB	X	X	X	X	X	X
	Hematocrit	X	X	X	X	X	X
	MCV	X	X	X	X	X	X
	MCH	X	X	X	X	X	X
	MCHC	X	X	X	X	X	X
	PLT	X	X	X	X	X	X
Differential		X	X	X	X	X	X
	Neutrophils	X	X	X	X	X	X
	LYMPH	X	X	X	X	X	X
	MONO	X	X	X	X	X	X
	EOS	X	X	X	X	X	X
	BANDS	X	X	X	X	X	X
	BASO	X	X	X	X	X	X
	BLAST	X	X	X	X	X	X
	RBC morphology		X	X	X	X	X
	Platelet observation		X	X	X	X	X
	Cells counted	X	X	X	X	X	X
Absolute differential							
	ABS SEGS		X	X	X	X	X
	ABS BANDS		X	X	X	X	X
	ABS LYMPHS		X	X	X	X	X
	ABS MONOS		X	X	X	X	X
	ABS EOS		X	X	X	X	X
	ABS BASOS		X	X	X	X	X
	RPR/VDRL/FTA	X	X	X	X	X	X
	ESR	X	X	X	X	X	X
	Glucose, 2HR PP	X	X	X	X	X	X
	Prothrombin time	X	X	X	X	X	X
Chemistry Routine							
	BUN	X	X	X	X	X	X
	Glucose fasting	X	X	X	X	X	X
	Cholesterol	X	X	X	X	X	X
	HDL cholesterol	X	X	X	X	X	X
	Triglycerides	X	X	X	X	X	X
	SGOT/AST	X	X	X	X	X	X
	SGPT/ALT	X	X	X	X	X	X

TABLE B-14 *Continued*

Cycle Examination Year	1 1982	2 1985	3 1987	4 1992	5 1997	6 2002
Gamma GT	X	X	X	X	X	X
Alkaline phosphatase	X	X	X	X	X	X
Total LDH	X	X	X	X	X	X
Creatinine serum	X			X	X	X
Creatine kinase	X	X	X	X	X	X
Amylase		X	X	X	X	X
Total bilirubin	X	X	X	X	X	X
Direct bilirubin	X	X	X	X	X	X
Chemistry Miscellaneous						
FSH	X	X	X	X	X	X
LH	X	X	X	X	X	X
Testosterone, free				X	X	X
Testosterone, total	X	X	X	X	X	X
Sex hormone binding globulin				X		
Estradiol				X	X	X
T4, free						X
T4, RIA	X	X	X	X	X	
T3, free						X
T3, uptake	X	X	X			
TSH	X	X	X	X	X	X
FTI	X					
PSA				X	X	X
Insulin, fasting						X
Glucagon @ 2 hr				X		X
Insulin, serum @ 2 hr				X	X	X
Glycated hemoglobin				X	X	X
C Peptide, serum				X		X
ACTH, serum				X		
Uric acid						X
Urinalysis Routine						
Color	X	X	X	X	X	X
Character	X	X	X	X	X	X
Glucose	X	X	X	X	X	X
pH	X	X	X	X	X	X
Ketone	X	X	X	X	X	X
Protein	X	X	X	X	X	X
Bile	X	X	X	X	X	X
Occult blood	X					X
Urobilinogen	X	X	X	X	X	X
Specific gravity	X	X	X	X	X	X
Epithelial cells	X	X	X	X	X	X

continues

TABLE B-14 *Continued*

Cycle Examination Year	1 1982	2 1985	3 1987	4 1992	5 1997	6 2002
Urinalysis Routine *(continued)*						
Bacteria	X	X	X	X	X	X
Mucus	X	X	X	X	X	X
WBC/HPF	X	X	X	X	X	X
Casts		X	X	X	X	X
Crystals		X	X	X	X	X
RBC		X	X	X	X	X
Nitrites		X	X	X	X	X
Leukocyte esterase					X	X
Other				X	X	X
Comments	X	X	X	X	X	X
Glucose, urine 2 hr	X	X	X	X	X	X
Urine 24 hr						
Coproporphyrin	X	X				
Uroporphyrin	X	X				
Porphobilinogen	X	X				
Heptacarboxyporphyrins		X				
Hexacarboxyporphyrins		X				
Pentacarboxyporphyrins		X				
Creatinine	X					
Aminolevulinic Acid	X					
Comments	X	X				
Cortisol Differential						
Cortisol 1	X	X				
Cortisol 2	X	X				
Protein Electrophoresis						
Total protein	X	X	X			
Prealbumin				X	X	X
Albumin	X	X	X	X	X	X
Alpha 1 globulin	X	X	X	X	X	X
Alpha 2 globulin	X	X	X	X	X	X
Beta globulin	X	X	X	X	X	X
Gamma globulin	X	X	X	X	X	X
IGA	X	X	X	X	X	X
IGG	X	X	X	X	X	X
IGM	X	X	X	X	X	X
Protein Profile						
Alpha 1 acid glycoprotein			X	X	X	X
Alpha 1 antitrypsin			X	X	X	X

TABLE B-14 *Continued*

Cycle / Examination Year	1 1982	2 1985	3 1987	4 1992	5 1997	6 2002
Alpha 2 macroglobulin			X	X	X	X
Apolipoprotein B			X	X	X	X
C3 complement			X	X	X	X
C4 complement			X	X	X	X
Haptoglobin			X	X	X	X
Transferrin			X	X	X	X
HI-RES Electrophoresis						
High-resolution bands						
IGG-Kappa				X		
IGG-Lambda				X		
IGG-No light chain				X		
IGA-Kappa				X		
IGA-Lambda				X		
IGA-No light chain				X		
IGM-Kappa				X		
IGM-Lambda				X		
IGM-No light chain				X		
KAPPA-No heavy chain				X		
LAMBDA-No heavy chain				X		
Hepatitis Panel						
HA Antibody	X		X	X	X	X
HBs Antigen	X	X	X	X	X	X
HBc Antibody	X		X	X	X	X
HBs Antibody	X	X	X	X	X	X
HC Antibody				X	X	X
HD Antibody					X	X
HIV-1 ELISA Screen			X	X	X	X
Semen Analysis						
Total count	X					
Volume	X					
Abnormal forms	X					
Immunology						
Mixed lymphocyte RX		X	X			
Cell surface markers		X	X			
Killer cell no interferon		X	X			
Killer cell interferon		X	X			
Mitogen PHA stimulate		X	X			
Mitogen pokweed stimulation		X	X			

continues

TABLE B-14 *Continued*

Cycle	1	2	3	4	5	6
Examination Year	1982	1985	1987	1992	1997	2002
Lymphocyte Phenotyping Panel						
WBC count				X	X	X
% Lymphocytes				X	X	X
Absolute lymphocytes				X	X	X
C45 total lymph (CD14–)				X	X	X
CD14 monocytes				X	X	X
Absolute CD14				X		
CD20 B cells				X		
Absolute CD20				X	X	X
CD5 T cells				X	X	X
Absolute CD5				X		
Absolute CD20 and CD5+				X		
CD4 helper T cells				X		
Absolute CD4				X	X	X
CD4+CD3				X	X	X
Absolute CD4+CD3					X	X
CD8 suppressor T cells					X	X
Absolute CD8				X	X	X
CD4+ & CD8+				X	X	X
Absolute CD4+ & CD8+				X		
Ratio CD4/CD8				X		
CD8+CD3				X		
Absolute CD8+CD3					X	X
CD3 T cells					X	X
Absolute CD3				X	X	X
CD16/56 NK cells				X	X	X
Absolute CD16/56				X	X	X
CD3+ & CD16/56+NK-like T cells				X	X	X
Absolute CD3+ & CD16/56+				X		
CD25 IL-2 receptor cells				X		
Absolute CD25				X		
CD25+ & CD3+ activated T cells				X		
Absolute CD25+ & CD3+				X		
(CD4 + CD8)/CD3				X		
(CD3 + CD20 + CD16)/CD45				X		
Occult Blood Panel—Fecal						
Occult blood 1				X		
Occult blood 2				X		
Occult blood 3				X		

TABLE B-14 *Continued*

Cycle	1	2	3	4	5	6
Examination Year	1982	1985	1987	1992	1997	2002
Mouse Stomach/Kidney Lupus Panel						
Antinuclear AB					X	X
Antimitochondrial AB				X	X	X
Antismooth Muscle AB				X	X	X
Antiparietal Cell AB				X	X	X
MSK other				X		
Thyroid microsomal AB				X	X	X
Rheumatoid factor latex				X	X	X
ANA on HEP-2 Cells						
Hep-2 cells				X		
Speckled				X		
Homogenous				X		
Nucleolar				X		
Centromere				X		
ANA Hep-2 other				X		
DNA antibodies (IFA)				X		
Anti Sm				X		
Anti RNP				X		
SSA antibody				X		
SSB antibody				X		
Lymphocyte phenotyping panel				X	X	X
Islet cell antibody				X	X	X
T-Cell clone						X
Anti-thyroid antibody				X		X
Fibrinogen					X	X
Microalbumin						
Microalbumin screen						X
Urine creatinine						X
Microalbumin quantity						X
Ratio						X
Diabetes Panel						
Hemoglobin A1c						X
Islet Cell AB						X
GAD Ab						X
C-Peptide						X
Proinsulin						X

TABLE B-15 Covariate Data Collected (Nonexhaustive List)

Age (years) (MIL)
Aminodiphenyl exposure (Q)
Anthracene exposure (Q)
Arsenic exposure (Q)
Asbestos exposure (Q)
Average lifetime residential history (Q)

Benzene exposure (Q)
Benzidene exposure (Q)
Body fat (percentage) (PE)
Body mass index (kg/m^2) (PE)

Chloromethylether exposure (Q)
Cholesterol (mg/dl) (LAB)
Chromate exposure (Q)
Coal tar exposure (Q)
Combat service (MIL)
Compliance to dietary restrictions (PE)
Composite carcinogen exposure (Q)
Composite exposure to heavy metals (Q)
Composite skin-reaction index (Q)
Creosote exposure (Q)
Cumulative degreasing chemical exposure (Q)
Cumulative herbicide exposure (Q)
Cumulative industrial chemical exposure (Q)
Cumulative insecticide exposure (Q)
Cumulative ionizing radiation exposure (Q)
Current alcohol use (drinks/day) (Q)
Current cigarette smoking (cigarettes/day) (Q)
Current employment
Current marital status (Q)
Current occupation (Q)
Current parental status (Q)
Current total household income (dollars) (Q)
Current wine consumption (drinks of wine/day) (Q)
Cutting oil exposure (Q)

Diabetes status (Q/LAB/MRV)
Diabetic severity (MRV)
Duration of diabetes (years) (LAB/MRV)

Ethnic background (Q)
Eye color (PE)

Family history of diabetes (Q)
Family history of heart disease (Q)
Family history of heart disease before age 45 (Q)

Hair color (PE)

Lifetime alcohol history (drink-years) (Q)
Lifetime cigarette smoking history (pack-years) (Q)
Lifetime wine history (drink-years of wine) (Q)

Maternal age (refers to partner in reproductive evaluation) (Q)
Maternal drinking habits (refers to partner in reproductive evaluation) (Q)
Maternal smoking (refers to partner in reproductive evaluation) (Q)
Military occupation (MIL)
Mustard gas exposure (Q)

Naphthyamine exposure (Q)
Nonmedical X ray (Q)

Personality type (PE)
Physical activity index (kcal/kg/day) (Q)
Presence of pre-SEA acne (Q)
Presence of PTSD (Q)

Race (MIL)

Skin color (PE)
Skin reaction to sun after first exposure (Q)
Skin reaction to sun after repeated exposure (Q)

Taking blood pressure medication (Q)
Time of conception relative to SEA tour (refers to reproductive evaluation) (Q/MRV)
Trichloroethylene exposure (Q)

UV light exposure (nonsolar) (Q)

Vinyl chloride exposure (Q)

Waist-to-hip ratio (PE)

NOTES: Data sources: (Q) questionnaires; (PE) physical examination; (LAB) laboratory tests; (MRV) medical records verified; (MIL) military records.

TABLE B-16 AFHS Questionnaire Data

Cycle	Subject Areas
1	Subject
	Demographic
	Employment history
	Marital/reproductive history
	Medical history
	Substance abuse history
	Psychological history
	Exposure to toxic substances
	Income
	Spouse
	Demographic
	Reproductive history
	Substance abuse history
	Next of Kin (Proxy)
	Demographic
	Employment history
	Marital/reproductive history
	Medical history
	Substance abuse history
	Leisure activities
	Mortality data
Additions to Interval Questionnaires	
2	Subject
	Skin cancer
	Personality type
	Birth marks
	Smoking habits
	Drinking habits
3	Subject
	Detailed drinking history
	Sleep disorders
	Interviewer remarks section added[a]
4	Subject
	Occupational exposures (heavy metals and vibrating power tools)
	Family health history (with particular reference to diabetes, heart trouble, and heart disease)
	Diabetes history (type, treatment received, and medications taken)
	Hepatitis B vaccination history
	Intermittent claudication and vascular insufficiency history
	Normal physical activity level
	Dietary survey[b]
5	Subject
	Percentage of herbicide spraying missions flown
	Intentional herbicide ingestion
6	Subject
	Drinking history 2 weeks prior to physical exam
	Current personal relationships
	Employment history 1 week prior to physical exam
	Children under 18 living at home (including children, grandchildren, stepchildren, foster or adopted children)
	History of mission volunteerism in SEA

[a]This section was added to the baseline questionnaire.

[b]The dietary survey was developed by Walter Willett at Harvard University and administered at the Cycle 4 follow-up only.

REFERENCES

AFHS. 1984. *An Epidemiologic Investigation of Health Effects in Air Force Personnel Following Exposure to Herbicides. Baseline Morbidity Study Results.* Brooks AFB, TX: USAF School of Aerospace Medicine. NTIS AD-A-138-340.

AFHS. 1987. *An Epidemiologic Investigation of Health Effects in Air Force Personnel Following Exposure to Herbicides. First Follow-up Examination Results.* 2 vols. Brooks AFB, TX: USAF School of Aerospace Medicine. USAFSAM-TR-87-27.

AFHS. 1990. *An Epidemiologic Investigation of Health Effects in Air Force Personnel Following Exposure to Herbicides.* 2 vols. Brooks AFB, TX: USAF School of Aerospace Medicine. USAFSAM-TR-90-2.

AFHS. 1992. *An Epidemiologic Investigation of Health Effects in Air Force Personnel Following Exposure to Herbicides. Reproductive Outcomes.* Brooks AFB, TX: Armstrong Laboratory. AL-TR-1992-0090.

AFHS. 1993. *An Epidemiologic Investigation of Health Effects in Air Force Personnel Following Exposure to Herbicides. Mortality Update: 1993.* Brooks AFB, TX: Armstrong Laboratory. AL/AO-TR-1993-0161.

AFHS. 1995. *An Epidemiologic Investigation of Health Effects in Air Force Personnel Following Exposure to Herbicides. 1992 Followup Examination Results.* Brooks AFB, TX: Epidemiologic Research Division. Armstrong Laboratory. AL-TR-920107.

AFHS. 1998. *An Epidemiologic Investigation of Health Effects in Air Force Personnel Following Exposure to Herbicides. Reproductive Outcome Update.* Brooks AFB, TX: Epidemiologic Research Division. Armstrong Laboratory. AFRL-HE-BR-TR-1998-0073.

AFHS. 2000. *An Epidemiologic Investigation of Health Effects in Air Force Personnel Following Exposure to Herbicides. 1997 Follow-up Examination Results.* Brooks AFB, TX: Human Systems Program Office. Armstrong Laboratory. AFRL-HE-BR-TR-2000-02.

AFHS. 2005. *An Epidemiologic Investigation of Health Effects in Air Force Personnel Following Exposure to Herbicides. 2002 Followup Examination Results.* Brooks AFB, TX: Epidemiologic Research Division. Armstrong Laboratory. AFRL-HE-BR-SR-2005-0003.

C

Epidemiologic Studies of Vietnam Veterans Health

Table C-1 provides an overview of design aspects of the epidemiologic studies related to Vietnam veterans' health reviewed in the Institute of Medicine's Veterans and Agent Orange report series (IOM, 1994, 1996, 1999, 2001, 2003, 2005). The summaries include the study's design type, the numbers of subjects in the study and comparison populations, and a synopsis of how subjects were selected, how data were collected, what inclusion criteria were used, and how exposure was determined. The table was excerpted from Appendix A of the *Veterans and Agent Orange: Update 2004* report. More information on these studies may be found in the reports referenced.

TABLE C-1 Epidemiologic Studies of Vietnam Veterans

Reference	Study Design	Description	Study Group (*N*)	Comparison Group (*N*)*
UNITED STATES STUDIES				
AFHS Studies Reviewed in *Update 2004*				
Akhtar et al., 2004	Cohort	Follow-up to Ketchum et al. (1999), comparing cancer incidence among Ranch Hands with Vietnam veterans who served in Southeast Asia but did not spray herbicides and with U.S. national cancer rates	1,189 net Ranch Hands for external analysis; 1,009 net Ranch Hands for internal analysis	1,776 net comparison subjects for external analysis; 1,429 net comparison subjects for internal analysis
Barrett et al., 2003	Cohort	Serum TCDD measurement and psychological functioning among Ranch Hand veterans	1,109	1,493
Michalek et al., 2003	Cohort	Correlation for TCDD elimination and Ranch Hands with diabetes	343	No comparison group
Pavuk et al., 2003	Cohort	Study to examine the relationship between serum TCDD and thyroid function in Ranch Hand veterans	1,009	1,429
AFHS Studies Reviewed in *Update 2002*				
Barrett et al., 2001	Cohort	Based on tests of cognitive functioning in 1982 and dioxin concentrations measured in 1987 and 1992, analyzed association between serum dioxin levels and cognitive functioning	937 Ranch Hands	1,052 Ranch Hand comparisons

Michalek et al., 2001a	Cohort	Based on physical examination through 1992 and medical records reviewed through March 1993, association between serum dioxin levels and hepatic abnormality	1,109 Ranch Hands	1,493 Ranch Hand comparisons
Michalek et al., 2001b	Cohort	Based on physical examination in 1982, 1985, 1987, 1992, and 1997, and medical records through 1997, association between serum dioxin and peripheral neuropathy	761 Ranch Hands	1,086 Ranch Hand comparisons
Michalek et al., 2001c	Cohort	Based on physical examination in 1982, 1985, 1987, and 1992, and medical records through 1997, association between serum dioxin and hematologic function	953 Ranch Hands	1,280 Ranch Hand comparisons
Steenland et al., 2001	Cohort	Reexamine and compare diabetes data from the NIOSH cohort and the United States Air Force (USAF) Ranch Hands in order to reconcile differences between the two study methods and protocols	267 NIOSH workers; 990 Ranch Hands	227 NIOSH comparisons 1,275 Ranch Hand comparisons
AFHS Studies Reviewed in *Update 2000*				
AFHS, 2000	Cohort	266 health-related endpoints, including assessments of 10 clinical areas: general health, neoplasia, neurologic, psychologic, gastrointestinal, cardiovascular, hematologic, endocrine, immunologic, pulmonary	995	1,299
Longnecker and Michalek, 2000	Cohort	Based on physical examination and medical records review through 1992, association between serum dioxin and diabetes mellitus among comparison group (no Ranch Hands)	—	1,197
Ketchum et al., 1999	Cohort	Based on physical examination and medical records review through 1992, association between serum dioxin and cancer, skin cancer, cancer other than skin cancer	980 Ranch Hands	1,275 Ranch Hand comparisons
Michalek et al., 1999a	Cohort	Further elucidate relationship between dioxin and diabetes mellitus, effect of dioxin body burden on sex-hormone-binding globulin and insulin and fasting glucose	871 Ranch Hands	1,121 Ranch Hand comparisons

continues

TABLE C-1 *Continued*

Reference	Study Design	Description	Study Group (*N*)	Comparison Group (*N*)*
Michalek et al., 1999b	Cohort	Based on physical examinations in 1982, 1985, 1987, and 1992, immunologic response and exposure to dioxin among Ranch Hand and comparison cohorts	914 Ranch Hands 372 (lymphocyte counts conducted)	1,186 Ranch Hand comparisons 491 (lymphocyte counts conducted)
Burton et al., 1998	Cohort	Based on physical examination and medical record review through 1992, association between serum dioxin and occurrence and timing (relative to Southeast Asia service) of chloracne and acne	930 Ranch Hands	1,200 Ranch Hand comparisons
Michalek et al., 1998b	Cohort	Updates, all-cause and cause-specific post-service mortality (through 1993) among veterans of Operation Ranch Hand, using standardized mortality ratios	1,261 Ranch Hands	19,080 Ranch Hand comparisons
Michalek et al., 1998c	Cohort	Prospective study, exposure and long-term health, survival, reproductive outcome	1,208 veterans; 903 offspring	1,549 veterans; 1,254 offspring
Michalek et al., 1998d	Cohort	Third report in a series investigating dioxin body burden and preterm birth, intrauterine growth retardation, infant death among offspring of Ranch Hand veterans	859	1,223
AFHS Studies Reviewed in *Update 1998*				
Michalek et al., 1998a	Cohort	Paternal serum dioxin levels and infant death among Ranch Hand offspring	859 children: 323 background exposure; 267 low exposure; 269 high exposure	1,223 children

Henriksen et al., 1997	Cohort	Relationship between serum dioxin and glucose, insulin, and diabetes mellitus in Ranch Hands through 1992	989	1,276
AFHS, 1996; Michalek et al., 1998b	Cohort	Mortality update, Ranch Hands through the end of 1993 in the AFHS cohort (1983, 1984b, 1985, 1986, 1989, 1991a, 1995)	1,261	19,080
Henriksen et al., 1996	Cohort	Serum dioxin and reproductive hormones in Ranch Hands, 1982, 1985, 1987, and 1992	1,045 participants (1982); 474 provided semen	1,224 participants (1982); 532 provided semen
AFHS Studies Reviewed in *Update 1996*				
AFHS, 1995	Cohort	Mortality updates of Ranch Hands who sprayed herbicides in Vietnam, compared with USAF C-130 air and ground crew veterans in Southeast Asia who did not spray herbicides	1,261, original cohort	19,101, original cohort
Wolfe et al., 1995	Cohort	Paternal serum dioxin and reproductive outcomes of Ranch Hand veterans, compared with USAF veterans from Southeast Asia who did not spray herbicides	932	1,202
AFHS Studies Reviewed in *VAO*				
AFHS, 1992	Cohort	Reproductive outcomes of AFHS participants	791	942
AFHS, 1984a, 1987, 1990, 1991b	Cohort	Baseline morbidity, follow-up examination results	1,208 baseline	1,668 baseline

continues

TABLE C-1 *Continued*

Reference	Study Design	Description	Study Group (*N*)	Comparison Group (*N*)*
AFHS, 1983, 1984b, 1985, 1986, 1989, 1991a	Cohort	Mortality updates, Ranch Hands who sprayed herbicides in Vietnam, compared with USAF C-130 air and ground crew veterans in Southeast Asia who did not spray herbicides	1,261 (original cohort)	19,101 (original cohort)
Michalek et al., 1990	Cohort	Mortality of Ranch Hands, compared with USAF C-130 air and ground crew veterans in Southeast Asia	1,261	19,101
Wolfe et al., 1990	Cohort	Health status of Ranch Hands at second follow-up, compared with USAF C-130 air and ground crew veterans in Southeast Asia	995	1,299
Centers for Disease Control and Prevention Studies Reviewed in *VAO*				
Decoufle et al., 1992	Cohort	Association between self-reported health outcomes and perception of exposure to herbicides based on Vietnam Experience Study	7,924	7,364
O'Brien et al., 1991	Cohort	Interview report and mortality for NHL based on Vietnam Experience Study	8,170	7,564
CDC, 1990a	Case-control	Selected Cancers Study: population-based case-control study of all men born 1921–1953; cases diagnosed area covered by eight cancer registries, controls selected by random-digit dialing	1,157 NHL; 342 STS; 310 HD; 48 nasal carcinoma; 80 nasopharyngeal carcinoma; 130 primary liver cancer	1,776

CDC, 1990b	Case-control	Selected Cancers Study: population-based case-control study of all men born 1921–1953; cases diagnosed in area covered by eight cancer registries, controls selected by random-digit dialing for NHL	1,157	1,776
CDC, 1990c	Case-control	Selected Cancers Study: STS	342	1,776
CDC, 1990d	Case-control	Selected Cancers Study: HD, nasal cancer, nasopharyngeal cancer, primary liver cancer	310 HD; 48 nasal carcinoma; 80 nasopharyngeal carcinoma; 130 primary liver cancer	1,776
CDC, 1989b	Cohort	Vietnam Experience Study: random sample, U.S. Army enlisted men, 1965–1971	2,490	1,972
CDC, 1988a	Cohort	Vietnam Experience Study: random sample, U.S. Army enlisted men, 1965–1971, psychosocial outcomes	2,490	1,972
CDC, 1988b	Cohort	Vietnam Experience Study: physical health outcomes	2,490	1,972
CDC, 1988c	Cohort	Vietnam Experience Study: reproductive outcomes	12,788 children	11,910 children
CDC, 1987; Boyle et al., 1987	Cohort	Vietnam Experience Study: mortality	9,324	8,989
Erickson et al., 1984 a,b	Case-control	CDC birth defects study, children born in the Atlanta, Georgia, area 1968–1980, comparing paternal Vietnam experience and potential Agent Orange exposure for birth defects cases and normal controls	7,133	4,246

continues

TABLE C-1 *Continued*

Reference	Study Design	Description	Study Group (*N*)	Comparison Group (*N*)*
Department of Veterans Affairs Studies Reviewed in *Update 2002*				
Kang et al., 2001	Cohort	Health of Army Chemical Corps Vietnam veterans, compared with Army Chemical Corps veterans who did not serve in Vietnam	2,872	2,737
Kang et al., 2000a	Cohort	Self-report pregnancy outcomes for female Vietnam veterans, compared with contemporary veterans not deployed to Vietnam; odds ratios calculated for reproductive history and various birth defects	3,392 women; 1,665 women with indexed pregnancy	3,038 women; 1,912 women with indexed pregnancy
Kang et al., 2000b	Cohort	Gynecologic cancers among female Vietnam veterans, compared with veteran controls	484	5,946
Department of Veterans Affairs Studies Reviewed in *Update 1998*				
Dalager and Kang, 1997	Cohort	Morbidity and mortality experience (1968–1987), Army Chemical Corps Vietnam veterans, compared with U.S. men; extension of Thomas and Kang (1990)	2,872	2,737
Mahan et al., 1997	Case-control	Lung cancer among Vietnam veterans (1983–1990)	329	269 111
McKinney et al., 1997	Cross-sectional	Tobacco use in veterans and nonveterans by 1987 NMES	15,000	—
Bullman and Kang, 1996	Cohort	Mortality of veterans with nonlethal (combat and noncombat) wounds sustained during the Vietnam war	34,534	—
Watanabe and Kang, 1996	Cohort	Mortality experience (1965–1988) of Army and Marine Corps Vietnam veterans; extension of Breslin et al. (1988) and Watanabe et al. (1991)	33,833	36,797

Dalager et al., 1995b	Case-control	HD cases diagnosed 1969–1985 among Vietnam-era veterans	283	404
Watanabe and Kang, 1995	Cohort	Postservice mortality among Marine Vietnam veterans	10,716	9,346
Department of Veterans Affairs Studies Reviewed in *Update 1996*				
Dalager et al., 1995a	Cohort	Update of Thomas et al. (1991) through Dec. 31, 1995	4,586	5,325
Bullman et al., 1994	Case-control	Association between testicular cancer and surrogate measures of exposure to Agent Orange in male Vietnam veterans	97	311
Department of Veterans Affairs Studies Reviewed in *VAO*				
Bullman et al., 1991	Case-control	PTSD cases in Vietnam veterans, compared with Vietnam veterans without PTSD, for association with traumatic combat experience	374	373
Dalager et al., 1991	Case-control	NHL cases diagnosed 1969–1985 among Vietnam-era veterans, compared with cases of other malignancies among Vietnam-era veterans, for association with Vietnam service	201	358
Eisen et al., 1991	Cohort	Health effects in male monozygotic twins serving in the armed forces during Vietnam era (1965–1975)	2,260	2,260
Thomas et al., 1991	Cohort	Mortality experience (1973–1987) among female Vietnam veterans, compared with female non-Vietnam veterans and for each cohort compared with U.S. women	4,582	5,324

continues

TABLE C-1 *Continued*

Reference	Study Design	Description	Study Group (N)	Comparison Group (N)*
Watanabe et al., 1991	Cohort	Mortality experience (1965–1984) in Army and Marine Corps Vietnam veterans, compared with: (1) branch-specific (Army and Marine) Vietnam-era veterans, (2) all Vietnam-era veterans combined, (3) the U.S. male population	24,145 Army 5,501 Marines	(1) 27,145 Army 4,505 Marines (2) 32,422 combined Vietnam era (3) U.S. male population
Bullman et al., 1990	Cohort	Mortality experience in Army I Corps Vietnam veterans, compared with Army Vietnam-era veterans	6,668 deaths	27,917 deaths
Farberow et al., 1990	Case-control	Psychological profiles, military factors associated with suicide and MVA fatalities in Los Angeles County Vietnam-era veterans (1977–1982)	22 Vietnam suicides; 19 Vietnam-era suicides	21 Vietnam MVA; 20 Vietnam-era MVA
Thomas and Kang, 1990	Cohort	Morbidity and mortality experience (1968–1987) in Army Chemical Corps Vietnam veterans compared with U.S. men	894	—
True et al., 1988	Cross-sectional	PTSD and Vietnam combat experience among Vietnam-era veterans	775	1,012
Breslin et al., 1988; Burt et al., 1987	Cohort	Mortality experience (1965–1982) in Army and Marine Corps Vietnam veterans, compared with Vietnam-era veterans who did not serve in Southeast Asia, standardized by age and race; nested NHL case-control study	24,235	26,685

Kang et al., 1987	Case-control	STS cases (1975–1980) diagnosed at the Armed Forces Institute of Pathology (AFIP), compared with controls identified from patient logs of referring pathologists or their departments, for association with Vietnam service and likelihood of Agent Orange exposure	217	599
Kang et al., 1986	Case-control	STS (1969–1983) in Vietnam-era veterans, for association with branch of Vietnam service as a surrogate for Agent Orange exposure	234	13,496
American Legion Studies Reviewed in *VAO*				
Snow et al., 1988	Cohort	PTSD in association with traumatic combat experience among American Legion members serving in Southeast Asia (1961–1975)	2,858	Study group subdivided for internal comparison
Stellman et al., 1988a	Cohort	Physical health, reproductive outcomes among American Legion members who served in Southeast Asia (1961–1975), for association with combat and herbicide exposure	2,858	3,933
Stellman et al., 1988b	Cohort	Social, behavioral outcomes among American Legion members who served in Southeast Asia (1961–1975), association with combat and herbicide exposure	2,858	3,933
State Studies Reviewed in *Update 1998*				
Clapp, 1997	Case-control	Selected cancers identified (1988–1993) among Massachusetts Vietnam veterans, compared with Massachusetts Vietnam-era veterans with cancers of other sites; update of Clapp et al., 1991	245	999
State Studies Reviewed in *Update 1996*				
Visintainer et al., 1995	Cohort	Mortality experience (1965–1971) in male Michigan Vietnam veterans, compared with non-Vietnam veterans from Michigan	3,364 deaths	5,229 deaths

continues

TABLE C-1 *Continued*

Reference	Study Design	Description	Study Group (*N*)	Comparison Group (*N*)*
State Studies Reviewed in *VAO*				
Fiedler and Gochfeld, 1992; Kahn et al., 1992a,b,c	Cohort	New Jersey: outcomes in select group of herbicide-exposed Army, Marine, and Navy Vietnam veterans, compared with veterans self-reported as unexposed	10 Pointman I 55 Pointman II	17 Pointman I 15 Pointman II
Clapp et al., 1991	Case-control	Massachusetts: selected cancers identified (1982–1988) among Vietnam veterans, compared with Massachusetts Vietnam-era veterans with cancers of other sites	214	727
Deprez et al., 1991	Descriptive	Maine: Vietnam veterans, compared with atomic test veterans and general population, for health status and reproductive outcomes	249	113 atomic test veterans
Levy, 1988	Cross-sectional	Massachusetts: PTSD in chloracne as indicator of exposure to TCDD; control Vietnam veterans	6	25
Anderson et al., 1986a	Cohort	Wisconsin: mortality experience, veterans compared with nonveterans (Phase 1); mortality experience of Vietnam veterans and Vietnam-era veterans, compared with nonveterans and other veterans (Phase 2)	110,815 white male veteran deaths; 2,494 white male Vietnam-era veteran deaths; 923 white male Vietnam veteran deaths	342,654 white male non-veteran deaths; 109,225 white male other veteran deaths

Anderson et al., 1986b	Cohort	Wisconsin: mortality experience in Vietnam-era veterans and Vietnam veterans, compared with U.S. men, Wisconsin men, Wisconsin nonveterans, and Wisconsin other veterans	122,238 Vietnam-era veterans; 43,398 Vietnam veterans	—
Goun and Kuller, 1986	Case-control	Pennsylvania: STS, NHL, selected rare cancer cases, compared with controls without cancer for Vietnam experience in men (1968–1983)	349	349 deceased
Holmes et al., 1986	Cohort	West Virginia: mortality experience (1968–1983) of veterans, Vietnam veterans, Vietnam-era veterans, compared with nonveterans; Vietnam veterans compared with Vietnam-era veterans	615 Vietnam veterans; 610 Vietnam-era veterans	—
Pollei et al., 1986	Cohort	New Mexico: chest radiographs of Agent Orange Registry Vietnam veterans, compared with radiographs of control USAF servicemen, for pulmonary and cardiovascular pathology	422	105
Kogan and Clapp, 1985, 1988	Cohort	Massachusetts: mortality experience (1972–1983) among white male Vietnam veterans, compared with non-Vietnam veterans and all other nonveteran white males in Massachusetts	840 deaths	2,515 deaths in Vietnam-era veterans
Lawrence et al., 1985	Cohort	New York: mortality experience in (1) Vietnam-era veterans, compared with nonveterans and (2) Vietnam veterans, compared with Vietnam-era veterans	(1) 4,558 (2) 555	17,936 941
Rellahan, 1985	Cohort	Hawaii: health outcomes in Vietnam-era (1962–1972) veterans residing in Hawaii, associated with Vietnam experience	232	186
Wendt, 1985	Descriptive	Iowa: health effects and potential exposure to Agent Orange among veterans who served in Southeast Asia	10,846	None

continues

TABLE C-1 *Continued*

Reference	Study Design	Description	Study Group (*N*)	Comparison Group (*N*)*
Greenwald et al., 1984	Case-control	New York: STS cases, compared with controls without cancer for Vietnam service and herbicide exposure including Agent Orange, dioxin, or 2,4,5-T	281	281 live controls; 130 deceased controls
Newell, 1984	Cross-sectional	Texas: preliminary (1) cytogenetic, (2) sperm, (3) immune response tests in Vietnam veterans, compared with controls	(1) 30; (2) 32; (3) 66	(1) 30; (2) 32; (3) 66
Other U.S. Veterans Studies Reviewed in *VAO*				
Tarone et al., 1991	Case-control	Testicular cancer (18–42 years old) cases, January 1976–June 1981, compared with hospital controls, for association with Vietnam service	137	130
Aschengrau and Monson, 1990	Case-control	Cases with late adverse pregnancy outcomes compared with normal control births, for association with paternal Vietnam service (1977–1980)	857 congenital anomalies 61 stillbirths; 48 neonatal deaths	998
Goldberg et al., 1990	Cohort	Male twin pairs who served in Vietnam era (1965–1975), for association between Vietnam service and PTSD	2,092	2,092
Aschengrau and Monson, 1989	Case-control	Association between husband's military service and spontaneous abortion at or by 27 weeks, compared with women delivering at 37 weeks	201	1,119

AUSTRALIAN VETERANS STUDIES				
Australian Studies Reviewed in *Update 2000*				
AIHW, 1999	Cohort	Validation of the male veterans study (CDVA, 1998a) by medical documents, doctors' certification, records on a disease or death registry	6,842	—
CDVA, 1998a	Cohort	Self-reported data on male members of the Australian Defence Force and the Citizen Military Force who landed in Vietnam or entered Vietnamese water. Questions on physical (including reproductive history) and mental health, and that of their partner(s) and children	49,944 mailed; 39,955 responded	—
CDVA, 1998b	Cohort	Self-reported data on female members of the Australian Defence Force and the Citizen Military Force who landed in Vietnam or entered Vietnamese water. Questions on physical (including reproductive history) and mental health, and that of their partner(s) and children	278 mailed 225 responded	—
Australian Studies Reviewed in *Update 1998*				
Crane et al., 1997a	Cohort	Mortality experience (through 1994) of Australian veterans who served in Vietnam	59,036 men 484 women	—
Crane et al., 1997b	Cohort	Mortality experience (through 1994) of Australian national servicemen who served in Vietnam	18,949	24,646
O'Toole et al., 1996a,b,c	Cross-sectional	Survey of self-reported health status (1989–1990) of Australian Army Vietnam veterans	641	—
Australian Studies Reviewed in *VAO*				
Field and Kerr, 1988	Cohort	Tasmanian Vietnam veterans, compared with neighborhood controls for adverse reproductive and childhood health outcomes	357	281

continues

TABLE C-1 *Continued*

Reference	Study Design	Description	Study Group (*N*)	Comparison Group (*N*)*
Fett et al., 1987a	Cohort	Mortality experience in Vietnam veterans, compared with Vietnam-era veterans through 1981	19,205	25,677
Fett et al., 1987b	Cohort	Cause-specific mortality experience in Vietnam veterans, compared with Vietnam veterans through 1981	19,205	25,677
Forcier et al., 1987	Cohort	Mortality in Vietnam veterans by job classification, location, time of service	19,205	Internal comparison
Donovan et al., 1983, 1984	Case-control	Congenital anomalies in children (1969–1979), compared with infants born without anomalies, for association with paternal Vietnam service	8,517	8,517
OTHER VIETNAM VETERANS' STUDIES				
Other New Vietnam Veterans' Studies Reviewed in *Update 2004*				
Kim H-A et al., 2003	Cohort	Immunotoxicologic effects of Agent Orange exposure on Korean Vietnam veterans	51 (24 veterans–patient; 27 veterans–normal)	36
Kim J-S et al., 2003	Cross-sectional	Agent Orange exposure and Korean Vietnam veterans	1,224	154
Mo et al., 2002	Cohort	Skin and general disease patterns among Korean Vietnam veterans	332	None

Other Vietnam Veterans Studies Reviewed in *Update 1998*

Chinh et al., 1996	Cohort	Antinuclear antibodies and sperm autoantibodies among Vietnamese veterans who served 5–10 years in a "dioxin-sprayed zone"	25	63; 36

NOTE: Abbreviations: 2,4,5-T, 2,4,5-trichlorophenoxyacetic acid; AFHS, Air Force Health Study; CDC, Centers for Disease Control and Prevention; CDVA, Commonwealth Department of Veterans' Affairs (Australia); HD, Hodgkin's disease; MVA, motor vehicle accidents; NIOSH, National Institute for Occupational Safety and Health; NHL, non-Hodgkin's lymphoma; NMES, National Medical Expenditure Survey; PTSD, post-traumatic stress disorder; SMR, standardized mortality ratio; STS, soft-tissue sarcoma; TCDD, 2,3,7,8-tetrachlorodibenzo-*p*-dioxin; *Update 2004*, *Veterans and Agent Orange: Update 2004* (IOM, 2005); *Update 2000*, *Veterans and Agent Orange: Update 2000* (IOM, 2001); *Update 1998*, *Veterans and Agent Orange: Update 1998* (IOM, 1999); *Update 1996*, *Veterans and Agent Orange: Update 1996* (IOM, 1996); USAF, United States Air Force; and *VAO*, *Veterans and Agent Orange: Health Effects of Herbicides Used in Vietnam* (IOM, 1994).

*Comparison group based on a population (e.g., U.S. white males, country rates); details are given in the text for population specifics.

REFERENCES

AFHS (Air Force Health Study). 1983. *An Epidemiologic Investigation of Health Effects in Air Force Personnel Following Exposure to Herbicides. Baseline Mortality Study Results.* Brooks AFB, TX: USAF School of Aerospace Medicine. NTIS AD-A130 793.

AFHS. 1984a. *An Epidemiologic Investigation of Health Effects in Air Force Personnel Following Exposure to Herbicides. Baseline Morbidity Study Results.* Brooks AFB, TX: USAF School of Aerospace Medicine. NTIS AD-A138 340.

AFHS. 1984b. *An Epidemiologic Investigation of Health Effects in Air Force Personnel Following Exposure to Herbicides. Mortality Update: 1984.* Brooks AFB, TX: USAF School of Aerospace Medicine. NTIS-AD-A-162-687.

AFHS. 1985. *An Epidemiologic Investigation of Health Effects in Air Force Personnel Following Exposure to Herbicides. Mortality Update: 1985.* Brooks AFB, TX: USAF School of Aerospace Medicine. NTIS-AD-A-163-237.

AFHS. 1986. *An Epidemiologic Investigation of Health Effects in Air Force Personnel Following Exposure to Herbicides. Mortality Update: 1986.* Brooks AFB, TX: USAF School of Aerospace Medicine. USAFSAM-TR-86-43.

AFHS. 1987. *An Epidemiologic Investigation of Health Effects in Air Force Personnel Following Exposure to Herbicides. First Follow-up Examination Results.* Brooks AFB, TX: USAF School of Aerospace Medicine.USAFSAM-TR-87-27.

AFHS. 1989. *An Epidemiologic Investigation of Health Effects in Air Force Personnel Following Exposure to Herbicides. Mortality Update: 1989.* Brooks AFB, TX: USAF School of Aerospace Medicine.USAFSAM-TR-89-9.

AFHS. 1990. *An Epidemiologic Investigation of Health Effects in Air Force Personnel Following Exposure to Herbicides.* Brooks AFB, TX: USAF School of Aerospace Medicine. USAFSAM-TR-90-2.

AFHS. 1991a. *An Epidemiologic Investigation of Health Effects in Air Force Personnel Following Exposure to Herbicides. Mortality Update: 1991.* Brooks AFB, TX: Armstrong Laboratory. AL-TR-1991-0132.

AFHS. 1991b. *An Epidemiologic Investigation of Health Effects in Air Force Personnel Following Exposure to Herbicides. Serum Dioxin Analysis of 1987 Examination Results.* Brooks AFB, TX: USAF School of Aerospace Medicine. AL-TR-91-0009.

AFHS. 1992. *An Epidemiologic Investigation of Health Effects in Air Force Personnel Following Exposure to Herbicides. Reproductive Outcomes.* Brooks AFB, TX: Armstrong Laboratory. AL–TR–1992–0090.

AFHS. 1995. *An Epidemiologic Investigation of Health Effects in Air Force Personnel Following Exposure to Herbicides. 1992 Follow-up Examination Results.* Brooks AFB, TX: Epidemiologic Research Division, Armstrong Laboratory. AL-TR-920107.

AFHS. 1996. *An Epidemiologic Investigation of Health Effects in Air Force Personnel Following Exposure to Herbicides. Mortality Update 1996.* Brooks AFB, TX: Epidemiologic Research Division, Armstrong Laboratory. AL/AO-TR-1996-0068.

AFHS. 2000. *An Epidemiologic Investigation of Health Effects in Air Force Personnel Following Exposure to Herbicides. 1997 Follow-up Examination Results.* Brooks AFB, TX: Human Systems Program Office. Armstrong Laboratory. AFRL-HE-BR-TR-2000-02.

AIHW (Australian Institute of Health and Welfare). 1999. *Morbidity of Vietnam Veterans: A Study of the Health of Australia's Vietnam Veteran Community: Volume 3: Validation Study.* Canberra: AIHW.

Akhtar FZ, Garabrant DH, Ketchum NS, Michalek JE. 2004. Cancer in US Air Force veterans of the Vietnam war. *Journal of Occupational and Environmental Medicine* 46(2):123–136.

Anderson HA, Hanrahan LP, Jensen M, Laurin D, Yick WY, Wiegman P. 1986a. *Wisconsin Vietnam Veteran Mortality Study: Proportionate Mortality Ratio Study Results.* Madison, WI: Wisconsin Division of Health.

Anderson HA, Hanrahan LP, Jensen M, Laurin D, Yick WY, Wiegman P. 1986b. *Wisconsin Vietnam Veteran Mortality Study: Final Report*. Madison, WI: Wisconsin Division of Health.

Aschengrau A, Monson RR. 1989. Paternal military service in Vietnam and risk of spontaneous abortion. *Journal of Occupational Medicine* 31:618–623.

Aschengrau A, Monson RR. 1990. Paternal military service in Vietnam and the risk of late adverse pregnancy outcomes. *American Journal of Public Health* 80:1218–1224.

Barrett DH, Morris RD, Akhtar FZ, Michalek JE. 2001. Serum dioxin and cognitive functioning among veterans of Operation Ranch Hand. *Neurotoxicology* 22:491–502.

Barrett DH, Morris RD, Jackson WG Jr, Stat M, Michalek JE. 2003. Serum dioxin and psychological functioning in US Air Force veterans of the Vietnam War. *Military Medicine* 168:153–159.

Boyle C, Decoufle P, Delaney RJ, DeStefano F, Flock ML, Hunter MI, Joesoef MR, Karon JM, Kirk ML, Layde PM, McGee DL, Moyer LA, Pollock DA, Rhodes P, Scally MJ, Worth RM. 1987. *Postservice Mortality Among Vietnam Veterans*. Atlanta: Centers for Disease Control and Prevention. CEH 86-0076.

Breslin P, Kang H, Lee Y, Burt V, Shepard BM. 1988. Proportionate mortality study of US Army and US Marine Corps veterans of the Vietnam War. *Journal of Occupational Medicine* 30:412–419.

Bullman TA, Kang HK. 1996. The risk of suicide among wounded Vietnam veterans. *American Journal of Public Health* 86(5):662–667.

Bullman TA, Kang HK, Watanabe KK. 1990. Proportionate mortality among US Army Vietnam veterans who served in Military Region I. *American Journal of Epidemiology* 132:670–674.

Bullman TA, Kang H, Thomas TL. 1991. Posttraumatic stress disorder among Vietnam veterans on the Agent Orange Registry: a case-control analysis. *Annals of Epidemiology* 1:505–512.

Bullman TA, Watanabe KK, Kang HK. 1994. Risk of testicular cancer associated with surrogate measures of Agent Orange exposure among Vietnam veterans on the Agent Orange Registry. *Annals of Epidemiology* 4:11–16.

Burt VL, Breslin PP, Kang HK, Lee Y. 1987. *Non-Hodgkin's lymphoma in Vietnam veterans*. Washington, DC: Department of Medicine and Surgery, Veterans Administration.

Burton JE, Michalek JE, Rahe AJ. 1998. Serum dioxin, chloracne, and acne in veterans of Operation Ranch Hand. *Archives of Environmental Health* 53(3):199–204.

CDC (Centers for Disease Control). 1987. Postservice mortality among Vietnam veterans. *Journal of the American Medical Association* 257:790–795.

CDC. 1988a. Health status of Vietnam veterans. I. Psychosocial characteristics. *Journal of the American Medical Association* 259:2701–2707.

CDC. 1988b. Health status of Vietnam veterans. II. Physical health. *Journal of the American Medical Association* 259:2708–2714.

CDC. 1988c. Health status of Vietnam veterans. III. Reproductive outcomes and child health. *Journal of the American Medical Association* 259:2715–2717.

CDC. 1989. *Health Status of Vietnam Veterans: Vietnam Experience Study*. Vols. I–V, Supplements A–C. Atlanta: US Department of Health and Human Services.

CDC. 1990a. *The Association of Selected Cancers with Service in the US Military in Vietnam: Final Report*. Atlanta: US Department of Health and Human Services.

CDC. 1990b. The association of selected cancers with service in the US military in Vietnam. I. Non-Hodgkin's lymphoma. *Archives of Internal Medicine* 150:2473–2483.

CDC. 1990c. The association of selected cancers with service in the US military in Vietnam. II. Soft-tissue and other sarcomas. *Archives of Internal Medicine* 150:2485–2492.

CDC. 1990d. The association of selected cancers with service in the US military in Vietnam. III. Hodgkin's disease, nasal cancer, nasopharyngeal cancer, and primary liver cancer. *Archives of Internal Medicine* 150:2495–2505.

CDVA (Commonwealth Department of Veterans' Affairs). 1998a. *Morbidity of Vietnam Veterans: A Study of the Health of Australia's Vietnam Veteran Community. Volume 1: Male Vietnam Veterans Survey and Community Comparison Outcomes*. Canberra: Department of Veterans' Affairs.

CDVA. 1998b. *Morbidity of Vietnam Veterans: A Study of the Health of Australia's Vietnam Veteran Community. Volume 2: Female Vietnam Veterans Survey and Community Comparison Outcomes*. Canberra: Department of Veterans' Affairs.

Chinh TT, Phi PT, Thuy NT. 1996. Sperm auto-antibodies and antinuclear antigen antibodies in chronic dioxin-exposed veterans. *Chemosphere* 32(3):525–530.

Clapp RW. 1997. Update of cancer surveillance of veterans in Massachusetts, USA. *International Journal of Epidemiology* 26(3):679–681.

Clapp RW, Cupples LA, Colton T, Ozonoff DM. 1991. Cancer surveillance of veterans in Massachusetts, 1982–1988. *International Journal of Epidemiology* 20:7–12.

Crane PJ, Barnard DL, Horsley KW, Adena MA. 1997a. *Mortality of Vietnam Veterans: The Veteran Cohort Study. A Report of the 1996 Retrospective Cohort Study of Australian Vietnam Veterans.* Canberra: Department of Veterans' Affairs.

Crane PJ, Barnard DL, Horsley KW, Adena MA. 1997b. *Mortality of National Service Vietnam Veterans: A Report of the 1996 Retrospective Cohort Study of Australian Vietnam Veterans.* Canberra: Department of Veterans' Affairs.

Dalager NA, Kang HK. 1997. Mortality among Army Chemical Corps Vietnam veterans. *American Journal of Industrial Medicine* 31(6):719–726.

Dalager NA, Kang HK, Burt VL, Weatherbee L. 1991. Non-Hodgkin's lymphoma among Vietnam veterans. *Journal of Occupational Medicine* 33:774–779.

Dalager NA, Kang HK, Thomas TL. 1995a. Cancer mortality patterns among women who served in the military: the Vietnam experience. *Journal of Occupational and Environmental Medicine* 37:298–305.

Dalager NA, Kang HK, Burt VL, Weatherbee L. 1995b. Hodgkin's disease and Vietnam service. *Annals of Epidemiology* 5(5):400–406.

Decoufle P, Holmgreen P, Boyle CA, Stroup NE. 1992. Self-reported health status of Vietnam veterans in relation to perceived exposure to herbicides and combat. *American Journal of Epidemiology* 135:312–323.

Deprez RD, Carvette ME, Agger MS. 1991. *The Health and Medical Status of Maine Veterans: A Report to the Bureau of Veterans Services, Commission of Vietnam and Atomic Veterans.* Portland, ME: Public Health Resource Group.

Donovan JW, Adena MA, Rose G, Battistutta D. 1983. *Case-Control Study of Congenital Anomalies and Vietnam Service: Birth Defects Study. Report to the Minister for Veterans' Affairs.* Canberra: Australian Government Publishing Service.

Donovan JW, MacLennan R, Adena M. 1984. Vietnam service and the risk of congenital anomalies: a case-control study. *Medical Journal of Australia* 140:394–397.

Eisen S, Goldberg J, True WR, Henderson WG. 1991. A co-twin control study of the effects of the Vietnam War on the self-reported physical health of veterans. *American Journal of Epidemiology* 134:49–58.

Erickson JD, Mulinare J, McClain PW, Fitch TG, James LM, McClearn AB, Adams MJ Jr. 1984a. Vietnam Veterans' Risks for Fathering Babies with Birth Defects. Atlanta: Centers for Disease Control.

Erickson JD, Mulinare J, McClain PW, Fitch TG, James LM, McClearn AB, Adams MJ Jr. 1984b. Vietnam veterans' risks for fathering babies with birth defects. *Journal of the American Medical Association* 252:903–912.

Farberow NL, Kang H, Bullman T. 1990. Combat experience and postservice psychosocial status as predictors of suicide in Vietnam veterans. *Journal of Nervous and Mental Disease* 178:32–37.

Fett MJ, Adena MA, Cobbin DM, Dunn M. 1987a. Mortality among Australian conscripts of the Vietnam conflict era. I. Death from all causes. *American Journal of Epidemiology* 126:869–877.

Fett MJ, Nairn JR, Cobbin DM, Adena MA. 1987b. Mortality among Australian conscripts of the Vietnam conflict era. II. Causes of death. *American Journal of Epidemiology* 125:878–884.

Fiedler N, Gochfeld M. 1992. *Neurobehavioral Correlates of Herbicide Exposure in Vietnam Veterans.* New Jersey Agent Orange Commission.

Field B, Kerr C. 1988. Reproductive behaviour and consistent patterns of abnormality in offspring of Vietnam veterans. *Journal of Medical Genetics* 25:819–826.

Forcier L, Hudson HM, Cobbin DM, Jones MP, Adena MA, Fett MJ. 1987. Mortality of Australian veterans of the Vietnam conflict and the period and location of their Vietnam service. *Military Medicine* 152:9–15.

Goldberg J, True WR, Eisen SA, Henderson WG. 1990. A twin study of the effects of the Vietnam war on posttraumatic stress disorder. *Journal of the American Medical Association* 263:1227–1232.

Goun BD, Kuller LH. 1986. *Final Report: A Case-Control Mortality Study on the Association of Soft Tissue Sarcomas, Non-Hodgkin's Lymphomas, and Other Selected Cancers and Vietnam Military Service in Pennsylvania Males.* Pittsburgh, PA: University of Pittsburgh.

Greenwald P, Kovasznay B, Collins DN, Therriault G. 1984. Sarcomas of soft tissues after Vietnam service. *Journal of the National Cancer Institute* 73:1107–1109.

Henriksen GL, Michalek JE, Swaby JA, Rahe AJ. 1996. Serum dioxin, testosterone, and gonadotropins in veterans of Operation Ranch Hand. *Epidemiology* 7(4):352–357.

Henriksen GL, Ketchum NS, Michalek JE, Swaby JA. 1997. Serum dioxin and diabetes mellitus in veterans of Operation Ranch Hand. *Epidemiology* 8(3):252–258.

Holmes AP, Bailey C, Baron RC, Bosanac E, Brough J, Conroy C, Haddy L. 1986. *West Virginia Department of Health Vietnam-Era Veterans Mortality Study, Preliminary Report.* Charleston, WV: West Virginia Health Department.

IOM (Institute of Medicine). 1994. *Veterans and Agent Orange: Health Effects of Herbicides Used in Vietnam.* Washington, DC: National Academy Press.

IOM. 1996. *Veterans and Agent Orange: Update 1996.* Washington, DC: National Academy Press.

IOM. 1999. *Veterans and Agent Orange: Update 1998.* Washington, DC: National Academy Press.

IOM. 2001. *Veterans and Agent Orange: Update 2000.* Washington, DC: National Academy Press.

IOM. 2003. *Veterans and Agent Orange: Update 2002.* Washington, DC: The National Academies Press.

IOM. 2005. *Veterans and Agent Orange: Update 2004.* Washington, DC. The National Academies Press.

Kahn PC, Gochfeld M, Lewis WW. 1992a. Dibenzodioxin and Dibenzofuran Congener Levels in Four Groups of Vietnam Veterans Who Did Not Handle Agent Orange. New Jersey Agent Orange Commission.

Kahn PC, Gochfeld M, Lewis WW. 1992b. *Immune Status and Herbicide Exposure in the New Jersey Pointman I Project.* New Jersey Agent Orange Commission.

Kahn PC, Gochfeld M, Lewis WW. 1992c. *Semen Analysis in Vietnam Veterans with Respect to Presumed Herbicide Exposure.* New Jersey Agent Orange Commission.

Kang HK, Weatherbee L, Breslin PP, Lee Y, Shepard BM. 1986. Soft tissue sarcomas and military service in Vietnam: a case comparison group analysis of hospital patients. *Journal of Occupational Medicine* 28:1215–1218.

Kang HK, Enzinger FM, Breslin P, Feil M, Lee Y, Shepard B. 1987. Soft tissue sarcoma and military service in Vietnam: a case-control study. *Journal of the National Cancer Institute* 79:693–699 [published erratum appears in *Journal of the National Cancer Institute* 79:1173].

Kang HK, Mahan CM, Lee KY, Magee CA, Mather SH, Matanoski G. 2000a. Pregnancy outcomes among US women Vietnam veterans. *American Journal Industrial Medicine* 38(4):447–454.

Kang HK, Mahan CM, Lee KY, Magee CA, Selvin S. 2000b. Prevalence of gynecologic cancers among female Vietnam veterans. *Journal of Occupational and Environmental Medicine* 42:1121–1127.

Kang HK, Dalager NA, Needham LL, Patterson DG, Matanoski GM, Kanchanaraksa S, Lees PSJ. 2001. US Army Chemical Corps Vietnam veterans health study: preliminary results. *Chemosphere* 43:943–949.

Ketchum NS, Michalek JE, Burton JE. 1999. Serum dioxin and cancer in veterans of Operation Ranch Hand. *American Journal of Epidemiology* 149(7):630–639.

Kim H-A, Kim E-M, Park Y-C, Yu J-Y, Hong S-K, Jeon S-H, Park K-L, Hur S-J, Heo Y. 2003. Immunotoxicological effects of Agent Orange exposure to the Vietnam War Korean veterans. *Industrial Health* 41:158–166.

Kim J-S, Lim H-S, Cho S-I, Cheong H-K, Lim M-K. 2003. Impact of Agent Orange Exposure among Korean Vietnam Veterans. *Industrial Health* 41:149–157.

Kogan MD, Clapp RW. 1985. *Mortality Among Vietnam Veterans in Massachusetts, 1972–1983.* Boston: MA. Massachusetts Office of the Commissioner of Veterans Services, Agent Orange Program.

Kogan MD, Clapp RW. 1988. Soft tissue sarcoma mortality among Vietnam veterans in Massachusetts, 1972–1983. *International Journal of Epidemiology* 17:39–43.

Lawrence CE, Reilly AA, Quickenton P, Greenwald P, Page WF, Kuntz AJ. 1985. Mortality patterns of New York State Vietnam veterans. *American Journal of Public Health* 75:277–279.

Levy CJ. 1988. Agent Orange exposure and posttraumatic stress disorder. *Journal of Nervous and Mental Disorders* 176:242–245.

Longnecker MP, Michalek JE. 2000. Serum dioxin level in relation to diabetes mellitus among Air Force veterans with background levels of exposure. *Epidemiology* 11(1):44–48.

Mahan CM, Bullman TA, Kang HK, Selvin S. 1997. A case–control study of lung cancer among Vietnam veterans. *Journal of Occupational and Environmental Medicine* 39(8):740–747.

McKinney WP, McIntire DD, Carmody TJ, Joseph A. 1997. Comparing the smoking behavior of veterans and nonveterans. *Public Health Reports* 112(3):212–217.

Michalek JE, Wolfe WH, Miner JC. 1990. Health status of Air Force veterans occupationally exposed to herbicides in Vietnam. II. Mortality. *Journal of the American Medical Association* 264:1832–1836.

Michalek JE, Rahe AJ, Boyle CA. 1998a. Paternal dioxin, preterm birth, intrauterine growth retardation, and infant death. *Epidemiology* 9(2):161–167.

Michalek JE, Ketchum NS, Akhtar FZ. 1998b. Postservice mortality of US Air Force veterans occupationally exposed to herbicides in Vietnam: 15-year follow-up. *American Journal of Epidemiology* 148(8):786–792.

Michalek JE, Rahe AJ, Boyle CA. 1998c. Paternal dioxin and the sex of children fathered by veterans of Operation Ranch Hand (2). *Epidemiology* 9(4):474–475.

Michalek JE, Albanese RA, Wolfe WH. 1998d. Paternal dioxin, preterm birth, intrauterine growth retardation, and infant death. *Epidemiology* 9(2):161–167.

Michalek JE, Akhtar FZ, Kiel JL. 1999a. Serum dioxin, insulin, fasting glucose, and sex hormone-binding globulin in veterans of Operation Ranch Hand. *Journal of Clinical Endocrinology and Metabolism* 84(5):1540–1543.

Michalek JE, Ketchum NS, Check IJ. 1999b. Serum dioxin and immunologic response in veterans of Operation Ranch Hand. *American Journal of Epidemiology* 149(11):1038–1046.

Michalek JE, Ketchum N, Longnecker MP. 2001a. Serum dioxin and hepatic abnormalities in veterans of Operation Ranch Hand. *Annals of Epidemiology* 11(5):304–311.

Michalek JE, Akhtar FZ, Arezzo JC, Garabrant DH, Albers JW. 2001b. Serum dioxin and peripheral neuropathy in veterans of Operation Ranch Hand. *Neurotoxicology* 22:479–490.

Michalek JE, Akhtar FZ, Longnecker MP, Burton JE. 2001c. Relation of serum 2,3,7,8-tetrachlorodibenzo-*p*-dioxin (TCDD) level to hematological examination results in veterans of Operation Ranch Hand. *Archives of Environmental Health* 56(5):396–405.

Michalek JE, Ketchum NS, Tripathi RC. 2003. Diabetes mellitus and 2,3,7,8-tetrachlorodibenzo-*p*-dioxin elimination in veterans of Operation Ranch Hand. *Journal of Toxicology and Environmental Health*, Part A, 66:211–221.

Mo HJ, Park HJ, Kim JH, Lee JY, Cho BK. 2002. A study about the skin and general disease patterns of the Vietnam veterans exposed to dioxin. *Korean Journal of Dermatology* 40(6):634–638.

Newell GR. 1984. *Development and Preliminary Results of Pilot Clinical Studies. Report of the Agent Orange Advisory Committee to the Texas Department of Health.* University of Texas System Cancer Center.

O'Brien TR, Decoufle P, Boyle CA. 1991. Non-Hodgkin's lymphoma in a cohort of Vietnam veterans. *American Journal of Public Health* 81:758–760.

O'Toole BI, Marshall RP, Grayson DA, Schureck RJ, Dobson M, French M, Pulvertaft B, Meldrum L, Bolton J, Vennard J. 1996a. The Australian Vietnam Veterans Health Study: I. Study design and response bias. *International Journal of Epidemiology* 25(2):307–318.

O'Toole BI, Marshall RP, Grayson DA, Schureck RJ, Dobson M, French M, Pulvertaft B, Meldrum L, Bolton J, Vennard J. 1996b. The Australian Vietnam Veterans Health Study: II. Self-reported health of veterans compared with the Australian population. *International Journal of Epidemiology* 25(2):319–330.

O'Toole BI, Marshall RP, Grayson DA, Schureck RJ, Dobson M, French M, Pulvertaft B, Meldrum L, Bolton J, Vennard J. 1996c. The Australian Vietnam Veterans Health Study: III. Psychological health of Australian Vietnam veterans and its relationship to combat. *International Journal of Epidemiology* 25(2):331–340.

Pavuk M, Schecter AJ, Akhtar FZ, Michalek JE. 2003. Serum 2,3,7,8-tetrachlorodibenzo-*p*-dioxin (TCDD) levels and thyroid function in Air Force veterans of the Vietnam War. *Annals of Epidemiology* 13(5):335–343.

Pollei S, Mettler FA Jr, Kelsey CA, Walters MR, White RE. 1986. Follow-up chest radiographs in Vietnam veterans: are they useful? *Radiology* 161:101–102.

Rellahan WL. 1985. *Aspects of the Health of Hawaii's Vietnam-Era Veterans.* Honolulu, HI: Hawaii State Department of Health, Research, and Statistics Office.

Snow BR, Stellman JM, Stellman SD, Sommer JF. 1988. Post-traumatic stress disorder among American Legionnaires in relation to combat experience in Vietnam: associated and contributing factors. *Environmental Research* 47:175–192.

Steenland K, Calvert G, Ketchum N, Michalek J. 2001. Dioxin and diabetes mellitus: an analysis of the combined NIOSH and Ranch Hand data. *Occupational and Environmental Medicine* 58:641–648.

Stellman JM, Stellman SD, Sommer JF. 1988a. Social and behavioral consequences of the Vietnam experience among American Legionnaires. *Environmental Research* 47:129–149.

Stellman SD, Stellman JM, Sommer JF Jr. 1988b. Health and reproductive outcomes among American Legionnaires in relation to combat and herbicide exposure in Vietnam. *Environmental Research* 47:150–174.

Tarone RE, Hayes HM, Hoover RN, Rosenthal JF, Brown LM, Pottern LM, Javadpour N, O'Connell KJ, Stutzman RE. 1991. Service in Vietnam and risk of testicular cancer. *Journal of the National Cancer Institute* 83:1497–1499.

Thomas TL, Kang HK. 1990. Mortality and morbidity among Army Chemical Corps Vietnam veterans: a preliminary report. *American Journal of Industrial Medicine* 18:665–673.

Thomas TL, Kang H, Dalager N. 1991. Mortality among women Vietnam veterans, 1973–1987. *American Journal of Epidemiology* 134:973–980.

True WR, Goldberg J, Eisen SA. 1988. Stress symptomatology among Vietnam veterans. Analysis of the Veterans Administration Survey of Veterans II. *American Journal of Epidemiology* 128:85–92.

Visintainer PF, Barone M, McGee H, Peterson EL. 1995. Proportionate mortality study of Vietnam-era veterans of Michigan. *Journal of Occupational and Environmental Medicine* 37(4): 423–428.

Watanabe KK, Kang HK. 1995. Military service in Vietnam and the risk of death from trauma and selected cancers. *Annals of Epidemiology* 5(5):407–412.

Watanabe KK, Kang HK. 1996. Mortality patterns among Vietnam veterans: a 24-year retrospective analysis. *Journal of Occupational and Environmental Medicine* 38(3):272–278.

Watanabe KK, Kang HK, Thomas TL. 1991. Mortality among Vietnam veterans: with methodological considerations. *Journal of Occupational Medicine* 33:780–785.

Wendt AS. 1985. Iowa Agent Orange Survey of Vietnam Veterans. Iowa State Department of Health.

Wolfe WH, Michalek JE, Miner JC, Rahe A, Silva J, Thomas WF, Grubbs WD, Lustik MB, Karrison TG, Roegner RH, Williams DE. 1990. Health status of Air Force veterans occupationally exposed to herbicides in Vietnam. I. Physical health. *Journal of the American Medical Association* 264:1824–1831.

Wolfe WH, Michalek JE, Miner JC, Rahe AJ, Moore CA, Needham LL, Patterson DG. 1995. Paternal serum dioxin and reproductive outcomes among veterans of Operation Ranch Hand. *Epidemiology* 6(1):17–22.

D

Calculation of Expected Number of Deaths in the U.S. Air Force Ranch Hand Morbidity Study Cohort over the Next 10 Years

As noted in Chapters 2 and 5, the latest Air Force Health Study (AFHS) mortality update (Ketchum and Michalek, 2005) reported an elevated relative risk for all-cause mortality among all Ranch Hand veterans and a statistically significant increase in the risk of death from circulatory system diseases among veterans with the highest serum dioxin levels. If confirmed by further follow-up, these trends could have implications for the cohort and possibly for Vietnam veterans in general. This appendix presents a calculation of the expected number of deaths over the next 10 years among the participants of the morbidity study and the statistical power to detect excess relative risks.

CALCULATION OF THE EXPECTED NUMBER OF DEATHS

One possible future application of the AFHS data assets is to further investigate associations between cause-specific mortality, herbicide exposure, and information on the various risk factors and characteristics of participants obtained during the course of the study. To determine the usefulness of continuing a mortality follow-up—through, for example, the U.S. National Death Index (NDI)—it is useful to estimate the estimated number of deaths that would occur for a fixed follow-up period and the resulting statistical power to identify excess relative risks.

Brookmeyer and colleagues (1985) provide one statistical framework for this calculation based on standard survival methods, in which rates of the cause of death of interest as well as other censoring mechanisms are included (i.e., deaths from other causes, losses to follow-up). This calculation requires knowledge of age-specific rates as well as censoring mechanisms.

An alternative approach—which has sufficient accuracy to make a rough estimate of statistical power[1]—is to calculate the expected number of deaths in the cohort over a given period of follow-up. For the purpose of this exercise, the committee chose a 10-year follow-up beginning in 2005 and ending in 2015. Calculations were made for each AFHS subject who was alive on January 1, 2005, by making use of the U.S. life table (NCHS, 2004c) for men. Specifically, for each subject we multiplied the age-specific probabilities of surviving in each age interval across the length of follow-up, subtracting this probability from unity to obtain the cumulative probability of dying, and then summing over all subjects. In equation form—for each AFHS subject alive on January 1, 2005—if one designates p_a as the probability of surviving through each 1-year age interval a, then the estimated probability of dying over a specified period of follow-up is:

$$1-\left\{\prod_{a=agealive_i}^{agefollowup_i} p_a\right\}$$

and e, the estimated number of deaths in the cohort, is the sum of each subject's contribution

$$e = \sum_{i=\{\text{subjects alive at beginning of follow-up}\}}^{n} \left[1-\left\{\prod_{a=agealive_i}^{agefollowup_i} p_a\right\}\right]$$

where *agealive* was the age of the subject on January 1, 2005, and *agefollowup* is the age of each subject in 2015. Calculations were truncated at age 99.

AFHS staff provided the committee with a denominalized file containing the relevant information to carry out this calculation (AFHS, 2005). The data comprised a randomly assigned ID number; an indicator for whether the subject was a Ranch Hand or comparison veteran; the year the subject was last known to be alive; age at that year; and an indicator of whether the subject participated in one or more cycle exams (*compliant* in the study's terminology) or not (*noncompliant*).

The calculations, which were performed on data for compliant subjects only, yield estimates for deaths from all causes combined. To partition these estimated deaths according to specific causes, the percentages of deaths from selected causes for ages 60–89 years (in 5-year intervals) were extracted from National Center for Health Statistics data (NCHS, 2004a) and averaged across the intervals. This exercise yielded the following estimates for the proportion of deaths for some of the most common causes of death:

- Malignant neoplasms: 33.9 percent of all deaths
- Diseases of the heart: 23.6 percent of all deaths
- Chronic lower respiratory diseases: 7.5 percent of all deaths

[1]Statistical power is the probability that a statistical test will produce a significant difference at a given significance level.

To estimate the statistical power for rarer health outcomes, the committee also carried out calculations for hypothetical endpoints that have proportions of 5 percent (for example, influenza) and 3 percent (diabetes mellitus) of total deaths. Standard formulas were used to calculate the power of observing specific relative risks (= observed number of events/expected number of events) with these estimated values.

RESULTS

Table D-1 shows the number of compliant subjects presently in the Ranch Hand and comparison cohorts and how those numbers would change over a 10-year (2005–2015) follow-up period if mortality followed the same pattern as the general U.S. population for the corresponding age range. Estimates of mortality were made using data from the U.S. 2002 life tables (NCHS, 2004c). The figures shown in Table D-2 indicate that there is at present (2005) sufficient statistical power to detect a relatively modest excess risk for all-cause mortality. Table D-3 extends this analysis to other causes of death, using the power to detect a relative risk of 1.5 as the benchmark and the expected percentage of cause-specific mortality listed above. The table shows that although there is sufficient power to detect a relative risk of 1.5 for *malignant neoplasms* and *diseases of the heart*, there is insufficient power to detect this excess risk for less common ailments, and that it is not possible to detect lower relative risks.

Tables D-4 through D-9 present rough estimates of the estimated numbers of deaths and statistical power to detect relative risks of 1.2, 1.5, and 2.0 for the hypothetical 10-year (2005–2015) mortality follow-up of the compliant members of the AFHS cohorts. All-cause mortality and selected causes of death are considered. The estimates suggest that a 10-year follow-up makes it possible to confidently detect small increases in the relative risk of health outcomes common to aging males and markedly increases the power of the study to detect larger risk increases for relatively rare outcomes.

A follow-up that included the much larger pool of noncompliant potential comparison subjects (9,500 persons in total[2]) would greatly increase the power of the calculations to detect differences in mortality rates between AFHS cohort veterans and the general population for less common health outcomes. However, it would do so at the expense of the detailed information on individuals that would allow in-depth empirical examination of the possible determinants of the differences.

It is relatively inexpensive to perform a periodic mortality update. Assuming that a National Death Index search is performed on the entire compliant cohort known to be alive at the time of the last update and that cause of death codes are

---

[2]This figure is the approximate number of compliant and noncompliant subjects alive on January 1, 2005, according to data provided by AFHS.

TABLE D-1 Summary Statistics for the Compliant Cohorts and Estimated Numbers of Deaths from 2005 until 2015

	Ranch Hand Cohort	Comparison Cohort
Number of subjects who died before 2005	199	258
Number of subjects alive in 2005	998	1,597
Mean age (std. dev.) of subject alive in 2005	64.8 (7.2)	64.4 (7.1)
Estimated number of deaths 2005–2015	281	436
Estimated percent of deaths 2005–2015	28%	27%
Estimated number of subjects alive in 2015	717	1,161

NOTE: Numbers may not add up because of independent rounding.

TABLE D-2 Power to Detect Various Relative Risks for All-Cause Mortality, if There Is No Further Follow-Up*

Relative Risk	Ranch Hand Cohort	Comparison Cohort
1.2	85.4	100
1.5	100	100
2.0	100	100

*Based on the number of subjects who died before 2005.

requested for subjects found to be deceased, it would cost ~$650 to obtain the data from NCHS exclusive of the labor to generate the request.[3] A survey of the entire compliant and non-compliant cohort would cost ~$2,100. To make meaningful use of these data, they would need to be reviewed and coded by a nosologist as part of whatever study was planned.

In sum, rough estimates suggest that the AFHS cohort is big enough to detect moderate to large associations in future mortality analyses of health outcomes of potential interest to Vietnam veterans, using a well-established and relatively inexpensive research approach.

[3]This estimate is based on a charge of $.21 per subject per year searched × 2,600 subjects, plus a service charge of $100 for a repeat user of the NDI (NCHS, 2004b).

TABLE D-3 Power to Detect Relative Risks of 1.5 by Cause of Death, if There Is No Further Follow-Up*

	Ranch Hand Cohort	Comparison Cohort
Malignant neoplasms	98.0	99.5
Diseases of the heart	92.5	96.9
Chronic lower respiratory diseases	54.0	63.3
A disease that contributes 5% to the total number of deaths	41.4	49.0
A disease that contributes 3% to the total number of deaths	29.5	34.7

*Based on the number of subjects who died before 2005.

TABLE D-4 All-Cause Mortality: Estimated Number of Deaths and Power to Detect Various Relative Risks with an Additional 10 Years of Follow-Up

	Ranch Hand Cohort	Comparison Cohort
Estimated* number of deaths in cohort by 2015	480	694
Power to detect relative risks of:		
1.2	99.5	100
1.5	100	100
2.0	100	100

*The number of deaths observed before 2005 plus estimated number of deaths between 2005–2015.

TABLE D-5 Malignant Neoplasms: Estimated Number of Deaths and Power to Detect Various Relative Risks with an Additional 10 Years of Follow-Up

	Ranch Hand Cohort	Comparison Cohort
Estimated* number of deaths in cohort by 2015	163	271
Power to detect relative risks of:		
1.2	78.7	93.4
1.5	100	100
2.0	100	100

*The estimated number of deaths from ailment before 2005 plus estimated number of deaths between 2005–2015.

TABLE D-6 Diseases of the Heart: Estimated Number of Deaths and Power to Detect Various Relative Risks with an Additional 10 Years of Follow-Up

	Ranch Hand Cohort	Comparison Cohort
Estimated* number of deaths in cohort by 2015	113	164
Power to detect relative risks of:		
1.2	65.1	79.0
1.5	99.1	100
2.0	100	100

*The estimated number of deaths from ailment before 2005 plus estimated number of deaths between 2005–2015.

TABLE D-7 Chronic Lower Respiratory Diseases: Estimated Number of Deaths and Power to Detect Various Relative Risks with an Additional 10 Years of Follow-Up

	Ranch Hand Cohort	Comparison Cohort
Estimated* number of deaths in cohort by 2015	36	52
Power to detect relative risks of:		
1.2	31.0	39.6
1.5	85.5	94.5
2.0	100	100

*The estimated number of deaths from ailment before 2005 plus estimated number of deaths between 2005–2015.

TABLE D-8 A Disease That Contributes 5 Percent to the Total Number of Deaths: Estimated Number of Deaths and Power to Detect Various Relative Risks with an Additional 10 Years of Follow-Up

	Ranch Hand Cohort	Comparison Cohort
Estimated* number of deaths in cohort by 2015	24	35
Power to detect relative risks of:		
1.2	24.1	30.5
1.5	71.3	83.6
2.0	99.2	99.9

*The estimated number of deaths from ailment before 2005 plus estimated number of deaths between 2005–2015.

TABLE D-9 A Disease That Contributes 3 Percent to the Total Number of Deaths: Estimated Number of Deaths and Power to Detect Various Relative Risks with an Additional 10 Years of Follow-Up

	Ranch Hand Cohort	Comparison Cohort
Estimated* number of deaths in cohort by 2015	15	21
Power to detect relative risks of:		
1.2	18.4	22.2
1.5	54.0	66.3
2.0	94.2	98.5

*The estimated number of deaths from ailment before 2005 plus estimated number of deaths between 2005–2015.

REFERENCES

AFHS (Air Force Health Study). 2005. Microsoft Excel file (04-12-05—IOM—Part 1—Q1.xls) provided in response to committee request. Brooks AFB, TX.

Brookmeyer R, Day N, Pompe-Kirn V. 1985. Assessing the impact of additional follow-up in cohort studies. *American Journal of Epidemiology* 121(4):611–619.

Ketchum NS, Michalek JE. 2005. Postservice mortality of Air Force veterans occupationally exposed to herbicides during the Vietnam War: 20-year follow-up results. *Military Medicine* 170(5): 406–413.

NCHS (National Center for Health Statistics). 2004a. *Deaths, Percent of Total Deaths, and Death Rates for the 15 Leading Causes of Death in 5-Year Age Groups, by Race and Sex: United States, 2001.* [Online]. Available: http://www.cdc.gov/nchs/data/dvs/LCWK1_2001.pdf [accessed October 11, 2005].

NCHS. 2004b. *National Death Index User Fees. Effective October 1, 2004.* [Online]. Available: www.cdc.gov/nchs/r&d/ndi/Users_Fees_Worksheet.pdf [accessed October 11, 2005].

NCHS. 2004c. *United States Life Tables, 2002.* [Online]. Available: http://www.cdc.gov/nchs/data/dvs/life2002.pdf [accessed October 11, 2005].

E

Comparison of Data Sharing Programs That Use Data Enclaves[a]

	Medical Expenditure Panel Survey (MEPS)	Census Research Data Centers (RDCs)
General Information on the Data Sharing Programs		
Type of Data	MEPS is the third (and most recent) in a series of national probability surveys conducted by Agency for Healthcare Research and Quality (AHRQ) on the financing and use of medical care in the United States. MEPS collects data on the specific health services that Americans use; how frequently they use them; the costs of the services; how they are paid for; and the cost, scope, and breadth of private health insurance held by and available to the U.S. population.	Census data include microdata and data that cannot be released publicly because they contain detailed information on geographic location and other characteristics about the firms or households that could be used to determine their identities.

Health and Retirement Study (HRS)	California Health Interview Survey (CHIS)	Vaccine Safety Datalink (VSD)[b]
The University of Michigan HRS surveys more than 22,000 Americans over the age of 50 every two years. The survey collects data on Americans' physical and mental health, insurance coverage, financial status, family support systems, labor-market status, and retirement planning. Registered users can download HRS public data products free. Restricted-release files contain sensitive information that can be made available only under specified conditions.	CHIS is a telephone survey of adults, adolescents, and children from all parts of the state of California. The survey is conducted every two years. Some of the data collected are prepared for public release as free public-use files. The files are designed to minimize the risk of respondent identification yet preserve the broadest range of descriptive demographic data. Restricted-use files at CHIS are available at the Data Access Center (DAC) and contain detailed geographic identifiers and full demographic descriptions for the survey respondents from the 2001 survey. The files also include responses to sensitive questions that are excluded from the public-use data files.	The VSD is a large linked database that was developed in 1991 by the collaborative efforts of CDC and several private MCOs. The VSD currently includes data from administrative records for more than 7 million members of eight MCOs. In the VSD, vaccination records, patient characteristics, and health outcomes are linked, allowing the VSD to serve as a unique and potentially powerful resource for the continuing evaluation of vaccine safety.

continues

	Medical Expenditure Panel Survey (MEPS)	Census Research Data Centers (RDCs)
Elements of Study Proposal		
Identification of Specific Variables to Be Studied	• Researchers must list data files which they would like access to. • Researchers will have access only to the variables identified in their approved proposals.	• Researchers must identify specific dataset to be analyzed.
Confidentiality Protection Measures in Study Design	• The proposed study must be done without compromising confidentiality of respondents. • Researchers must read and comply with the CFACT-DC User Guide.	• Researchers must obtain Special Sworn Status. • Researchers can use confidential data only for the purpose for which the data are supplied.
Feasibility of Study and Data-Resource Assessment	Decision Criteria: • Can the research be conducted with the available data?	• The proposal must show that the research can be conducted successfully with the proposed method and available data. • The proposal should show the need for and importance of using confidential data.

Health and Retirement Study (HRS)	California Health Interview Survey (CHIS)	Vaccine Safety Datalink (VSD)[b]
• A specific dataset must be chosen from the list of restricted-use datasets. • Researchers must state why the unrestricted data would not be adequate for their research purpose.	• Researchers must request variables using the DAC variable lists.	• Researchers must provide a list detailing data requested: data system, files, years, and variables. • Only variables needed to conduct the proposed analyses will be included in the analytic file.
• Researchers must submit a Restricted Data Protection Plan to HRS. • Risk of disclosure of restricted information is considered based on the users' description of expected analysis and results. • The confidentiality agreement restricting disclosure and use of data from the Michigan Center on the Demography of Aging Data Enclave must be read and signed by the researchers. • All users will be periodically audited by HRS to ensure that all conditions of the restricted data agreement are being met. Various data from 1992–2004 are available.	Decision Criteria: • Is there a risk of disclosure of confidential information? • Does the project propose to merge user-supplied data with CHIS data? • What additional risks of disclosure are associated with the merged dataset? • Researchers must sign a Nondisclosure Affidavit and Data Access Confidentiality Agreement before starting their work.	• All users must sign an affidavit of confidentiality promising not to attempt to identify respondents. • Researchers can use confidential data only for the purpose for which the data are supplied.
• Scientific and technical feasibility of the project, including availability of data files being requested, is considered.	Decision Criteria: • Is sample size sufficient? • Are CHIS data appropriate for answering the research questions proposed? • Are the variables requested related to the proposed analyses?	• No criteria specified for review of VSD proposals. • No publicly available data.

continues

	Medical Expenditure Panel Survey (MEPS)	Census Research Data Centers (RDCs)
Consistency with Mission of the Organization	• The proposed study must be in accordance with the mission of AHRQ (this is specified in its authorizing legislation).	• All projects must provide a benefit to Census Bureau programs. The benefit requirement is an explicit proposal criterion and is required by law (Title 13, Sec. 23, U.S.C.).
IRB Approval	(Information not available.)	• The need for IRB approval is based on where the confidential data come from, and the researchers must follow the rules and regulations of that agency.
Other Guidelines		
Costs and Fees	• At the data center: To cover technical assistance, simple file construction, and up to 2 hours of programming support, there is a $150.00 fee. Additional programming support can cost $80.00 an hour.	• $3,125/month for a full-time seat • A project that requires a 40% level of access (about 2 days/week) for a period of 1 year would cost $15,000. • Additional fees may be charged to projects that use datasets outside the core or that impose other special costs on CES, the Census Bureau, or the RDC.
Who Reviews Researchers' Application and Proposal?	• The manager at the CFACT-DC coordinates the review of each proposal.	• Both the RDC and the Census Bureau must approve the proposal. • The RDC administrator reviews the preliminary proposal and suggests ways to improve or refine it. The RDC administrator must approve the preliminary proposal before the researchers can submit the final proposal.

Health and Retirement Study (HRS)	California Health Interview Survey (CHIS)	Vaccine Safety Datalink (VSD)[b]
• Proposed project must be in accordance with the mission of the MiCDA.	• Study must be compatible with the purpose of CHIS.	• Not specified for VSD data.
• Researchers must be affiliated with an institution with an NIH-certified human subjects review process. • A signed form from the researchers' institution certifying Human Subjects Review was done is necessary.	• Copy of approval or exemption by home institution's IRB is necessary.	• Researchers must obtain IRB approval from each MCO whose data they would need to undertake the analyses.
• Academic (faculty members of accredited institutions of higher education) or government (federal, state, or local): \$200/day. • Student (currently enrolled in an accredited graduate or undergraduate program): \$50/day. • Other: \$500/day.	Costs are developed on an individual basis and include • \$500 initial set-up fee • \$65/hour for guest research access • \$140/hour for programming services • \$120/hour to run programs. • \$1,000 minimum fee per project Charges are determined by actual time spent on project.	• Set-up charge of \$500/day for merging files or creating custom file formats. • Guest researchers at \$200/day (2-day minimum, 10-day maximum).
• The HRS DCC-WG reviews the application. When the application is adequate, the DCC-WG will contact the researchers and let them know that they can submit the application to their local IRB for review. Once the researchers have IRB approval, their application is complete, and they can submit it for review by the DCC for review and final approval.	• DAC staff prepares a summary of the application. The CHIS Data Disclosure Review Committee meets biweekly, reviews the application, and makes a recommendation to the CHIS PI to approve or reject the application or to request further information from the researchers.	• Completed proposals are sent to the NCHS RDC for review by a committee consisting of the director of NCHS RDC, the RDC staff liaison, the NCHS confidentiality officer, and the director of the NCHS data division whose data are included in the proposal. • Approval for use of the VSD requires approval by the MCOs' IRBs.

continues

	Medical Expenditure Panel Survey (MEPS)	Census Research Data Centers (RDCs)
Response Time	• Applications are accepted continuously. • About 4–6 weeks after a proposal is approved, researchers can go into the CFACT-DC.	• There is at least a 6-month period between the deadline for the final proposal submission and the commencement of research.
Assistance from Program Staff	• Currently, there are limited staff resources to help at the CFACT-DC, so extensive programming support must be contracted ahead of time for a fee.	• Researchers work closely with the RDC administrator to develop a preliminary proposal.
Available Data Programs	SAS, Stata, SPSS, and SUDAAN are the software packages most suitable for analyzing MEPS data.	(Information not available.)

Health and Retirement Study (HRS)	California Health Interview Survey (CHIS)	Vaccine Safety Datalink (VSD)[b]
• When HRS receives an application, it is logged and review is scheduled.	• The CHIS PI will respond to the request within 21 days after receiving the application. • Computer programs that are e-mailed to the DAC staff will be run within five working days.	• Response time varies but NCHS tries to respond to the initial proposal as soon as possible. • The time it takes between securing proposal approval and using the RDC varies as well (depends on the complexity of the work, how long it will take to prepare the data files, and what other work is already scheduled at the RDC).
At the MiCDA data center: • Enclave users are responsible for developing and implementing all data-management procedures necessary to produce datasets to be used for analysis. • Enclave staff provide assistance with dataset installation, software installation, operating-system problems, statistical-package operation, backups, and user-interface issues. • Staff members do not provide assistance in carrying out statistical analysis.	• Researchers are encouraged to consult the DAC manager while developing their proposals. • Researchers are provided with limited technical assistance on CHIS variables, weighting, and variance calculation. • A senior programmer contact is assigned to the project. • Dummy data files are sent to the researchers.	• Researchers are encouraged to check with RDC staff before writing their proposals to ensure that the data of interest can be made available to them. • Researchers must be able to conduct their analyses with the software specified in their research proposal.
STATA (v6.0), SAS (v6.12), SPSS (v9.0).	SAS, SPSS, State, STAT/Transfer, SUDAAN, and Wesvar; custom software is installed on request.	Hardware: Pentium computers with Windows 2000. SAS is the standard program for use of VSD data, but other languages can be made available with sufficient lead time.

continues

	Medical Expenditure Panel Survey (MEPS)	Census Research Data Centers (RDCs)
Where Data Can Be Accessed	• Public-use datasets can be downloaded from the MEPS web site (http://www.meps.ahrq.gov). • Restricted data can be accessed by approved researchers at the CFACT-DC, in Rockville, MD. • Researchers may also choose to contract with the AHRQ data-processing contractor (Social and Scientific Systems) to develop and run their programs.	• All analysis must be done on site in the RDC.
Disclosure Review Before Material Leaves the RDC	• All materials must be reviewed by AHRQ staff before they can be removed from the data center.	• Researchers cannot remove any confidential data from the RDC on any medium. All output must be submitted to Census Bureau personnel for disclosure review.
Other Requirements	Researchers must also provide: • List of publication plans and other intended uses of data in the proposal • Sources of funding • Estimated timeframe for viewing data and completing their work • Resumes or CVs for all persons who will access the data center	Researchers must provide: • Purpose of the research • Funding source • CVs for all investigators • Abstract of the proposal • Project description • Statement of benefits to Census Bureau Preliminary and final proposals are completed through the Census Bureau web site.

Health and Retirement Study (HRS)	California Health Interview Survey (CHIS)	Vaccine Safety Datalink (VSD)[b]
• Public-use files can be accessed through the HRS web site (http://hrsonline.isr.umich.edu/data/avail.html). • Restricted-use data can be viewed by approved researchers at the MiCDA data enclave in the Institute for Social Research.	• Public-use files can be accessed through the CHIS web site by registering free (http://www.chis.ucla.edu/main/default.asp?page=puf). • Restricted data can be viewed at the DAC at the UCLA Center for Health Policy Research after submitting and gaining approval of a proposal. • Researchers can also gain access to restricted files after proposal approval by e-mailing computer programs to DAC staff, who will run them and send results to the researchers.	• All analyses must be done on site in the RDC in Hyattsville, MD. • A maximum of three collaborating researchers can sit at a computer station at the RDC.
• Users are allowed to remove results of statistical analysis from the data enclave only after enclave staff have conducted a disclosure-limitation review to protect respondent confidentiality.	• DAC manager or senior programmer conducts a disclosure review for all output before it is removed from the DAC.	• All output and materials removed from the RDC are subject to disclosure-limitation review. • Researchers must provide a list of the table shells, equations, and test statistics of statistical output they plan to take out of the RDC.
• If institutional or physical circumstances of the researchers change, HRS is to be contacted to modify the underlying agreement. • Yearly recertification of the certification and data agreement is required. • Researchers must submit a renewal request if the initial agreement expires and they want continued access to the data.	If there are many small cells, the programmer recommends the recoding of variables so that this does not occur. If there are few small cells in the output, the programmer must suppress small cells and do complementary suppression. DAC applications include: • DAC application forms. • Personal and organizational information • Service request • Abstract	Researchers must provide: • Current resumes or CVs • Dates of proposed use of the RDC • Source of funding • Summary of proposed study • Background of the study • Data dictionary NCHS complies with 308(d) Confidentiality Statute.

continues

	Medical Expenditure Panel Survey (MEPS)	Census Research Data Centers (RDCs)
Other Requirements (continued)		
Post Use Application Activities	(Information not available.)	• Once a proposal is approved, all researchers must go through a background investigation. • Researchers are asked (but not required) to work with the RDC administrator before releasing final output.

NOTE: Sources: AHRQ, 2004a,b,c,d; CDC, 2004; Census Bureau, 2004a,b; CHIS, 2003, 2004a,b; HRS, 2004a,b.

[a]Excerpted from *Vaccine Safety Research, Data Access, and Public Trust* (IOM, 2005).

[b]Based on 2004 *Federal Register* Notice (69FR 67854, et seq.).

Health and Retirement Study (HRS)	California Health Interview Survey (CHIS)	Vaccine Safety Datalink (VSD)[b]
Researchers must also provide: • Current resumes or CVs • Dates of proposed tenure at the data enclave • Funding sources for user project and for data enclave cost recovery	Supplemental materials include: • Biographic sketch or resume • List of CHIS variables requested • Detailed description of any user-supplied files	
(Information not available.)	Researchers must also: • Acknowledge CHIS in their manuscript for publication • Submit copies of publications to DAC	• External researchers are required to submit a copy of the data-sharing guidelines and a copy of the signed confidentiality agreement with any manuscript submitted to a journal. • Must include certain disclaimers in their manuscript.

REFERENCES

AHRQ (Agency for Healthcare Research and Quality). 2004a. *CFACT Data Center (CFACT-DC).* [Online]. Available: http://www.meps.ahrq.gov/datacenter.htm [accessed June 30, 2004].

AHRQ. 2004b. *CFACT Data Center (CFACT-DC): User Guide/Application Information.* [Online]. Available: http://www.meps.ahrq.gov/datacenter/dcuserguide.htm [accessed June 30, 2004].

AHRQ. 2004c. *Overview of the Medical Expenditure Panel Study.* [Online]. Available: http://www.meps.ahrq.gov/WhatIsMEPS/Overview.HTM [accessed June 30, 2004].

AHRQ. 2004d. *FAQs about the Data Center.* [Online]. Available: http://www.meps.ahrq.gov/FAQs/FAQ_DataCenter.HTM [accessed May, 2004].

CDC (Centers for Disease Control and Prevention). 2004. Procedures and Costs for Use of the Research Data Center. *Notice and Request for Action. Federal Register* 69:222.

Census Bureau. 2004a. *CES RDC Research Proposal Guidelines.* [Online]. Available: http://148.129.75.160/ces.php/guidelines [accessed July 8, 2004].

Census Bureau. 2004b. *The Research Data Center Program.* [Online]. Available: http://148.129.75.160/ces.php/research [accessed July 8, 2004].

CHIS (California Health Interview Survey). 2003. *CHIS Research Clearinghouse.* [Online]. Available: http://www.chis.ucla.edu/rc/ [accessed November 3, 2004].

CHIS. 2004a. *About the California Health Interview Survey.* [Online]. Available: http://www.chis.ucla.edu/about.html [accessed June 28, 2004].

CHIS. 2004b. *The Data Access Center at the UCLA Center for Health Policy Research.* [Online]. Available: http://www.chis.ucla.edu/chis_dac.html [accessed June 28, 2004b].

HRS (Health and Retirement Study). 2004a. *Background Information.* [Online]. Available: http://hrsonline.isr.umich.edu/intro/sho_intro.php?hfyle=uinfo [accessed June 16, 2004].

HRS. 2004b. *HRS Restricted Data: Application Processing Overview.* [Online]. Available: http://hrsonline.isr.umich.edu/rda/rdanarrative.htm [accessed July 1, 2004].

IOM (Institute of Medicine). 2005. *Vaccine Safety Research, Data Access, and Public Trust.* Washington, DC: The National Academies Press.

F

Committee on the Disposition of the Air Force Health Study

David Tollerud, M.D., M.P.H. *(Chair)*, is Professor and Associate Director of the Institute for Public Health Research, School of Public Health/Health Information Sciences, University of Louisville, Kentucky. He has extensive clinical training, with specialty board certifications in internal medicine, pulmonary and critical care medicine, and occupational medicine. Dr. Tollerud has research expertise in environmental and occupational health, epidemiology, and immunology, and consulting experience in the areas of occupational and environmental respiratory disease, medical surveillance, and workplace injury prevention programs. He currently serves on the IOM's Board on Population Health and Public Health Practices and the Committee on the Assessment of Wartime Exposure to Herbicides in Vietnam, and has served on a number of other IOM committees since 1992.

Dan G. Blazer, III, M.D., Ph.D., M.P.H. (IOM member), is the JP Gibbons Professor of Psychiatry and Behavioral Sciences at Duke University Medical Center. During Dr. Blazer's tenure as Dean of Medical Education, he expanded a Master of Public Health program for medical school students that now attracts over 20 percent of the medical school class. Dr. Blazer is the author or editor of over 20 books and author or co-author of over 250 peer-reviewed articles on topics including depression, epidemiology, and consultation liaison psychiatry. He is a fellow of the American College of Psychiatry and the American Psychiatric Association and is a member of the IOM with expertise in medical education, religion and medicine, and preventive medicine and public health. He was elected to the IOM in 1995.

Ellen Wright Clayton, M.D., J.D., is the Rosalind E. Franklin Professor of Genetics and Health Policy; Co-Director, Center for Biomedical Ethics and Society; Senior Fellow, Institute for Public Policy Studies; Professor of Law; and Professor of Pediatrics at Vanderbilt University. Dr. Clayton has been studying and teaching the ethical, legal, and social implications of developments in genetics for more than a quarter of a century and has published two books and more than 75 peer-reviewed articles and book chapters. She has been an active participant in policy debates advising the National Human Genome Research Institute as well as numerous other federal and international bodies on an array of topics, ranging from issues in children's health, including newborn screening, to the ethical conduct of research involving human subjects. In these roles, she has helped develop policy for numerous national and international organizations. Dr. Clayton is a member of the Health Sciences Policy Board of the Institute of Medicine, and has served on a number of other IOM committees.

Manning Feinleib, M.D., M.P.H., Dr.P.H. (IOM member), is Professor in the Department of Epidemiology at the Bloomberg School of Public Health of The Johns Hopkins University. He was Director of the National Center for Health Statistics from 1983 to 1995. His research interests include epidemiology of cardiovascular diseases with emphasis on demographic and secular trends, international comparisons, and effects of socioeconomic factors, nutrition, and prevention; vital statistics, population surveys, and linkage of data bases with emphasis on confidentiality issues, improving data quality, and facilitating research uses of large data bases. Dr. Feinleib is on the editorial board of the *American Journal of Epidemiology*. He is the recipient of the 2004 American College of Epidemiology Abraham Lilienfeld award for lifetime contributions to the field. Among his contributions to National Academies studies is his service on a recent IOM Panel on Gulf War and Health.

Mark S. Goldberg, Ph.D., is Associate Professor in the Department of Medicine, McGill University, Montreal, and Associate Member in their joint Departments of Epidemiology and Biostatistics and Occupational Health, and in the Department of Oncology. He is also Medical Scientist in the Royal Victoria Hospital, McGill University Health Centre. Dr. Goldberg is an occupational and environmental epidemiologist and holds an Investigator Award from the Canadian Institutes of Health Research. His current research interests include the investigation of occupational and environmental risk factors for cancer and the health effects associated with exposures to ambient air pollution. In addition to being a member of grant review panels, Dr. Goldberg was also a member of the McGill University Institutional Review Board, and is a member of Health Canada's Science Advisory Board. He has also served on a number of other National Academies committees.

Susan E. Hankinson, Sc.D., M.P.H., is Associate Professor of Epidemiology at the Harvard School of Public Health. Dr. Hankinson's research interests include the use of biomarkers in epidemiologic studies; the relationships between hormones (endogenous and exogenous) and subsequent risk of breast, endometrial, and ovarian cancers; and risk factors for eye disease. Her primary research base is the Nurses' Health Study (NHS) and Nurses' Health Study II (NHSII), two large prospective cohort studies that have been ongoing since 1976 and 1989 respectively. Similarly, Dr. Hankinson is currently conducting a range of studies on premenopausal endogenous hormones and breast cancer risk in the NHSII cohort. Her study evaluates lifestyle factors in relation to ovarian, endometrial, and breast cancers in women, and she is starting several new projects to assess potential biochemical and genetic predictors of risk of these cancers.

David A. Kalman, Ph.D., is Chair and Professor in the Department of Environmental and Occupational Health Sciences at the University of Washington School of Public Health and Community Medicine. He is an organic chemist by training and is interested in several aspects of chemical behavior as they relate to environmental health, including integrated human exposure assessment using chemical biomarkers of exposure. Among his current research projects is an ongoing assessment of exposures, health status, and possible mechanistic or genetic susceptibility aspects of diseases associated with arsenic poisoning via drinking water. Other research is elucidating the role of personal factors in governing toxicokinetics of inhaled solvents and evaluating biomarkers of exposure to inhaled particulate matter. In the early 1990s, he served on the National Academies' Committee on National Monitoring of Human Tissues.

De Juran Richardson, Ph.D., is a Professor at Lake Forest College, and Senior Adjunct Professor at the University of Illinois at Chicago and the University of Wisconsin-Madison. Dr. Richardson received his Ph.D., M.S., and B.A. degrees from Northwestern University. His professional activities include appointments on the ECOG Data Monitoring Committee (since 1994) and the National Institute of Neurological Disorders and Stroke (NINDS) Initial Grant Review Panel (through 2005) and Advisory Board for the Harvard School of Public Health, Department of Biostatistics, Summer Program in Biostatistics. Dr. Richardson has research interests in the design and analysis of large, multi-center, clinical trials; issues involving the recruitment and retention of underrepresented minorities in clinical trials; and performing statistical survival analyses in the presence of informative censoring. Dr. Richardson's research articles have appeared in several scientific journals: *Statistics in Medicine*, *Communications in Statistics*, *Journal of the National Technical Association*, *Journal of the National Medical Association*, *Neuroepidemiology*, *Journal of Stroke and Cerebrovascular Diseases*, *Clinical Oncology*, and *Journal of Acquired Immune Deficiency Syndromes*.

Regina M. Santella, Ph.D., is Professor of Environmental Health Sciences at the Mailman School of Public Health at Columbia University and serves as director for the National Institute of Environmental Health Sciences Center for Environmental Health in Northern Manhattan, the Carcinogenesis Program and Biomarkers Core Facility of the Cancer Center, and the Jean Sindab African American Breast Cancer Project. Dr. Santella's research involves the development of laboratory methods for the detection of human exposure to environmental and occupational carcinogens, and their use in molecular epidemiology studies to identify causative factors, susceptible populations, and preventive interventions. Dr. Santella has a M.S. in organic chemistry from the University of Massachusetts and a Ph.D. in biochemistry from the City University of New York. She has served as a member of the Metabolic Pathology Study Section as well as ad hoc reviewer for the American Cancer Society and NIEHS. She is currently a Senior Editor of *Cancer Research*; Past Chairperson of the Molecular Epidemiology Working Group of the American Association for Cancer Research, and Chair of the Molecular Epidemiology Subcommittee of the Southwest Oncology Group.

Consultants

James Hodge, J.D., L.L.M., is Associate Professor at Johns Hopkins Bloomberg School of Public Health, where he teaches international human rights, bioethics, and health information privacy. He also serves as Executive Director of the Center for Law and the Public's Health at Georgetown and Johns Hopkins universities. Dr. Hodge explores issues in public health law, health policy, bioethics, health information privacy, and genetics. As an Adjunct Professor of Law at Georgetown, he has lectured on constitutional law, public health law, medical ethics, international human rights, and health law and policy. Dr. Hodge consults with multiple governmental and private organizations and speaks extensively at national and regional conferences on a variety of health topics.

Victor Pontes, M.S., is a Senior Data Manager of the Nurses Health Study at the Channing Laboratory in the Harvard School of Public Health. Mr. Pontes is responsible for the management of biorespository data for several million biospecimens from approximately 100,000 participants. He has seven years of experience using the SAS system for data manipulation and analysis. Mr. Pontes received his masters in software engineering from Brandeis University.

Staff

Rose Marie Martinez, Sc.D., is Director of the Institute of Medicine (IOM) Board on Population Health and Public Health Practices. Before joining IOM, she was Senior Health Researcher at Mathematica Policy Research, where she studied the effects of health-system change on the public-health infrastructure, access to care for vulnerable populations, managed care, and the health care workforce. Dr. Martinez is former Assistant Director for Health Financing and Policy with the U.S. General Accounting Office, for which she directed evaluations and policy analysis on national and public health issues. Dr. Martinez received her doctorate from the Johns Hopkins School of Hygiene and Public Health.

David A. Butler, Ph.D., is a senior program officer in the Institute of Medicine (IOM) Board on Population Health and Public Health Practices. He received his B.S. and M.S. in engineering from the University of Rochester and Ph.D. in public policy analysis from Carnegie-Mellon University. Before joining IOM, Dr. Butler served as an analyst for the U.S. Congress Office of Technology Assessment and was Research Associate in the Department of Environmental Health at the Harvard School of Public Health. He has directed several IOM studies on environmental-health and risk-assessment topics, resulting in the reports *Veterans and Agent Orange: Update 1998*, and . . . *Update 2000*; the report series *Characterizing the Exposure of Veterans to Agent Orange and Other Herbicides Used in Vietnam*; *Clearing the Air: Asthma and Indoor Air Exposures*; and *Damp Indoor Spaces and Health.*

Amy R. O'Connor, M.P.H. candidate, is a research associate in the Institute of Medicine (IOM) Board on Population Health and Public Health Practices. She will complete her M.P.H. in Environmental and Occupational Health at the George Washington University School of Public Health in May 2006. She is a recipient of the George Washington University Ruhland Fellowship for outstanding applicant. She graduated from George Mason University magna cum laude with a B.A. in chemistry in 2003. She is also a first Gulf War-era Army veteran during which time she served as combat photographer. *Disposition of the Air Force Health Study* is her first report with IOM.

Sonia J. Cheruvillil, M.P.H., is a senior program assistant in the Institute of Medicine (IOM) Board on Population Health and Public Health Practices. She recently graduated with a masters in public health from the George Washington University School of Public Health. She received her undergraduate degrees in English literature (B.A.) and microbiology (B.S.) from the University of Iowa. She is involved with the IOM Report *Veterans and Agent Orange: Update 2005* as well *Update 2007*. *Disposition of the Air Force Health Study* is Sonia's second report with IOM.

Michael Saulle, B.S., is a clinical trials researcher at Memorial Sloan-Kettering Cancer Center's Department of Medicine in New York City. He received his BS in health studies/premed from Georgetown University. He interned at the Institute of Medicine (IOM) in the spring of his senior year where he worked as a research assistant on the *Disposition of the Air Force Health Study*.